Disorders of the Respiratory Tract

CURRENT ◊ CLINICAL ◊ PRACTICE

NEIL S. SKOLNIK, MD • SERIES EDITOR

Disorders of the Respiratory Tract: *Common Challenges in Primary Care,* MATTHEW L. MINTZ, 2006

The Handbook of Contraception: *A Guide for Practical Management,* DONNA SHOUPE AND SIRI L. KJOS, 2006

Obstetrics in Family Practice: *A Practical Guide,* PAUL LYONS, 2006

Psychiatric Disorders in Pregnancy and the Postpartum: *Principles and Treatment,* VICTORIA HENDRICK, 2006

Sexually Transmitted Diseases: *A Practical Guide for Primary Care,* edited by ANITA NELSON AND JOANN WOODWARD, 2006

Cardiology in Family Practice: *A Practical Guide,* STEVEN M. HOLLENBERG AND TRACY WALKER, 2006

Bronchial Asthma: *A Guide for Practical Understanding and Treatment, Fifth Edition,* edited by M. ERIC GERSHWIN AND TIMOTHY E. ALBERTSON, 2006

Dermatology Skills for Primary Care: *An Illustrated Guide,* DANIEL J. TROZAK, DAN J. TENNENHOUSE, AND JOHN J. RUSSELL, 2006

Thyroid Disease: *A Case-Based and Practical Guide for Primary Care,* EMANUEL O. BRAMS, 2005

Type 2 Diabetes, Pre-Diabetes, and the Metabolic Syndrome: *The Primary Care Guide to Diagnosis and Management,* RONALD A. CODARIO, 2005

Chronic Pain: *A Primary Care Guide to Practical Management,* DAWN A. MARCUS, 2005

Bone Densitometry in Clinical Practice: *Application and Interpretation, Second Edition,* SYDNEY LOU BONNICK, 2004

Cancer Screening: *A Practical Guide for Physicians,* edited by KHALID AZIZ AND GEORGE Y. WU, 2001

Hypertension Medicine, edited by MICHAEL A. WEBER, 2001

Allergic Diseases: *Diagnosis and Treatment, Second Edition,* edited by PHIL LIEBERMAN AND JOHN A. ANDERSON, 2000

Disorders of the Respiratory Tract

Common Challenges in Primary Care

By

Matthew L. Mintz, MD

Department of Medicine
The George Washington University School of Medicine
Washington, DC

HUMANA PRESS ✻ TOTOWA, NEW JERSEY

© 2006 Humana Press Inc.
999 Riverview Drive, Suite 208
Totowa, New Jersey 07512

humanapress.com

All rights reserved. No part of this book may be reproduced, stored in a retrieval system, or transmitted in any form or by any means, electronic, mechanical, photocopying, microfilming, recording, or otherwise without written permission from the Publisher.

All papers, comments, opinions, conclusions, or recommendations are those of the author(s), and do not necessarily reflect the views of the publisher.

Due diligence has been taken by the publishers, editors, and authors of this book to assure the accuracy of the information published and to describe generally accepted practices. The contributors herein have carefully checked to ensure that the drug selections and dosages set forth in this text are accurate and in accord with the standards accepted at the time of publication. Notwithstanding, as new research, changes in government regulations, and knowledge from clinical experience relating to drug therapy and drug reactions constantly occurs, the reader is advised to check the product information provided by the manufacturer of each drug for any change in dosages or for additional warnings and contraindications. This is of utmost importance when the recommended drug herein is a new or infrequently used drug. It is the responsibility of the treating physician to determine dosages and treatment strategies for individual patients. Further it is the responsibility of the health care provider to ascertain the Food and Drug Administration status of each drug or device used in their clinical practice. The publisher, editors, and authors are not responsible for errors or omissions or for any consequences from the application of the information presented in this book and make no warranty, express or implied, with respect to the contents in this publication.

This publication is printed on acid-free paper. ∞
ANSI Z39.48-1984 (American Standards Institute) Permanence of Paper for Printed Library Materials.

Cover design by Patricia F. Cleary

Production Editor: Amy Thau

For additional copies, pricing for bulk purchases, and/or information about other Humana titles, contact Humana at the above address or at any of the following numbers: Tel.: 973-256-1699; Fax: 973-256-8314; E-mail: orders@humanapr.com, or visit our Website: http://humanapress.com

Photocopy Authorization Policy:
Authorization to photocopy items for internal or personal use, or the internal or personal use of specific clients, is granted by Humana Press Inc., provided that the base fee of US $30.00 per copy is paid directly to the Copyright Clearance Center at 222 Rosewood Drive, Danvers, MA 01923. For those organizations that have been granted a photocopy license from the CCC, a separate system of payment has been arranged and is acceptable to Humana Press Inc. The fee code for users of the Transactional Reporting Service is: [1-58829-556-7/06 $30.00].

Printed in the United States of America. 10 9 8 7 6 5 4 3 2 1
eISBN: 1-59745-041-3
Library of Congress Cataloging in Publication Data
Disorders of the respiratory tract : common challenges in primary care / [edited] by Matthew L. Mintz.
   p. ; cm. -- (Current clinical practice)
  Includes bibliographical references and index.
  ISBN 1-58829-556-7 (alk. paper)
  1. Respiratory organs--Diseases. 2. Primary care (Medicine)
  [DNLM: 1. Respiratory Tract Diseases. 2. Respiratory Physiology.
3. Respiratory System--anatomy & histology. WF 140 D6126 2006] I.
Mintz, Matthew L. II. Series.
  RC731.D58 2006
  616.2--dc22
                    2005029431

Series Editor's Introduction

Disorders of the Respiratory Tract: Common Challenges in Primary Care by Dr. Matthew Mintz provides a well-written, concise overview of respiratory illness that is aimed at the busy primary care physician. Dr. Mintz is director of the ambulatory care rotation for the department of Internal Medicine at George Washington University in Washington, D.C., and through his experience as a clinician and teacher, he has developed a sharp eye for the learning needs of physicians practicing primary care. *Disorders of the Respiratory Tract: Common Challenges in Primary Care* covers the range of knowledge needed to provide excellent care for patients with respiratory disease from the basics of pulmonary function testing to understanding and caring for common respiratory illnesses including chronic obstructive pulmonary disease, asthma, allergic rhinitis, and pneumonia, and includes discussion of some less common illnesses including sarcoidosis and lung cancer. The chapters in this volume use a case-based approach to clarify the clinical questions that need to be answered, provide clear learning objectives for each topic, and then review the respiratory condition discussed in the chapter, with attention to answering the relevant information that a primary care physician will want to know when taking care of patients. The physicians who read *Disorders of the Respiratory Tract: Common Challenges in Primary Care* will understand and be able to treat more than 95% of the respiratory illnesses that will present in a busy primary care practice. For this accomplishment, Dr. Mintz deserves our thanks.

Neil Skolnik, MD
Temple University School of Medicine
Philadelphia, PA
and
Family Medicine Residency Program
Abington Memorial Hospital
Abington, PA

Introduction

I am pleased that you have chosen to read *Disorders of the Respiratory Tract: Common Challenges in Primary Care*. I am hopeful that this will be a worthwhile experience, and that you will not only use this book to improve your knowledge of respiratory disorders, but will also use it as a reference should patients with respiratory symptoms present to your clinic.

Disorders of the Respiratory Tract: Common Challenges in Primary Care was written exclusively for primary care practitioners. Respiratory symptoms are one of the most common presentations to a primary care setting. Although complex respiratory cases can be challenging for the primary care provider, even common diseases such as asthma and allergic rhinitis can prove difficult. What are the best approaches to these common disorders? How and to what degree do you need to work up a patient for a more severe condition? Unfortunately, many of the most up-to-date treatments and guidelines are published in multiple subspecialty journals, to which primary care providers rarely have access. Hopefully, *Disorders of the Respiratory Tract: Common Challenges in Primary Care* will provide primary care providers with answers to these and many other questions.

Disorders of the Respiratory Tract: Common Challenges in Primary Care begins with a section containing the basic approach to a patient with respiratory disorders ("The Basics"), reviews the anatomy and physiology of the respiratory tract, and offers a review of pulmonary function testing. The remainder of the book is divided into three sections: "Disorders of the Upper Airway," "Disorders of the Lower Airway," and "Non-Airway Disorders That Present With Respiratory Symptoms," respectively.

Each chapter follows an almost identical format, beginning with a clinical case that a primary care physician would typically see. Next, several key clinical questions that a primary care provider might ask are presented. Prior to the discussion of the topic, the learning objectives of the chapter are reviewed so that readers can orient themselves to the material. The chapter then sequentially reviews the epidemiology of the disease, the pathophysiology, and the diagnosis, differential diagnosis, and treatment of the disorder. Finally, because texts are usually out of date once they are printed, most chapters end with a section on future directions so that the primary care provider can be aware of the most up-to-date advances. Please also keep in mind that this book is available as a personal digital assistant (PDA) product for easy and efficient clinical use. To obtain the PDA, please contact the publisher, Humana Press (ISBN: 1-58829-919-8; www.humanapress.com).

I want to personally thank all of my coauthors who worked so hard to bring the most up-to-date reviews of common topics in respiratory medicine to *Disorders of the Respiratory Tract: Common Challenges in Primary Care*.

Matthew L. Mintz, MD

Contents

Series Editor's Introduction v
Introduction vii
Contributors xi

Part I. The Basics

1. Approach to the Patient With a Respiratory Disorder 3
   Nirav Patel and Matthew L. Mintz
2. Anatomy and Physiology of the Respiratory Tract 11
   Anna Person and Matthew L. Mintz
3. Pulmonary Function Testing 17
   Shyam Parkhie and Matthew L. Mintz

Part II. Disorders of the Upper Airway

4. Allergic Rhinitis 31
   Holly Bergman Sobota, Trissana Emdadi, and Matthew L. Mintz
5. Non-Allergic Rhinitis 47
   Cardin Bell and Matthew L. Mintz
6. Sinusitis 65
   Neelam Gor and Matthew L. Mintz
7. Pharyngitis 77
   David Jager and Matthew L. Mintz
8. Laryngitis and Hoarseness 89
   Matthew Chandler and Matthew L. Mintz

Part III. Disorders of the Lower Airway

9. Croup 103
   Jeremy Spencer and Matthew L. Mintz
10. Pediatric Asthma 115
    Katrina Dafnis and Matthew L. Mintz
11. Adult Asthma 131
    Dharti Patel and Matthew L. Mintz
12. Exercise-Induced Bronchospasm 147
    Khalid Jaboori and Matthew L. Mintz

13. Acute Cough 159
    Karen J. Scheer and Matthew L. Mintz
14. Chronic Cough 173
    Clara Peck and Matthew L. Mintz
15. Chronic Obstructive Pulmonary Disease 189
    Anna Person and Matthew L. Mintz
16. Lung Cancer 205
    Mohammad A. Raza and Matthew L. Mintz
17. Sarcoidosis 221
    Danielle Davidson and Matthew L. Mintz
18. Pneumonia 235
    Mohamed Al-Darei and Matthew L. Mintz
19. Bronchiolitis 249
    *Elizabeth A. Valois Asser, Alexander S. Asser,
    and Matthew L. Mintz*

*Part IV. Non-Airway Disorders That Present
With Respiratory Symptoms*

20. Obstructive Sleep Apnea 263
    Vikram Bakhru and Matthew L. Mintz
21. Obesity 273
    Rebecca Chatterjee and Matthew L. Mintz
22. Vocal Cord Dysfunction 279
    Amy Humfeld and Matthew L. Mintz
23. Pulmonary Embolism 289
    Eric Wollins and Matthew L. Mintz
24. Hemoptysis 307
    Samantha McIntosh and Matthew L. Mintz
25. Gastroesophageal Reflux Disease, Cough, and Asthma 317
    Niral Shah and Matthew L. Mintz

Index 325

Contributors

Following is a list of the contributing authors for this volume, all of whom are from The George Washington University School of Medicine in Washington, DC.

MOHAMED AL-DAREI
ALEXANDER S. ASSER, MD
CARDIN BELL
VIKRAM BAKHRU, MD
MATTHEW CHANDLER, MD
REBECCA CHATTERJEE, MD
KATRINA DAFNIS, MD
DANIELLE DAVIDSON, MD
TRISSANA EMDADI, MD
NEELAM GOR, MD
AMY HUMFELD, MD
KHALID JABOORI
DAVID JAGER, MD
SAMANTHA MCINTOSH, MD
MATTHEW L. MINTZ, MD
SHYAM PARKHIE, MD
DHARTI PATEL, MD
NIRAV PATEL, MD
CLARA PECK, MD
ANNA PERSON, MD
MOHAMMAD A. RAZA
KAREN J. SCHEER, MD, RSM
NIRAL SHAH, MD
HOLLY BERGMAN SOBOTA, MD
JEREMY SPENCER, MD
ELIZABETH A. VALOIS ASSER, MD
ERIC WOLLINS, MD

I The Basics

1 Approach to the Patient With a Respiratory Disorder

Nirav Patel and Matthew L. Mintz

CONTENTS

> INTRODUCTION
> HISTORY OF THE PRESENT ILLNESS
> ADDITIONAL HISTORY
> PHYSICAL EXAM
> DIAGNOSTIC TESTING
> SOURCES

INTRODUCTION

Patients with respiratory illness typically present with characteristic symptoms. The most common symptoms include dyspnea (shortness of breath) and cough. Less common symptoms include hemoptysis (coughing up blood) and chest pain. Regardless of which symptoms may be present, a stepwise approach must be taken so that an underlying etiology may be determined. A proper approach always begins with a detailed history regarding the nature of present symptoms, followed by information regarding the patient's past medical, family, and social history, on which a differential diagnosis can be entertained. A careful physical examination and appropriate diagnostic testing can help narrow the differential so that a diagnosis can be made and a plan for therapy initiated.

HISTORY OF THE PRESENT ILLNESS

When taking a history, the nature of questioning varies depending on the underlying symptom(s).

From: *Current Clinical Practice: Disorders of the Respiratory Tract:
Common Challenges in Primary Care*
By: M. L. Mintz © Humana Press, Totowa, NJ

Dyspnea

Shortness of breath is a common symptom of both respiratory and cardiac disease. Elements of the history including timing and onset, exacerbating and alleviating factors, and extent of physical impairment are essential to formulating a likely diagnosis. The length of time over which the dyspnea has arisen is particularly helpful in leading toward a differential as various disease processes present with different levels of acuity. For instance, a previously healthy patient developing an acute onset of shortness of breath (over hours to days) may be suffering from an acute process of the airways (such as asthma), a disease of the lung parenchyma (such as pneumonia), a disorder involving the pulmonary vasculature (such as a pulmonary embolism), or a disease process involving the pleural space (such as a pneumothorax). All of these disorders can give rise to an acute onset of dyspnea. Subacute (over days to weeks) and chronic (over weeks to months) presentations of dyspnea point more toward longer-standing disease processes, such as chronic obstructive pulmonary disease (COPD), interstitial lung disease, pleural effusion, neuromuscular disease, or chronic cardiac disease (congestive heart failure).

Questions regarding exacerbating and alleviating factors can help focus on the differential for dyspnea. Shortness of breath made worse when immediately lying flat (orthopnea) and improved when sitting up, for instance, is commonly seen in severely obstructive lung disease, diaphragmatic paralysis, and neuromuscular disease. This occurs secondary to the reduction in vital capacity stimulated by the supine position. Shortness of breath made worse after lying flat for several hours, such as with sleep (paroxysmal nocturnal dyspnea), and improved with sitting up is more consistent with cardiac causes of dyspnea, such as congestive heart failure. In this scenario, the supine increase in venous return combined with the reduction in cardiac output seen in congestive heart failure causes a slow engorgement of the pulmonary vasculature resulting in edema and subsequent dyspnea.

Cough and Hemoptysis

Cough occurs secondary to irritation of the mucous membrane along the respiratory tract. It is typically classified into one of two categories: acute cough (lasting <3 weeks) and chronic cough (lasting >3 weeks). Although there are a host of triggers that can stimulate cough, certain conditions are more likely to cause it. Acute cough typically develops secondary to such processes as viral upper respiratory tract infection, bacterial sinusitis, COPD exacerbation, allergic rhinitis, and environmental exposure. The three most common causes of chronic cough (accounting for >90% of cases in nonsmokers) include postnasal drip, followed by asthma and gastroesophageal reflux; however, chronic bronchitis should always be considered in patients with a long-standing history of smoking.

A proper approach to cough thus begins with determining how long the symptom has been present because there are different diagnostic possibilities to consider.

The presence or absence of sputum is also an important consideration in the history. In particular, specific questions regarding the quantity, color, timing, and presence or absence of blood in the sputum can help narrow the differential to specific disorders. Chronic bronchitis, for instance, presents clinically as a productive cough occurring on most days in at least 3 consecutive months over at least 2 years; sputum volume can exceed 50 mL per day. Patients with bacterial infections of the respiratory tract often present with green- or yellow-colored sputum. Blood-tinged sputum is also particular to certain conditions and can be a worrisome finding. In otherwise healthy nonsmokers, hemoptysis can usually be attributed to a mild airway infection, such as bronchitis. In individuals with smoking histories, however, more serious conditions need to be considered, the most worrisome of which is cancer. Less common but serious causes of hemoptysis in both smokers and nonsmokers include bronchiectasis, pulmonary embolus, pneumonia, and tuberculosis. When dealing with a complaint of bloody sputum, it is important to ensure that the blood is originating from the respiratory tract and not elsewhere. The nose, back of the throat, and gastrointestinal (GI) tract are all potential sources of expectorated blood. When the GI tract is involved, the condition is known as hematemesis rather than hemoptysis; it is important to distinguish the two because prognosis and treatment are markedly different.

Chest Pain

Chest pain is a nonspecific symptom that can occur from a host of disease processes involving the respiratory, cardiac, GI, musculoskeletal, and neurological systems. Chest pain of respiratory origin can be distinguished from most nonrespiratory causes of chest pain in that it is almost always respirophasic in nature (i.e., increases with forced inhalation or exhalation or during spontaneous breathing), or when increased as pressure is applied to the chest wall. Sometimes this is referred to as pleuritic pain, which, as the name implies, results from disease or inflammation of the pleura and can be caused by pleural and pulmonary vascular disorders, such as pneumothorax, infection, and pulmonary embolus. It can also result from certain musculoskeletal disorders and associated symptoms. For example, hemoptysis and acute onset of shortness of breath, which may present with the pleuritic pain of pneumothorax, are helpful clues in leading one toward a likely diagnosis.

ADDITIONAL HISTORY

Elements of the past medical history can help elucidate the etiology of the presenting complaint. For instance, a patient with a known history of chronic bronchitis presenting with dyspnea and cough productive of sputum is likely to be with an exacerbation of his COPD. A patient with HIV presenting with a similar complaint may be with *Pneumocystis carinii* pneumonia. Information regarding past medical history is thus essential in guiding one's clinical suspicion. Obtaining a good family history is also important. For instance, a patient presenting with recurrent respiratory disease and copious sputum production with a family history of cystic fibrosis may raise suspicion for cystic fibrosis. Asthma also has a high genetic predisposition.

Components of the social history can prove to be very useful in the approach to the patient with a respiratory disorder. In particular, information regarding smoking, occupational/environmental exposure, and risk factors for AIDS should be obtained because all can contribute to the onset of respiratory disease. The smoking history is particularly important because tobacco from cigarette smoke is associated with a variety of respiratory ailments, the most worrisome of which are COPD and lung cancer. Questions regarding smoking history should be focused on determining the intensity (i.e., number of packs smoked per day), duration (i.e., number of years spent smoking), a combination of the two (pack-years is equal to the number of packs per day multiplied by the number of years one has smoked), as well as the time of first cigarette, which is a marker of severity of addiction (the sooner the patient smokes the first cigarette after awakening, the heavier the addiction to nicotine). If the patient has stopped smoking, the interval since smoking cessation should be determined because the risk for developing a complication, such as lung cancer, does not improve much until the decade following the discontinuation of smoking. Finally, one cannot forget to ascertain any exposure to second-hand smoke because this significantly increases one's risk of respiratory disorders, although to a lesser degree than first-hand smoking.

Detailed information regarding environmental and occupational hazards, such as exposure to inorganic dusts (particularly asbestos and silica dust), organic antigens (molds and animal proteins), environmental allergens (dust, pet dander, and pollen) and air-borne pathogens (*Mycobacterium tuberculosis*), should be obtained because all are potential sources of a variety of respiratory illnesses. Asbestos exposure, for instance, can lead to mesothelioma, whereas asthma can be triggered by a host of environmental allergens. In these cases, an environmental and occupational investigation can certainly be useful. The history should begin by determining the patient's field of work followed by specifics regarding the potential exposure (i.e., which agent[s], how much, how long). Environmental sources, such as those related to personal hobbies or the home environment, can then be sought.

Although certain conditions may directly cause pulmonary damage and precipitate disease, others may indirectly predispose a patient to developing a respiratory disorder. People with AIDS, for instance, are at increased risk for various infections secondary to their immunocompromised state; the lungs, in particular, are a common site for infection to occur. Some respiratory disorders commonly associated with AIDS include *P. carinii* pneumonia, tuberculosis, and *Mycobacterium avium* complex. Risk factors for AIDS should thus be identified because a person at high risk presenting with respiratory complaints may have an opportunistic disease. Questions regarding sexual history (i.e., sexual orientation, nature of engaged behavior [oral, anal, or vaginal sex], number of lifetime partners, and use of barrier protection), history of intravenous drug use, and history of blood transfusions should all be ascertained because all can give insight into the patient's relative risk for AIDS and associated pulmonary disease.

PHYSICAL EXAM

The general appearance is important for the physical exam in any patient, especially one who presents with respiratory symptoms. Distress displayed by a patient with a respiratory condition can be a sign of a life-threatening illness. Although complaints of shortness of breath can be subjective, looking for signs of respiratory distress, such as cyanosis or the inability to speak in complete sentences, is critical. A patient's body habitus can also be telling. Obesity is associated with a number of respiratory conditions, and cachexia can be a sign of cancer or AIDS, both of which are associated with respiratory disorders. In children with serious respiratory disorders, such as severe chronic asthma and cystic fibrosis, growth and development can be delayed. Finally, smelling alcohol or cigarette smoke can aid in diagnosis of the patient with respiratory complaints.

Examination of the thorax should be approached in an organized sequence: inspection, palpation, percussion, and auscultation. On inspection, the rate and pattern of breathing should be observed and the chest wall should be examined for signs of deformities or asymmetry. Abnormalities, such as kyphoscoliosis, pectus excavatum (funnel chest), and ankylosing spondylitis, can lead to restrictive ventilatory disease secondary to the thoracic cavity compression caused by these disorders. Any impairment in respiratory movement on one or both sides should be noted, and the interspaces should be checked for abnormalities of retraction. Retractions are commonly seen in severe asthma, COPD, or upper airway obstruction, whereas a unilateral impairment or lagging of respiratory movement is suggestive of underlying lung or pleural disease (e.g., fibrosis, lobar pneumonia, pleural effusion, and so on).

On palpation, the chest wall should be palpated for tenderness and fremitus. Intercostal tenderness results from inflammation of the pleura and can result from both pulmonary (e.g., pleuritis secondary to lower respiratory tract infection) and nonpulmonary causes (e.g., costochondritis). Fremitus refers to the palpable vibration transmitted along the bronchopulmonary tree during speech; it can be tested for by placing the edge of each hand along the patient's chest wall while the patient speaks. In normal patients, fremitus should be felt symmetrically along the chest wall. A decreased vibratory sense can be seen in conditions such as pleural effusion in which the accumulation of fluid in the pleural space causes a dampening of vibration. Fibrosis, COPD, and pneumothorax are other conditions that can cause a decrease in fremitus. Fremitus is increased when the transmission of sound is increased as in the consolidated lung of pneumonia.

Percussion of the chest wall allows the physician to determine whether the underlying tissue is air- or fluid-filled or solid. In the normal lung, the underlying tissue is air-filled and should produce a resonant sound to percussion. In conditions, such as pleural effusion or lobar pneumonia, in which fluid replaces the air-containing lung and dullness replaces the resonant sound. Dullness to percussion can also be heard when solid tissue replaces the air-filled lung, such as with pulmonary fibrosis or lung cancer. Hyperresonance can be heard bilaterally in the hyperinflated lung, such as with emphysema or asthma, whereas unilateral hyperresonance suggests the presence of a large pneumothorax.

On auscultation, the quality, intensity, and presence of adventitious (extra) breath sounds should be determined. The quality of breath sounds in normal lungs are characterized as bronchial, vesicular, or bronchovesicular. Bronchial breath sounds are loud, high-pitched, and characteristically heard over the central airways with expiratory sounds lasting longer than inspiratory sounds. Vesicular breath sounds are soft, low-pitched, and heard best at the periphery and at the base of the lungs; they are heard through inspiration and continue without pause through expiration. Bronchovesicular breath sounds are a combination of both bronchial and vesicular breath sounds and are heard best over medium-sized airways; inspiratory and expiratory sounds are about equal in length and, at times, separated by a silent interval. If bronchial or bronchovesicular breath sounds are heard in sites distant from their typical location, the air-filled lung has likely been replaced by fluid-filled or solid lung tissue.

The intensity of the breath sounds should be noted. Breath sounds vary depending on the region being auscultated but are typically heard loudest in the posterior lung fields. They may be decreased when airflow is decreased, as with obstructive lung disease, or they may be decreased when the transmission of sound is decreased, as with pleural effusion, pneumothorax, or emphysema.

The most common adventitious (extra) breath sounds not heard in normal lungs include wheezes, rales, and rhonchi. Wheezes are relatively high-pitched sounds that have a hissing or shrill-like quality and can be heard in respiratory disorders in which the airways have narrowed or become obstructed, such as with asthma, obstructive lung disease, and even congestive heart failure. Rales, or "crackles," are described as either fine or coarse. Fine crackles are soft, high-pitched sounds that are brief in duration and heard most commonly at the lung bases. They are produced on inspiration from the opening of collapsed alveoli as in the patient with atelectasis, pulmonary edema, and interstitial fibrosis. Coarse crackles are loud, low-pitched, and longer in duration; they result from the presence of mucus in the airways and can be seen in conditions such as bronchiectasis and bronchitis in patients who are unable to effectively expectorate these secretions. Rhonchi are relatively low-pitched sounds that have a snoring quality and result from the presence free liquid in the airway lumen. Other adventitious breath sounds include friction rubs and stridor. The sound of a friction rub is likened to the sound of rubbing two pieces of leather against each other and results from inflamed pleural surfaces sliding against one another. Stridor results from narrowing of the upper airways and is heard most prominently during inspiration; it is seen most commonly in infants with croup.

Finally, extrathoracic examination should be considered. Because cardiac and GI causes can be related to respiratory complaints, these systems should be examined. Examination of the oropharynx and nasal cavity is obligatory in any patient presenting with respiratory symptoms, especially cough. The tympanic membranes should be inspected in patients complaining of congestion and other upper respiratory symptoms because enlarged nasal turbinates can block Eustachian tubes leading to serous and/or otitis media. Clubbing of the nail beds can be seen in severe hypoxic disorders.

DIAGNOSTIC TESTING

Chest radiography (chest X-ray) is often the initial diagnostic study of choice in patients presenting with symptoms of respiratory disease. Diagnostic possibilities vary depending on the nature of underlying findings: nodules, for instance, may suggest neoplasia, whereas a localized opacification may suggest pneumonia. Another test commonly employed is computed tomography (CT) of the chest. Findings on chest CT are more sensitive than plain radiography. The reason for this lies with the fact that, although a chest X-ray only shows two views of the chest, a CT scan shows cross-sectional images and thus subtle abnormalities are more easily seen. CT testing is particularly useful in cases of trauma, evaluation of pulmonary embolism (spiral CT), and in the diagnosis of primary and secondary neoplasia. The drawback of CT is its cost, and thus chest radiography continues to remain the initial study of choice in patients with respiratory disease.

Other tests commonly utilized in the evaluation of patients with respiratory disease include pulmonary function testing, arterial blood gas analysis, pulse oximetry, and bronchoscopy. Pulmonary function testing is useful in the evaluation of obstructive or restrictive lung disease, whereas arterial blood gas and pulse oximetry are useful in evaluating acid–base disorders (which may be of either respiratory or metabolic origin).

Bronchoscopy can be useful when tissue samples are required from the lung parenchyma, as with evaluation of infection or neoplasm, or when visualization of the airways is necessary, as in the case of foreign body obstruction. Whichever diagnostic method is utilized, it should be guided by clinical suspicion because appropriate testing can provide much insight into the nature of the underlying illness.

SOURCES

Albert RK, Spio SG, Jett JR. Comprehensive Respiratory Medicine. Mosby, London, 1999.

Brigham KL, Slovis BS. Approach to the patient with respiratory disease. In: Andreoli TE, Carpenter CCJ, Griggs R, Loscalzo J, eds. Cecil Essentials of Medicine, 5th Ed. W.B. Sauders, Philadelphia, 2001, 167–171.

Cole RB, Mackay AD. Essentials of Respiratory Disease. Churchill Livingstone, New York, 1990.

Drazen JM, Weinberger SE. Approach to the patient with disease of the respiratory system. In: Kasper DL, Braunwald E, Fauci AS, et al., eds. Harrison's Principles of Internal Medicine. McGraw Hill, New York, 2005, 1495–1498.

Irwin RS, Madison JM. The diagnosis and treatment of cough. N Engl J Med 2000;343:1715–1721.

2 Anatomy and Physiology of the Respiratory Tract

Anna Person and Matthew L. Mintz

CONTENTS
  INTRODUCTION
  ANATOMY
  PHYSIOLOGY
  SOURCES

INTRODUCTION

The anatomy and physiology of the respiratory tract is quite complex. Each anatomic segment performs in concert with the others and is accountable for a wide variety of physiological responsibilities. These responsibilities vary with rest or exercise, disease or health. Throughout this book, the reader will discover that the respiratory tract is a delicate and complicated system that can be involved in a number of disease processes. An understanding of the anatomy and physiology of the respiratory tract is critical to understanding this elaborate system to maintain respiratory health and treat respiratory diseases.

ANATOMY

The respiratory system is comprised of several elements including the central nervous system, the chest wall, the pulmonary circulation, and the respiratory tract. The respiratory tract can be divided into four distinct segments: the naso-oropharynx, the conducting airways, the respiratory bronchioles, and the alveoli. The lungs can also be divided into the conducting airways and the units of respiration. The trachea, bronchi, and bronchioles conduct and transport air from the outside world and deliver it to the respiratory units—the alveoli. Gas

From: *Current Clinical Practice: Disorders of the Respiratory Tract: Common Challenges in Primary Care*
By: M. L. Mintz © Humana Press, Totowa, NJ

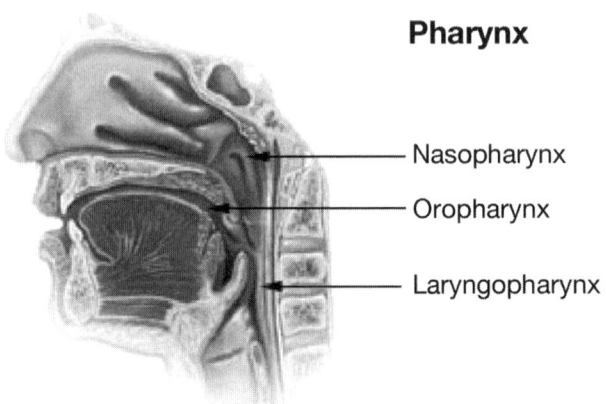

Fig. 1. The nasopharynx.

exchange occurs at the level of the alveoli, providing the necessary oxygen for the body's daily functions. Malfunction of any of these components can lead to the myriad respiratory disorders discussed in this book.

The first segment of the respiratory tract is the naso-oropharynx (*see* Fig. 1), which begins with the nostrils and lips, and includes the nasal passage, sinuses, and glottis until reaching the trachea. The purpose of the naso-oropharynx is to filter out any large particles and to humidify and warm the air that is delivered to the respiratory units. The epiglottis and muscles of the larynx coordinate the passage of food and air, and generally assure that food reaches the esophagus and air reaches the trachea.

The next segment is the conducting airways, beginning with the trachea, which branches repeatedly to form approximately 14 generations of conduits for air reaching several distinct pulmonary segments. The trachea bifurcates at the carina into the right and left mainstem bronchi. Aspiration occurs more commonly at the right main bronchus because of its gentler angle off the trachea. The right lung is divided into upper, middle, and lower lobes, each of which is further subdivided into segments and each with its own conducting airway. The upper lobe contains three segments: the apical, posterior, and anterior. The middle lobe consists of the lateral and medial segments. The lower lobe has five segments: the superior, medial basal, anterior basal, lateral basal, and posterior basal. The right lung has 10 segments, as opposed to 8 found in the left lung. The left main bronchus has two divisions serving the left upper lobe. The superior division of the bronchus leads to the apical–posterior and anterior segments. The inferior division of the bronchus leads to the superior and inferior lingular segments. The left lower lobe consists of the superior, anteromedial basal, lateral basal, and posterior basal segments. Each bronchopulmonary segment is supplied by an individual branch of the pulmonary artery.

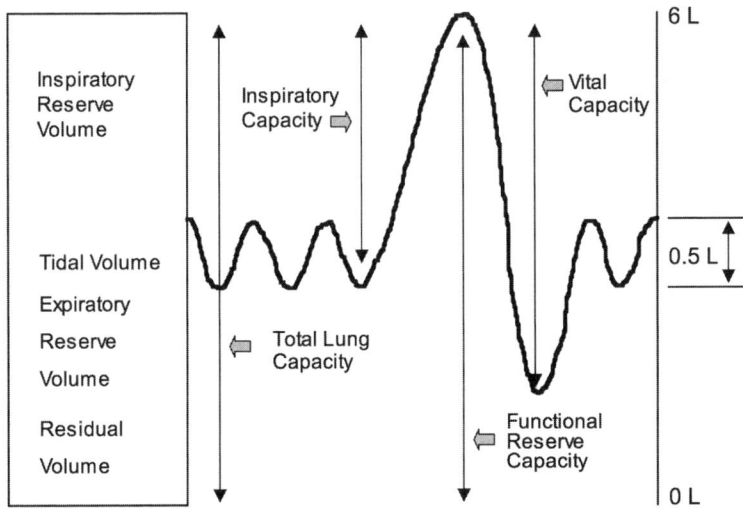

Fig. 2. Lung volumes.

The respiratory bronchioles are the last bronchioles before reaching the alveoli. Smaller foreign particles may be trapped here, and lymphatic channels are found as well. The solitary layer of epithelial cells that compose the surface of the respiratory tract gives way to the cells that comprise the lining of alveoli. The warriors of the immune system are found at this level; macrophages, neutrophils, and eosinophils are poised to act should unknown antigens be found. Once the air reaches the alveoli, type I epithelial cells allow for gas exchange, and create a total surface area of around 130 sq ft among all alveoli. The millions of alveoli are embedded among capillaries to create an air–blood interface.

PHYSIOLOGY

The physiological makeup of the lungs maintains the delicate balance between these disparate anatomic entities. Several terms have been developed to describe the various physiological capacities of the respiratory tract (Fig. 2). Total lung capacity is defined as the volume of gas in the lungs following maximal inspiration. Functional residual capacity is the volume of gas in the lungs at the end of normal expiration. The functional residual capacity is comprised of the expiratory reserve volume (the amount of air that can be expelled with maximal expiratory effort) and the residual volume (the volume of air in the lungs after maximal expiration). Tidal volume is the volume of gas in any normal breath (generally around 500–800 mL), whereas vital capacity is the maximal volume of air that can be expelled following maximal inspiration. These volumes can be measured by spirometry (*see* Chapter 3).

The three main physiological functions of the respiratory tract are ventilation, perfusion, and diffusion. Ventilation is the process of procuring air from the external environment via inspiration to supply the alveolus, after which it is subsequently returned to the outside of the body through expiration. The elastic nature of the lungs and chest wall permit pressure differentials without which inspiration and expiration could not occur. The lungs are distended by pressure exerted by the airways and alveoli (positive internal pressure) or by pressure outside the lungs (negative external pressure). The chest wall's elasticity allows it to act as a spring. When the pressures exerted on it are altered, the chest wall moves and breathing occurs. The stimulus for respiration comes mainly from the medulla and pons, which constantly receive neural inputs from several sources. The carotid bodies detect changes in PaO_2, $PaCO_2$, and pH, whereas the medulary chemporeceptor monitors $PaCO_2$ and pH alone. Muscle spindles and Golgi tendon organs monitor chest wall muscles and stretch. All of this information is combined to determine ventilatory needs, which increase in illness, exercise, or other physiological states in which tissue oxygen needs are increased. The responses of these receptors can be blunted and lead to decreased ventilation as well. This can occur with obesity, severe chronic bronchitis, or severe metabolic alkalosis.

The ventilatory drive is stimulated by PaO_2 and $PaCO_2$ levels, although the body demonstrates far greater sensitivity to $PaCO_2$ levels. In normal individuals at rest, the $PaCO_2$ level is tightly controlled. If the $PaCO_2$ level raises slightly, to 42 mmHg, the rate of ventilation quickly increases. However, the PaO_2 generally must decrease to around 65 mmHg for a similar ventilatory response to be initiated via hypoxemic stimulus. Hypercapnia is therefore the primary drive for ventilation.

Distribution of inhaled air also varies. In a normal, upright individual intrapleural pressure is most negative at lung apices and least negative at lung bases. At rest, therefore, the alveoli are least distended at the bases of the lungs, and this area receives greater ventilation as a result.

Another main physiological responsibility of the respiratory tract is diffusion (Fig. 3). This is measured by diffusion capacity for carbon monoxide, which tests how well the gas in inspired air can cross the wall of the alveolus and enter the capillary. This entails crossing the alveolar type 1 epithelial cells, the interstitial space, and the vascular endothelial cells. Carbon monoxide is used for measuring the diffusing capacity of the lung, generally by use of the single breath determination. Adjustments must be made for those with altered lung volumes, those with increased carbon monoxide levels (such as smokers), and those who are anemic or who are being tested at high altitudes. Elevated values may be found in asthmatics or those with pulmonary hemorrhage, whereas decreased values are found in emphysema, interstitial lung diseases, or any other process that may disturb the integrity of the alveoli.

Chapter 2 / The Respiratory Tract

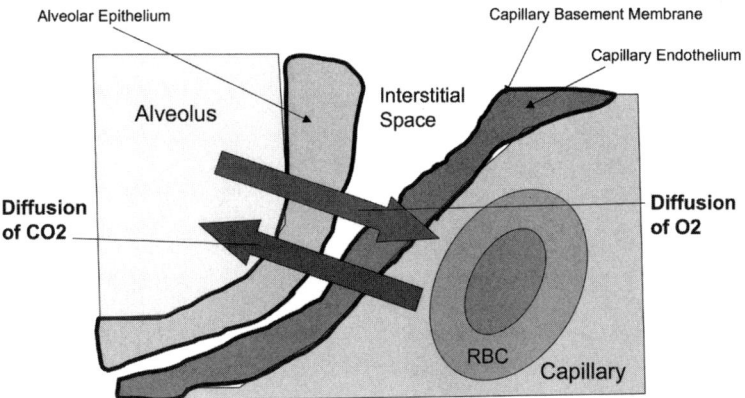

Fig. 3. Diffusion of gases across the alveolar–capillary membrane. RBC, red blood cell.

Perfusion is the final responsibility of the respiratory tract, and is necessary to maintain ventilation and diffusion of its anatomical components. Each division and subdivision of the respiratory tract has its own blood supply. Perhaps most valuable, however, are the pulmonary artery capillaries that surround the alveoli and provide the physiological proximity necessary for the transport of oxygen and other gases into the blood supply and carbon dioxide from the blood back into the lungs for expulsion. Because of gravitational forces, perfusion is greater at the lung bases than at the lung apices, leading to a slight normal physiological mismatch of perfusion compared with ventilation.

SOURCES

Kochar R. Anatomy, physiology and pulmonary function testing. In: Kutty K, Kochar MS, Schapira R, Van Ruiswyk J. Kochar's Concise Textbooks of Medicine, 4th Ed. Baltimore, MD, Lippincott, Williams and Wilkins, 2002, p. 481.

Myers AR. Pulmonary function studies. In: National Medical Series for Independent Study: Medicine, 4th ed. Lippincott, Williams and Wilkins, Baltimore, MD, 2001; pp. 63–69.

Reynolds HY. Respiratory structure and function. In: Goldman L, Ausiello D, eds. Cecil Textbook of Medicine, 22nd ed. W. B. Saunders, Philadelphia, 2004, pp. 485–501.

Weinberger SE, Drazen JM. Distrubances of respiratory function. In: Kasper DL, Braunwald E, Fauci AS, et al., eds. Harrison's Principles of Internal Medicine, 16th Ed. McGraw-Hill, New York, 2005, pp. 1498–1521.

3
Pulmonary Function Testing

Shyam Parkhie and Matthew L. Mintz

CONTENTS
>   INTRODUCTION
>   OBSTRUCTION
>   RESTRICTION
>   TYPES OF LUNG FUNCTION TESTS
>   BRONCHOPROVICATION TESTING
>   CARBON MONOXIDE DIFFUSION
>   SUMMARY
>   KEY POINTS
>   REFERENCES

INTRODUCTION

Pulmonary function tests (PFTs) refer to a panel of tests including spirometry, measurement of lung volumes, and diffusion capacity for carbon monoxide (DLCO). We first review the basic types of pulmonary disorders (obstructive versus restrictive), and then discuss the main types of PFTs. An algorithm for the use of PFTs is given at the end of this chapter.

OBSTRUCTION

Obstructive lung diseases have in common decreased airflow during expiration. The three classic obstructive diseases are asthma, chronic bronchitis, and emphysema. They are defined on spirometry as having a volume of air in the first second of forced expiration (FEV_1), which is less than 70 to 80% of the predicted value matched for age and gender.

From: *Current Clinical Practice: Disorders of the Respiratory Tract:
Common Challenges in Primary Care*
By: M. L. Mintz © Humana Press, Totowa, NJ

RESTRICTION

Decreased lung volumes characterize restrictive lung diseases. They are defined as having a total lung capacity (TLC) less than 80% of predicted. Extrinsic causes include decreased chest wall compliance (e.g., obesity, kyphoscoliosis, concentric chest wall burns) and weakening of the muscles of respiration (e.g., neuromuscular disorders). Intrinsic defects are within the lung itself (e.g., interstitial lung disease, congestive heart failure).

TYPES OF LUNG FUCTION TESTS

Spirometry

Spirometry measures changes in lung volume over time during forced breathing maneuvers (Fig. 1). The patient is instructed to take a full inspiration and then exhales as forcefully as possible for as long a possible. The total volume of expired air is the forced vital capacity (FVC) (Table 1). Air expired in the first second of that maneuver is the FEV_1. Spirometry is one of the easiest and inexpensive PFTs. For most breathing disorders, it is best to start with spirometry and order further testing as warranted.

TEST ACCEPTABILITY

The first step in interpreting spirometry is making sure the test is of good quality because results are dependent on the patient's effort and cooperation. The American Thoracic Society has published guidelines regarding acceptability. When viewing a graph of expired volume over time, the exhalation should start at time zero, there should be a smooth curve (no hesitation or cough), and a plateau of at least 1 second at the end of the maneuver (no air movement). A minimum of three attempts should be made. The absolute value between the two largest FVC measurements and the two largest FEV_1 measurements should be within 0.2 L of each other *(1)*.

INTERPRETING RESULTS

FEV_1 and FVC are expressed as both absolute volumes and percent predicted. The predicted values are based on healthy volunteer data and are matched to the patient's age, height, sex, and race. FEV_1:FVC is the direct ratio of the patient's own values.

An FEV_1 of less than 70 to 80% of predicted suggests obstruction. The FVC may be normal or decreased, but to a lesser degree than the FEV_1. An FEV_1:FVC ratio of less than 0.7 is characteristic of obstruction. Classically, FEV_1 and FVC are both reduced in restriction, but the ratio of FEV_1:FVC is normal or increased. An FEV_1:FVC ratio of more than 0.7 suggests restriction *(2)* (Table 1).

The slow vital capacity (SVC) can be used to differentiate restriction from obstruction in patients in which both FEV_1 and FVC are decreased. Patients with

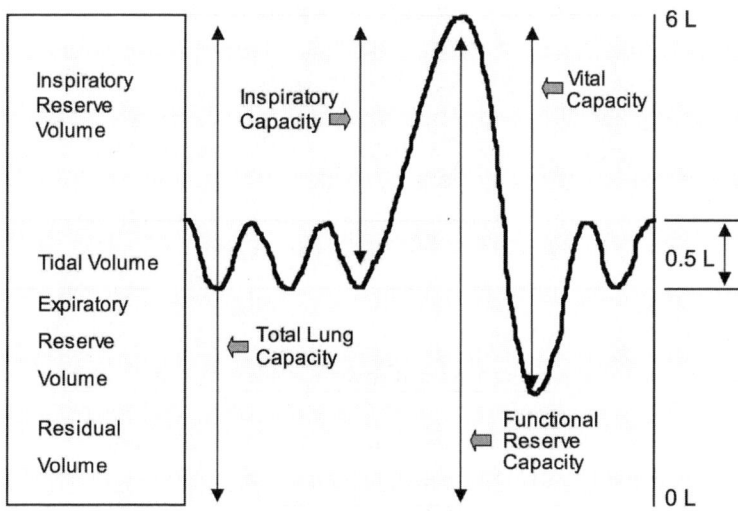

Fig. 1. Lung volumes.

Table 1
Spirometry Terms

	Obstruction	Restriction
Forced expiratory volume (FEV)$_1$ is the volume of air that is forcefully exhaled in 1 second.	Decreased, <0.7–0.8 predicted	Normal, decreased, or increased
Forced vital capacity (FVC) is the volume of air that can be maximally forcefully exhaled.	Normal or decreased	Decreased
FEV$_1$:FVC is ratio of FEV$_1$ to FVC, expressed as a percentage.	<0.7	>0.7
Forced expiratory flow (FEF)$_{25-75}$ is the average volume of air during the mid-25 to 75% portion of the FVC.	Decreased	N/A
Slow vital capacity is maximal volume of air exhaled nonforcibly.	Normal or increased	Decreased
Peak expiratory flow rate is the peak flow rate during expiration.	Lability: >30% in children >20% in adults	N/A

N/A, not applicable.

severe obstruction may have a falsely low FVC because of collapsed airways during forceful expiration. An SVC will be more normal in this obstructed patient. In restrictive disease, both the SVC and FVC are decreased. Use of SVC plus FVC may obviate the need for static lung volumes to diagnose restriction *(3)*.

The forced expiratory flow $(FEF)_{25-75\%}$, when decreased, is used as an indicator of small airways disease. When it is the only abnormality seen on spirometry, it suggests early obstruction. However, this value is highly variable among normal volunteers and many experts caution against using it to diagnose obstructive lung disease *(4)*.

BRONCHODILATOR RESPONSE

If obstruction is suspected by initial spirometry, the test can be repeated 10 minutes after administration of a bronchodilator, such as albuterol. Patient education is crucial to ensure proper use of the metered-dose inhaler.

An improvement in FEV_1 of more than 12% or 0.2 L postbronchodilator indicates acutely responsive airway constriction. This is most consistent with asthma, but reversible airway constriction can be seen in chronic bronchitis and emphysema. A negative test does not exclude the diagnosis of asthma or any obstructive disease. If obstructive disease is suspected, the patient should be considered for a 6- to 8-week trial of bronchodilators and/or inhaled corticosteroids. This is especially important in the case of asthma, when bronchoconstriction is intermittent, and thus a response to bronchodilators may not be appreciated during testing in the clinic.

BRONCHOPROVICATION TESTING

Broncopulmonary hyperresponsiveness, as seen in asthma, can be diagnosed or excluded by spirometry before and after inhalation of a known bronchial irritant. Bronchoprovication testing (i.e., methacholine challenge) is *not* required to make the diagnosis of asthma. It should be done only in a monitored environment. Again, this test is particularly useful in patients that have intermittent symptoms, who may have normal spirometry in between episodes.

An alternative to this is ambulatory monitoring of peak flow or FEV_1. Measurements are taken intermittently over 2 weeks. Variability in values is evidence for airway hyperreactivity and reversible bronchoconstriction. Peak-flow variability of more than 30% in children and more than 20% in adults suggests asthma.

Flow–Volume Loops

Plotting flow (*y*-axis) versus volume (*x*-axis) during forced maximal inspiration and expiration can be helpful in determining the site of lung obstruction. Restrictive lung disease also gives a distinctive flow–volume loop pattern, but

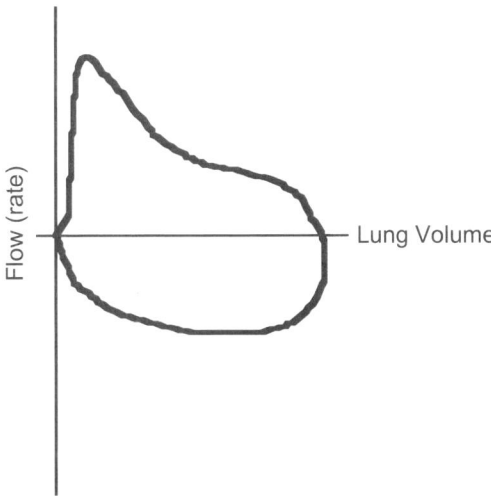

Fig. 2. Chronic obstructive pulmonary disease flow–volume loop.

these plots are generally not helpful in differentiating between types of restrictive lung disease.

In general, flow loops are evaluated qualitatively by the pattern of flow. However, the data can be quantified as a ratio of expiratory to inspiratory flow at 50% of vital capacity, $FEF_{(50\%)}$:forced inspiratory flow $(FIF)_{(50\%)}$. An obstruction symptomatic primarily with expiration would have a $FEF_{(50\%)}/FIF_{(50\%)}$ of less than 1, and an inspiratory obstruction of greater than 1.

Following are six classic patterns of obstruction:

1. Obstructive pulmonary disease: asthma and chronic obstructive pulmonary disease (COPD) have obstruction on the level of the intrathoracic airways. The "scooped-out" pattern. In COPD, this "scooped-out" pattern is secondary to premature closure of the major airways secondary to loss of the tethering effect of the surrounding parenchyma (Fig. 2).
2. Upper airway obstruction: defined as obstruction between the mouth and lower trachea and are divided into intra- and extrathoracic, based on proximity to thoracic inlet. Some lesions are either small or compliant enough to present only when a positive pressure is exerted on them. In these cases, their anatomic location can be suggested by the variable obstruction on the flow–volume loop. Large or firm lesions will present as a fixed obstruction on flow–volume loop. The flow–volume loop will not indicate location with respect to the thoracic inlet (Fig. 3).
    a. Variable (or dynamic) extrathoracic obstruction: the inspiratory limb is flattened, whereas the expiratory limb is relatively normal. This pattern should

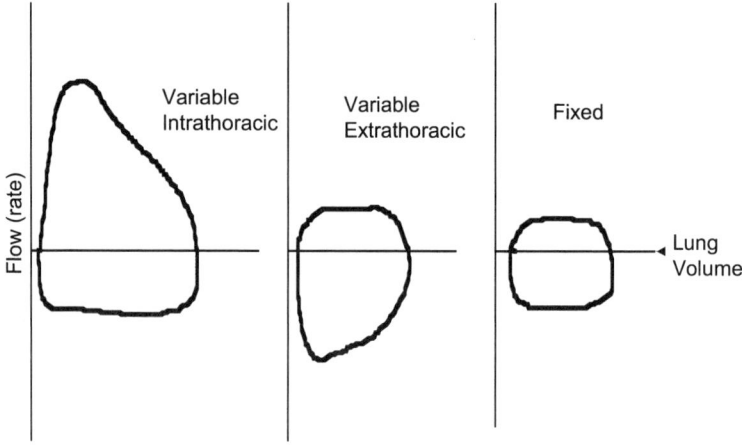

Fig. 3. Upper airway obstruction.

make the clinician think of trachemalacia of the upper trachea or vocal cord lesions.

b. Variable (or dynamic) intrathoracic obstruction: the expiratory limb is flattened and the inspiratory limb is relatively unaffected. Examples include tracheamalacia of the lower trachea or tracheal lesions. Intrathoracic lesions are more commonly malignant processes than extrathoracic lesions.

c. Fixed lesion: obstruction is present regardless of the pressure changed associated with respiration. Both the inspiratory and expiratory limbs are flattened.

d. Variable obstruction at the thoracic inlet: in the case of an obstruction that lies at the thoracic inlet (i.e., a low posttracheotomy scar) the obstruction may move from intrathoracic to extrathoracic during expiration. The classic "double hump" is seen. Spirometry can be repeated in these patients with flexion and extension in the neck. A variable intrathoracic then extrathoracic pattern may be seen, respectively (Fig. 4).

e. Obstructive sleep apnea (OSA): flow–volume loops have been evaluated for a test for OSA. Inspiratory and expiratory "saw-tooth" oscillations have been described, and the $FEF_{(50\%)}:FIF_{(50\%)}$ would be expected to be greater than one. However, the sensitivity of both results is low for diagnosing OSA. Specificities for the saw-tooth pattern and $FEF_{(50\%)}:FIF_{(50\%)}$ greater than one are reported as 94 and 86% percent, respectively *(5,6)* (Fig.5).

CARBON MONOXIDE DIFFUSION

Also called the "transfer function," the diffusion capacity (DLCO) measures the ability of the alveolar capillary membrane to diffuse gases. The patient is required to inhale a harmless, composite gas (usually 10% helium and 0.3% CO)

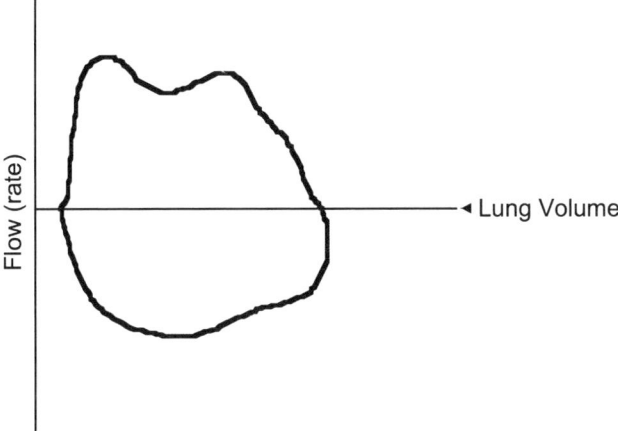

Fig. 4. Variable obstruction at the thoracic inlet.

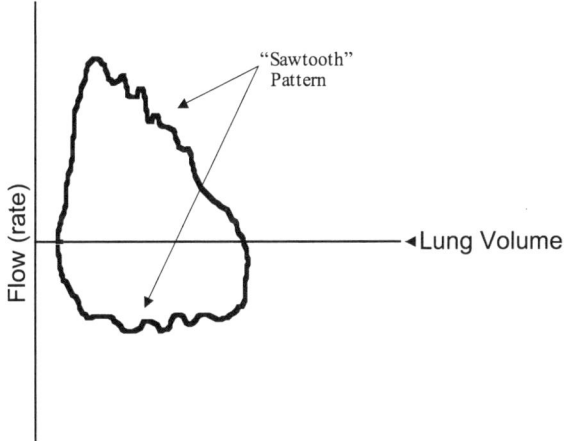

Fig. 5. Obstructive sleep apnea.

and hold their breath for 10 seconds. The exhaled breath is then analyzed for dilution of helium and uptake of CO. A DLCO of less than 74% predicted is considered mild impairment. Severe impairment is defined as less than 40% predicted *(7)*. DLCO of less than 30% predicted is central to the US Social Security Disability definition of respiratory impairment *(8)*.

1. Obstruction: DLCO is decreased in obstruction when there is anatomic destruction of the alveoli (emphysema). This makes DLCO measurement a good way to differentiate chronic bronchitis and asthma from emphysema. A low DLCO correlates well with low mean density of the lung on computed tomography scan *(9)*.

2. Restrictive disease: DLCO is most useful in differentiating intrinsic restrictive lung disease from extrinsic disease. A decreased DLCO is seen in significant interstitial lung disease (intrinsic), whereas normal values are typically seen in other causes of decreased lung volume, such as obesity, neuromuscular diseases, kyphoscoliosis, and pleural scarring.

Interstitial lung disease is often iatrogenic and DLCO is often used to follow patients at risk. This may be helpful in patients receiving chemotherapy (e.g., bleomycin), radiation to the chest, or amiodarone. Likewise, disease progression of sarcoidosis can be checked with DLCO monitoring.

An abnormal DLCO may be a clue to pulmonary vascular disease in the patient with normal spirometry and dyspnea *(10)*. This includes chronic recurrent pulmonary emboli, primary pulmonary hypertension, and vasculitis with pulmonary involvement (as seen in rheumatoid arthritis, systemic lupus erythematosus, and irritable bowel syndrome).

It is important to note that DLCO can be abnormally low in patients with anemia or who have been recently smoking (secondary to increased carboxyhemoglobin levels). It can be abnormally high in polycythemia, severe obesity, mild heart failure (increased blood in the pulmonary capillaries without pulmonary edema), and if the patient has exercised just before the test (increased cardiac output) *(11)*.

Lung Volumes

Lung volumes are most useful in diagnosing restriction by demonstrating decreased TLC. In most cases, restriction can be diagnosed by spirometry, as detailed in subheading entitled "Spirometry." Lung volumes can be helpful in diagnosing restriction superimposed in a patient with obstruction and a low vital capacity.

There are four methods for obtaining TLC. Nitrogen washout and helium dilution are relatively easy to do, but can underestimate TLC in a patient with moderate to severe COPD. Body plethesmography is the gold standard for TLC measurement but involves complex equipment and is expensive. A rough estimate of TLC can be made with measurement taken from a chest X-ray taken at maximal expiration. TLC values by this method are typically within 15% of body plethesmography readings *(12)*.

Maximal Expiratory Pressure/Maximal Inspiratory Pressure

Neuromuscular disease affecting respiration presents as a restrictive defect. The strength of the respiratory muscles can be assessed using maximal inspiratory pressure and maximal expiratory pressure. Both are measured with a simple pressure transducer placed on a mouthpiece. Maximal expiratory pressure is the maximal force generated against a blocked mouthpiece with cheeks bulging after full inspiration and maximal inspiratory pressure is a similar value measured after full expiration. Both measurements are useful in detecting a neuromuscular disease and in tracking disease progression.

Preoperative Testing

PFTs are often used preoperatively to determine risks of pulmonary complications from surgery and to evaluate a patient for lung resection surgery. The primary care physician often does the latter. Unfortunately, there is no single standardized way to use PFTs in preoperative evaluation *(13)*. Some general guidelines include *(14)* the following:

1. PFTs should be used to assess need for intervention to minimize pulmonary complications of surgery, but not to deny surgery to certain patients.
2. PFTs are only useful preoperatively in persons with lung disease suggested on history and physical.
3. In patients with moderate or severe obstruction, delay in elective surgery may be considered for smoking cessation, chest physiotherapy, weight reduction, or a course of bronchodilators, antibiotics, and/or steroids. Significant reduction in postoperative pulmonary complications is seen within 8 weeks of smoking cessation *(15)*.
4. Risk of the procedure relates to proximity to the diaphragm and the degree of anesthesia.

SUMMARY

PFTs are invaluable tools in evaluating respiratory disorders. PFTs provide more than percent predicted for certain values; they can be of added value when flow–volume loops are interpreted and other components, such as DLCO and bronchoprovocative challenges, are utilized. In evaluation of dyspnea, one needs to determine whether or not the patient has an obstructive or a restrictive disorder (Fig. 6). Methacholine challenge can assist establishing asthma as a diagnosis and DLCO can help define intrinsic or extrinsic restrictive disease.

KEY POINTS

1. There are many different types of PFTs. Individual tests should be ordered based on the patient's symptoms. Ordering comprehensive testing for all patients with breathing problems may yield misleading results.
2. Spirometry is a good first test to order for dyspnea.
3. DLCO is useful in differentiating the etiology of a restrictive disorder and distinguishes emphysema from chronic bronchitis and asthma.
4. Flow–volume loops are most useful in delineating extrathoracic from intrathoracic obstruction.

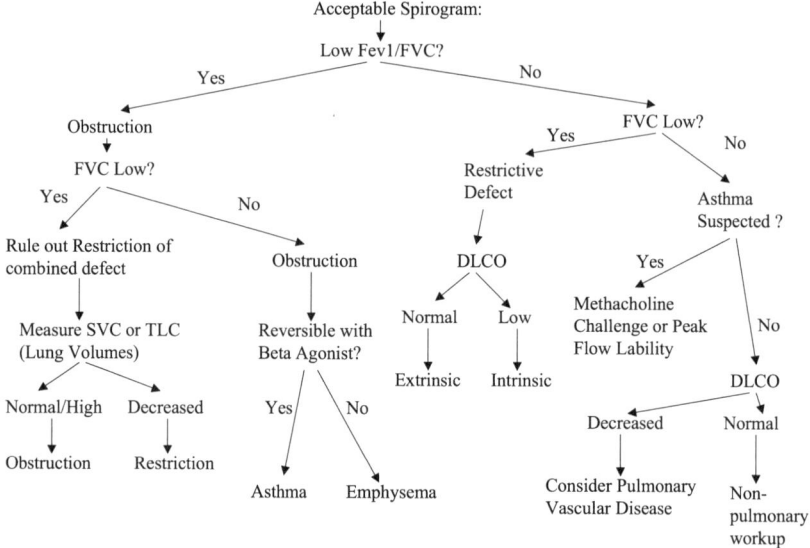

Fig. 6. Dyspnea algorithm.

5. PFTs can be used in preoperative evaluations to predict pulmonary risk, but should not be used to deny surgery.

REFERENCES

1. American Thoracic Society. Standardization of spirometry. Am J Respir Crit Care Med 1195;152:1107–1136.
2. West JB. Restriction and obstruction. In: Respiratory Physiology, 4th ed. Lippincott, Williams and Wilkins, Baltimore, MD, 1990; pp. 147–151.
3. Aaron SD, Dales RE, Cardinal P. How accurate is spirometry at predicting restrictive pulmonary impairment? Chest 1999;115:869–873.
4. Petty TL. Simple office spirometry. Clin Chest Med 2001;22:845–859.
5. Sanders MH, Martin RJ, Pennock BE, Rogers RM. The detection of sleep apnea in the awake patient. The saw tooth sign. JAMA 1981;245:2414–2418.
6. Hoffstein V, Wright S, Zamel N. Flow volume curves in snoring patients with and without obstructive sleep apnea. Am Rev Respir Dis 1989;139:957–960.
7. Becklake MR, Crapo RO. Lung function testing: selection of reference values and interpretative strategies. Official Statement of the American Thoracic Society. Am Rev Respir Dis 1991;144:1202–1218.
8. Social Security Administration. Disability evaluation under social security. Blue Book, 2003, section 3.02.
9. Gould GA, Redpath AT, Ryan M, et al. Lung CT density correlates with measurement of airflow limitation and diffusing capacity. Eur Respir J 1991;4:141–146.
10. Waxman AB. Pulmonary function test abnormalities in pulmonary vascular disease and chronic heart failure. Clin Chest Med 2001;22:751–758.

11. American Thoracic Society. Single breath carbon monoxide diffusing capacity: recommendations for standard technique 1995 update. Am J Resp Crit Care Med 1995;152:2185–2198.
12. Dull WL, Bonnassis JB, Teculescu D, Sadoul P. The place of the chest radiograph in estimating total lung capacity (author's translation). Bull Physiopath Respir 1980;16:777–784.
13. Powell CA, Caplan CE. Pulmonary function tests in pre-operative pulmonary evaluation. Clin Chest Med 2001;22:703–714.
14. Doyle RL. Assessing and modifying the risk of postoperative pulmonary complications. Chest 1999;115:77–81.
15. Warner MA, Divertie MB, Tinker JH. Preoperative cessation of smoking an pulmonary complications in coronary bypass patients. Anesthiology 1984;60:380–383.

II Disorders of the Upper Airway

4 Allergic Rhinitis

Holly Bergman Sobota, Trissana Emdadi, and Matthew L. Mintz

CONTENTS
>   CASE PRESENTATION
>   KEY CLINICAL QUESTIONS
>   LEARNING OBJECTIVES
>   EPIDEMIOLOGY
>   PATHOPHYSIOLOGY
>   DIFFERENTIAL DIAGNOSIS
>   DIAGNOSIS
>   TREATMENT
>   FUTURE DIRECTIONS
>   REFERENCES

CASE PRESENTATION

T. L. is a 29-year-old female who presents to her primary care physician in August complaining of a stuffy, itchy nose; sneezing; intermittent headache; and daytime somnolence for the past several months. She notes that since moving to Washington, DC 3 years ago, these same symptoms seem to bother her every spring and summer. She has tried over-the-counter pseudoephedrine with mild relief of congestion. She feels her symptoms are interfering with her ability to exercise outdoors and her performance at work. Her past medical history is significant for eczema as a child. Her father has had "hay fever" for years. She lives alone in an apartment and has no pets. Physical exam is remarkable for a bilaterally indurated, erythematous nasal mucosa, a clear, watery anterior and posterior nasal discharge, an erythematous oropharynx, and bilateral tenderness over the frontal sinuses.

> From: *Current Clinical Practice: Disorders of the Respiratory Tract:
> Common Challenges in Primary Care*
> By: M. L. Mintz © Humana Press, Totowa, NJ

KEY CLINICAL QUESTIONS

1. How does one confirm the diagnosis of allergic rhinitis?
2. How does one rule out alternative diagnosis, such as cold or flu?
3. When would one consider allergy testing and/or immunotherapy in this patient?
4. What is the best initial pharmacotherapeutic agent to use in this patient?

LEARNING OBJECTIVES

- Distinguish allergic rhinitis from other forms of rhinitis and from other respiratory diseases.
- Become familiar with the pathophysiology of allergic rhinitis.
- Classify and guide treatment by the severity and type of allergic rhinitis.
- Identify evidence-based treatment strategies.
- Recognize when further allergy testing and/or referral to a specialist are indicated.

EPIDEMIOLOGY

Allergic rhinitis, commonly referred to as "hay fever" or "grass fever," is an immunoglobulin (Ig)E-mediated type 1 hypersensitivity response of the nasal mucus membranes following exposure to an allergen in a sensitized individual. Resulting symptoms include rhinorrhea, nasal congestion, nasal pruritus, and sneezing. The inflammation and associated symptoms may be relieved either spontaneously or with appropriate treatment.

Allergic rhinitis has traditionally been subclassified as seasonal or perennial, depending on the temporal pattern of the symptoms. Seasonal allergic rhinitis is generally caused by outdoor allergens including pollens of trees, grasses, and weeds, and fungi, such as *Cladosporium, Alternaria, Penicillium,* and *Aspergillus*. Conversely, perennial allergic rhinitis is often caused by indoor allergens, such as dust mite feces, cockroach residues, cats, dogs, and molds.

The World Health Organization (WHO) has recently proposed an alternative subdivision of allergic rhinitis into intermittent and persistent, with further subclassification of symptoms as mild or moderate-severe *(1)* (Table 1).

The severity and frequency of symptoms caused by allergic rhinitis are highly variable, leading many persons with mild and/or intermittent symptoms to remain undiagnosed by a medical professional. Prevalence data are therefore difficult to establish, but estimates range between 10 and 25% of Americans, with rates rising by approximately 3.5% every 10 years *(2)*.

The Centers for Disease Control and Prevention estimates that during 2002, 9% of US adults (18.2 million) and 10.3% of US children (7.5 million) were diagnosed with allergic rhinitis. Among these patients, the overwhelming majority were Caucasian (84% of adults and 79% of children) and living above the

Table 1
Proposed Reclassification of Allergic Rhinitis

Intermittent	*Persistent*
Symptoms <4 days/week or <4 weeks/year	Symptoms ≥4 days/week and >4 weeks/year
Mild *None of the following is present:*	*Moderate-severe* *One or more of the following are present:* Sleep disruption Impairment of activities of daily living Impairment of performance at school or work Troublesome symptoms

Adapted from ref. *1*.

poverty level (61% of adults and 59% of children) *(3,4)*. In addition, 14 million physician office visits that year were attributable to the disease, making allergic rhinitis one of the top 10 reasons for primary care office visits *(1,4)*. Direct and indirect clinical costs fall between $1.2 and $5.3 billion annually *(5)*.

PATHOPHYSIOLOGY

A review of the relevant nasal anatomy and physiology is helpful in understanding the pathogenesis, diagnosis, complications, and comorbidities of allergic rhinitis.

The nasal cavity is formed by the superior, middle, and inferior turbinates bilaterally, the cribiform plate superiorly, and the hard palate inferiorly (Fig. 1). The cavity is further divided in half by the nasal septum, composed of bone proximally and cartilage distally. The external pyramidal nose opens via two nasal vestibules formed by the nasal bones proximally and cartilage distally. Posteriorly, the nasal cavity is contiguous with the pharynx, forming the nasopharynx. The frontal, ethmoidal, and maxillary sinuses each drain into the nasal cavity.

The majority of the nasal cavity is lined by a pseudostratified columnar, ciliated epithelium with goblet cells. The submucosa contains serous and seromucus glands, nerves, cellular elements, and an extensive vasculature. The structure of the nasal turbinates increases total mucosal surface area to 300 cm^2, thereby enhancing the humidification, particle removal, and temperature modulation of inspired air. A thin layer of mucus, formed from goblet cell and mucus gland secretion as well as exudation from vasculature, normally coats the nasal mucosa. Most inhaled particles are trapped in this mucus layer then moved via ciliary action

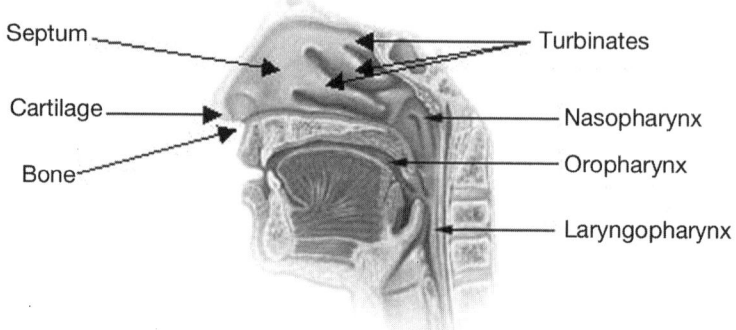

Fig. 1. Nasal cavity.

to the nasopharynx for swallowing. A second type of epithelium lines the vestibules. This keratinized, stratified squamous epithelium with numerous hairs functions to trap large inhaled particles as air is funneled inward. Finally, the olfactory mucosa, serving smell and taste functions, lines the portion of the nasal cavity just beneath the cribiform plate.

The extensive vasculature of the nasal cavity functions to humidify and regulate the temperature of inspired air. Among these vessels are capacitance vessels that modify the volume of the nasal mucosa: when constricted, they leave the nasal passages open, and when dilated, they lead to congestion. The nasal cavity is supplied both by autonomic and somatic sensory nerves. Nasal blood vessels dilate with parasympathetic stimulation and constrict with sympathetic stimulation, opening up the nasal passages. Parasympathetic stimulation also induces glandular secretion.

Particles are inhaled and deposited in the mucus layer overlying the nasal mucosa. Here, water-soluble proteinaceous particles, in picogram to nanogram quantities, undergo elution and diffusion into the nasal tissues. These proteins are cleaved by antigen-presenting cells into smaller peptides that can bind to receptors on certain major histocompatibility complex (MHC) class II molecules. For an allergic response to occur, sensitization must take place. It is the particular polymorphic MHC II molecules expressed by an individual that determines whether or not sensitization to a given peptide will occur *(6)*.

If the expressed MHC II molecules favor allergy development, the peptide (or antigen) will be presented to $CD4^+$ T-lymphocytes and, in turn, to B-cells. $CD4^+$ cells then release various cytokines including interleukin (IL)-3, IL-4, IL-5, IL-13, and granulocyte-macrophage colony-stimulating factor. These cytokines promote B-cell synthesis of allergen-specific IgE that then binds to receptors on the surface of mast cells and basophils.

Once sensitized, subsequent exposures to the particular antigen lead to an immediate allergic response. Cross-linking of IgE molecules by the allergen causes release of preformed mediators from mast cells and basophils via degranulation and stimulates *de novo* synthesis of other mediators. Histamine, tryptase, prostaglandin D_2, prostaglandin F_2, various leukotrienes, and bradykinin are rapidly released within minutes of the allergen exposure. These mediators stimulate mucus secretion, vasodilation, vascular leakage with plasma extravasation, and pooling of blood in the cavernous sinusoids, leading to congestion. Histamine specifically causes pruritis, rhinorrhea, and sneezing. This series of events constitutes the early phase of the allergic response, with mast cell activation being the crucial inciting event *(6)*. Patients with allergic rhinitis have been shown to have greatly increased numbers of mast cells in their nasal mucosa *(1)*.

The mediators and cytokines of the early-phase response initiate release of cytokines and chemokines that sustain the inflammatory infiltrate for hours, causing the late-phase response. Symptomatically, congestion predominates during the late phase. At the tissue level, eosinophils, recruited chiefly by IL-5, accumulate in the mucosa *(2)*. In addition to changes in the nasal mucosa, hypersensitivity of the turbinates develops. This leads to less and less allergen needed to produce symptoms, also referred to as "priming." Continued exposure to the allergen results in the mast cells developing increased numbers of IgE receptors and surface-bound IgE, which results in the ability to release more histamine. Chronically, nasal congestion and obstructed nasal passageways cause disruption in sleep quality and daytime somnolence, with a consequent impairment in quality of life, productivity, and cognition *(7)*.

In addition to being hyperresponsive to specific antigens, patients with allergic rhinitis often suffer from hyperresponsiveness to nonspecific stimuli, such as pollutants, strong odors, cigarette smoke, viral infection, and cold air. Although the exact mechanism is not known, studies have shown that nasal mucosal production of IgE and cytokines, such as IL-4 and IL-5, increases after exposure to diesel exhaust *(8,9)*. Other nonspecific triggers may act similarly as immune enhancers in the allergic patient.

DIFFERENTIAL DIAGNOSIS

The differential diagnosis for allergic rhinitis is wide, but a thorough history and physical exam can help narrow the list considerably (Table 2). Rhinitis can be caused by infection, vasomotor reaction, vagally mediated gustatory reaction, medications (decongestants, antihypertensives, cocaine abuse), hormones (e.g., pregnancy, hypothyroid, oral contraceptive use), mechanical obstruction (e.g., deviated septum, adenoid hypertrophy), non-allergic rhinitis with eosinophilia

Table 2
Differential Diagnosis of Rhinitis

Allergic	*Seasonal or perennial versus intermittent or persistent*
Hormonal	Pregnancy, hypothyroidism, oral contraceptives, hormone replacement therapy (HRT)
Drug-induced	Angiotensin-converting enzyme inhibitors, β-blockers, oral contraceptives, HRT, rebound effects of topical α-adrenergic decongestants, aspirin, nonsteroidal anti-inflammatory drugs
Mechanical	Polyposis, septal deviation, adenoidal hypertrophy, foreign body, tumor (benign or malignant), ciliary defects
Non-allergic	Vasomotor (idiopathic), non-allergic rhinitis with eosinophilia syndrome
Infectious	Viral, bacterial, fungal
Other	Atrophic rhinitis, gustatory rhinitis, Wegener's granulomatosis

syndrome, immotile cilia syndrome, cerebrospinal fluid leak, nasal polyps, or a granulomatous condition (e.g., Wegener granulomatosis, sarcoidosis) *(13)*.

Nasal pruritus is highly suggestive of allergy. This is further supported by coincident findings conjunctivitis. Unilateral nasal findings are suggestive of a mechanical etiology. New onset of allergic rhinitis is rare in elderly populations, in which atrophic rhinitis is more common. Finally, nasal polyps are rare in children and their presence should prompt suspicion of cystic fibrosis.

DIAGNOSIS

Patients with allergic rhinitis most commonly report symptoms of runny nose, sneezing, sniffing, loss of smell, nasal congestion, itchy nose, mouth breathing, and postnasal drip, all of which are nonspecific *(10)*. The hallmark of allergic rhinitis is the temporal relationship between such symptoms and exposure to an allergen. An exhaustive history that examines possible triggers and symptom pattern is therefore paramount to the correct diagnosis of allergic rhinitis. Patients should also be asked specifically about symptoms related to common comorbid conditions, including allergic conjunctivitis, asthma, and sinusitis (Table 3).

Physical exam should focus on the ear, nose, and throat exam, with visualization of the nasal cavity being most important. Anterior rhinoscopy may be adequate in cases in which there is no impedance to adequate visualization and a low suspicion for pathology in the sinuses or posterior nasal cavity. Nasal endoscopy is used when further visualization is deemed necessary.

Table 3
Key Points in the History

HPI	Past medical	Family	Social/environmental
Congestion	Facial trauma	Asthma	Occupation/exposures
Rhinorrhea	Facial/sinus surgery	Rhinitis	Living conditions
Sneezing	Drug sensitivities	Atopic	Smoking exposures
Fatigue		dermatitis	Illicit drug exposures
Mouth breathing	Relevant medical		Animal/pet exposures
Snoring	conditions:		
Nasal pruritus	• Asthma (shortness		
Frequent throat clearing, coughing	of breath, cough, chest tightness,		
Hyposmia, anosmia	wheezing)		
Pattern of symptoms	• Sinusitis (sinus		
Triggers	pain/pressure,		
Pregnancy	headache, purulent		
Current medications	nasal discharge)		
Response to prior treatment, including non-Rx	• Dermatitis • Conjunctivitis (lacrimation, pruritus, conjunctival injection)		

HPI, history of present illness.

On exam, nasal mucosa may appear pale and blue in the acute setting of allergic rhinitis, whereas chronically it is usually erythematous. Turbinates may be swollen or "boggy." A clear discharge may be seen in the nasal cavity as well as in the oropharynx. Dark circles beneath the eyes, or "allergic shiners," signify chronic venous stasis and congestion. A high-arched palate owing to mouth breathing and a nasal crease or "nasal salute" because of rubbing of the nose are signs more commonly seen in children. Signs of the common comorbidities should also be sought, including tenderness over the sinuses, purulent nasal drainage, wheezes, prolonged expiratory phase, conjunctival injection, and watery ocular drainage.

Definitive diagnosis of allergic rhinitis requires demonstration of the cause–effect relationship between an allergen and atopic response by skin tests, in vitro IgE assays, and nasal provocation tests. Skin-prick-puncture testing is the preferred immediate hypersensitivity skin test, recommended by the US Joint Council of Allergy Asthma and Immunology for diagnosis of IgE-mediated allergy and for research *(1)*. Skin testing carries a risk of systemic reaction and should therefore be avoided in patients with severe and/or ongoing symptoms, unstable asthma, or who are pregnant.

Approximately 20 allergens can be tested in the skin-prick test. The allergen and a negative control saline solution are introduced into the skin via needle prick. The most common places used for testing are the patient's back or arm. The saline control is used to ensure the patient's reaction is not merely a result of dermatographism. Once the allergen is injected, it will bind to any mast cell that has the specific IgE receptor, causing the mast cell to degranulate and release histamine, causing a wheal to form. The diameter of the wheal is measured after 15 to 20 minutes and the test is considered positive if the wheal created by the antigen is 3 mm larger than the wheal created by the saline control and has surrounding erythema. Establishing the sensitivity and specificity of skin testing is difficult because there is no widely accepted gold standard for defining a true allergic reaction, and because only five allergen extracts have been standardized in the United States, including ragweed pollen, cat dander, house dust mites, hymenoptera venom, and some grasses. All other allergen extracts tested are not necessarily reproducible. The skin-prick test results can be affected by certain medications, such as antihistamines or medications with antihistamine properties, such as tricyclic antidepressants. For the best possible results, such medications should be stopped at least 4 days before first-generation antihistamine testing and at least 10 days before second-generation antihistamine testing. Most other medications can be withheld only for the day of testing.

Intradermal skin testing is more specific, but less sensitive than skin-prick tests. It is usually done when skin-prick test results were negative, but there is still a high clinical suspicion of an allergy. Most often, it is done for venom and penicillin allergy testing. In this case, 0.01 to 0.02 mL of an allergen is injected intracutaneously with a small needle, and again the wheal is measured in 15 to 20 minutes.

Alternatively, allergen-specific serum IgE may be measured in vitro without the risk of systemic reaction and without inhibition by medication. In vitro testing is also preferable for patients with severe skin conditions. Evidence shows that skin puncture tests and properly performed in vitro tests are comparable in their diagnostic performance *(11)*. Limitations of in vitro testing include its cost and limited allergen profile of available assays. Furthermore, a 2001 study found that results from different commercial assays for a given type of IgE were not equal *(12)*. It is therefore recommended that physicians correlate the exact type of assay used by the laboratory with performance and standardization data of that assay *(11)*. The first-generation in vitro tests were called radioallergosorbent and enzyme-linked allergosorbent test. These worked by having a specific allergen bound to cellulose disk. Human serum would be added to the disk, if there was any specific IgE to the allergen it would bind to the disk. Then a radioactive enzyme-labeled antihuman IgE detection antibody would be added and the resulting radioactive count per minute could be done to determine the amount of specific IgE in the human serum. The amount of specific IgE produced to an allergen approximately correlates with the allergic sensitivity to that substance. Improvements have led to second-generation in vitro tests called ImmunoCAP™ and Phadiatop™, which have higher sensitivities and specificities but still work by measuring the specific IgE present to an allergen.

Nasal provocation is an alternative test that can demonstrate allergy used mainly when there is diagnostic doubt based on other tests *(1)*. Plain radiography, computed tomography, and magnetic resonance imaging are of limited use in the diagnosis of allergic rhinitis. Computed tomogaphy scan may be useful when the diagnosis is in doubt, but should only be performed after specialist referral *(1)*.

Despite the availability of allergy tests, their use is not always indicated in the diagnosis of allergic rhinitis. Evidence supports the use of allergy tests when the patient has a low to intermediate pretest probability of allergic rhinitis because the positive likelihood ratios in such circumstances have been shown to be high across multiple studies, meaning allergy testing in such patients is likely to change the posttest probability significantly, thereby affecting the decision to treat *(11)*. When a patient has an intermediate to high pretest probability of allergic rhinitis, empiric treatment is an appropriate first step, with frequent re-evaluation of the response to therapy. Allergy testing is also useful when patients fail to respond to medication. In this circumstance, testing helps to both confirm the diagnosis and inform the patient and physician of specific sensitivities, thereby allowing a more targeted approach to therapy *(11)*.

TREATMENT

Treatment of allergic rhinitis includes pharmacological therapy, immunotherapy, and avoidance of common environmental allergens (Table 4). Studies demonstrating beneficial effects of avoidance on asthma symptoms abound. However, there are only a few such studies on avoidance therapy for allergic rhinitis that have shown significant reductions in environmental allergen load; these studies have been unable to demonstrate clear clinical benefit *(13–19)*. Despite the lack of data demonstrating its efficacy, the WHO states that allergen avoidance in the treatment of rhinitis is always indicated *(1)*. Based on results from asthma studies, it is clear that allergen avoidance can improve allergy symptoms *(20)*. Appropriate targeting of avoidance measures requires knowledge of specific triggers that are often hard to identify without skin testing. Furthermore, many patients are sensitive to multiple allergens, requiring a range of avoidance strategies and making total avoidance nearly impossible. When implementing avoidance therapy, it is important to combine multiple strategies for maximal benefit *(1)*.

Antihistamines were the original medication used for allergic rhinitis. They reduce the symptoms of rhinorrhea, sneezing, and ocular injection, but have no affect on nasal congestion. The first-generation antihistamines easily cross the

Table 4
Allergen Avoidance Strategies

Dust mite	Animal dander	Cockroach	Indoor mold
Wash bedding in water over 55°C weekly[a] (14)	Weekly bathing[a] (19)	Control of damp areas	Maintain hygienic environment
Use impermeable casings for all bedding[a] (15)	Frequent vacuuming of carpets, upholstery, drapery	Extermination or chemical control[b] (20)	Reduce indoor humidity
Replace carpets with hard floors[b] (16)	Removal of the animal from the environment	Caulk/seal cracks and other openings in the home	Inspect humid areas, ventilation, and heating ducts regularly
Steam clean carpets regularly[b] (16) or treat with acaricides or tannic acid[b] (13)		Limit exposed food	
Wash curtains in water hotter than 55°C frequently or replace with blinds			
Vacuum with HEPA vacuum[b] (17) preferably bagless, regularly			
Reduce indoor humidity[b] (18)			
Minimize upholstered furniture or treat with acaricides or tannic acid[b] (13)			

Adapted from ref. 1.
[a]Evidence shows symptom improvement for asthma.
[b]Evidence shows reduction of allergen load in the environment.

blood–brain barrier and bind not only to H1 histamine receptors, but also to dopaminergic, serotinergic, and cholinergic receptors *(21)*. The adverse central nervous system effect (sedation, fatigue, and dizziness) and anticholinergic effect (dry mucous membranes) can be explained by the additional receptors that the antihistamine binds to. The central nervous system effects of first-generation antihistamines further decrease the cognitive function of the patient; therefore, first-generation antihistamines should be avoided unless used strictly at night.

The second- and third-generation antihistamines bind specifically to the H1 histamine receptors. These drugs are more lipophobic and large enough that they do not readily cross the blood–brain barrier. This more specific action means that they do not cause sedation or other anticholinergic effects and are as effective in decreasing the symptoms of allergic rhinitis as first-generation antihistamines. One of these nonsedating antihistamines, loratidine, is now sold over the counter, and is available in brand or generic form.

Intranasal medications include topical antihistamines, such as azelastine and intranasal corticosteroids. Azelastine can be used when patients are unable to tolerate oral antihistamines, because it is minimally absorbed into the bloodstream. However, when choosing a nasal medication, results from several studies have shown that intranasal corticosteroids are far more effective in reducing total nasal symptoms, including nasal congestion than topical antihistamines.

Intranasal corticosteroids are the most effective pharmacotherapy approved for the treatment of allergic rhinitis *(22)*. They inhibit the release of mediators from inflammatory cells in addition to regulating gene expression. Nasal inflammation in both the early- and late-phase reaction is prevented. No adverse systemic effects have been seen in adults. In children, there has been some concern with growth suppression; however, there has been no conclusive evidence to indicate that growth suppression occurs with use of intranasal corticosteroids.

Leukotriene receptor antagonists prevent the action of leukotrienes released from inflammatory cells by blocking the receptor. Only montelukast is approved in the United States for the treatment of allergic rhinitis. Montelukast appears to be as effective as loratadine *(23)*, a nonsedating antihistamine, but has not show equivalence to other antihistamines or superiority to other agents. Unlike the nonsedating antihistamines, which are now available over the counter and generically, montelukast requires a prescription and remains expensive.

Decongestants primarily address nasal congestion symptoms, but do not have any affect on sneezing or itching. They cause vasoconstriction by activating the α-adrenergic receptors on the respiratory mucosa. Decongestants are available in an oral and intranasal form. The oral medications have many side effects, such as tachycardia, increased blood pressure, insomnia, nervousness, and increased intraocular pressure. These oral decongestants should be used cautiously in the elderly. Intranasal decongestants cause vasoconstriction in the turbinates. They should not be used for more than 5 days in a row because they can lead to rebound congestion when stopped. If intranasal decongestants are used for an extended amount of time, a form of rhinitis (rhinitis medicamentosa) that is difficult to treat can develop.

The pharmacotherapeutic approach put forth by the WHO and its expert panel is summarized in Table 5. It should be noted that second-generation antihistamines are preferred over first-generation drugs because of their improved side-effect profile and associated improved patient tolerance *(24)*. Furthermore, a 2003 review of randomized, controlled clinical trials concluded that intranasal corticosteroids provide better relief in allergic rhinitis than antihistamines, particularly for nasal congestion *(25)*. The WHO and its expert panel therefore recommend that intranasal corticosteroids be first-line therapy for patients with moderate-severe and/or persistent allergic rhinitis, whereas mild and/or intermittent allergic rhinitis may be adequately managed with antihistamines as first-line therapy *(1)*. When adequate treatment of any form of allergic rhinitis fails to produce improvement after 3 months, the WHO recommends referral to a specialist *(1)*. A somewhat different approach to pharmacotherapy comes from a 1998 meta-analysis of 16 randomized, controlled trials that found that intranasal corticosteroids produce superior relief of congestion, rhinorrhea, sneezing, nasal pruritis, and postnasal drip when compared with antihistamines. Recommendations out of this study favored the use of intranasal corticosteroids as first-line therapy, with antihistamines used adjunctively for persistent nasal itch and/or ocular symptoms *(26)*. Thus, there is some controversy over the best first-line therapy for mild allergic rhinitis. Clearly, inhaled steroids should be used in moderate to severe disease. For patients with mild symptoms, there are multiple factors to take into consideration, including patient preference, cost of medications, and out-of-pocket cost to patients.

Specific immunotherapy is the only available treatment that can alter the natural history of allergic rhinitis. Immunotherapy, which is also referred to as desensitization, is recommended for those patients who fail to respond to both allergen avoidance and medications. Immunotherapy consists of subcutaneous injections of allergen for at least 3 to 5 years. These injections are usually done on a weekly basis and gradually the amount of allergen injected is increased. It usually takes 6 months of treatment to have any noticeable effects and typically 2–3 years to reach maximum effectiveness. It is thought that the efficacy derived from immunotherapy is related to the development of a specific IgG to the specific allergen.

A double-blind, placebo-controlled study published in 1999 in the *New England Journal of Medicine* showed at least a 3-year persistence of symptomatic relief following 3 to 4 years of grass pollen immunotherapy *(27)*, although other studies have shown decreased symptoms up to 6 years after discontinuation *(28)*. The

Table 5
Therapeutic Approach Based on Classification of Allergic Rhinitis

Classification	Medication	Follow-up
Mild intermittent	Oral or intranasal antihistamines Intranasal decongestants (for a maximum of 10 days twice monthly) Oral decongestants	
Moderate-severe intermittent	Oral or intranasal antihistamines Oral decongestants Intranasal glucocorticosteroids Intranasal cromolyn	
Mild persistent	Oral or intranasal antihistamines Oral decongestants Intranasal glucocorticosteroids Intranasal cromolyn	Re-assess in 2–4 weeks for: *Symptom improvement:* continue treatment, consider halving the dose of intranasal corticosteroids *Persistent mild symptoms on antihistamine or cromolyn therapy:* switch to intranasal corticosteroid *Moderate-severe symptoms:* Step up
Moderate-severe persistent	Intranasal glucocorticosteroids are first-line treatment With severe nasal blockage: add a 7- to 14-day course of oral glucocorticosteroids or Add intranasal decongestants (for a maximum of 10 days)	Re-assess in 2–4 weeks for: *No improvement:* assess compliance, consider additional pathology or alternative diagnosis, double the intranasal glucocorticosteroid dose if congestion predominates, add antihistamines if rhinorrhea, sneezing, itching predominate *Improvement:* Step down, but maintain treatment at least 3 months

Adapted from ref. *1*.

WHO and its expert panel argues for the use of immunotherapy when there has been an insufficient response to pharmacotherapy, if the patient cannot tolerate medication side effects, or the patient suffers from severe, prolonged allergic rhinitis, particularly when there is associated asthma *(1)*.

FUTURE DIRECTIONS

The relationship between allergic rhinitis and asthma is indisputable. A recently published longitudinal case–control study found that subjects with allergic rhinitis had more than a threefold risk of subsequent asthma development *(29)*. A 2003 review found that among patients with both allergic rhinitis and asthma, the effective management of allergic rhinitis decreases acute care service utilization for asthma symptoms and exacerbations *(30)*. Given the high costs of both allergic rhinitis and asthma, further research as to whether interventions for allergic rhinitis have preventive effects on asthma is needed, and if so, which interventions work best.

From a treatment perspective, further research is needed to determine whether multi-agent pharmacotherapy produces better results than single-agent therapy, differences in single agents for mild symptoms, as well as new agents in treating the disease. Regarding immunotherapy, one new potential option is sublingual immunotherapy, which has been shown to be effective in seasonal allergic rhinitis and asthmatic children with allergic rhinoconjunctivitis *(31,32)*.

One new therapy being used for asthma, which may have a role in allergic rhinitis is omalizumab. Omalizumab is a recombinant humanized monoclonal anti-IgE antibody that selectively binds to the Cε3 domain of IgE, which inhibits free IgE from binding to the mast cell FcεR1 receptor, thereby preventing activation and subsequent release of cellular mediators. There are potential benefits because this agent works earlier in the allergic-inflammatory cascade. Omalizumab is currently indicated for adults and adolescents (12 years of age and older) with moderate to severe persistent asthma who have positive skin tests and whose symptoms are inadequately controlled with inhaled corticosteroids. There is some preliminary data in allergic rhinitis that shows that combination of sublingual immunotherapy plus omalizumab was clinically superior to each treatment alone during the first year of observation, as well as data showing that omalizumab improves asthma-related quality of life in patients with severe allergic asthma. Currently, the product is injectable only and extremely expensive. However, monoclonal antibodies seem to show promise in the treatment of allergic disease, including allergic rhinitis *(33,34)*.

REFERENCES

1. Bousquet J, van Cauwenberge P, Khaltaev N. Allergic rhinitis and its impact on asthma. J Allergy Clin Immunol 2001;108:S147–S334.

2. Kramer MF, Ostertag P, Pfrogner E, Rasp G. Nasal interleukin-5, immunoglobulin E, eosinophillic cationic protein, and soluble intercellular adhesion molecule-1 in chronic sinusitis, allergic rhinitis, and nasal polyposis. Laryngoscope 2000;110:1056–1062.
3. Dey AN, Schiller JS, Tai DA. Summary health statistics for U.S. children: National Health Interview Survey, 2003. National Center for Health Statistics. Vital Health Stat 2005;223:1–78.
4. Lethbridge-Cejku M, Schiller JS, Bernadel L. Summary health statistics for U.S. adults: National Health Interview Survey, 2002. National Center for Health Statistics. Vital Health Stat 2004;10: 27–28.
5. Conner SJ. Evaluation and treatment of the patient with allergic rhinitis. J Fam Practice 2002;51:883–884, 887–890.
6. Baraniuk JN. Pathogenesis of allergic rhinitis. J Allergy Clin Immunol 1997;99:763–772.
7. Kakumanu S, Glass C, Craig T. Poor sleep and daytime somnolence in allergic rhinitis: significance of nasal congestion. Am J Resp Med 2002;1:195–200.
8. Diaz-Sanchez D, Tsien A, Casillas A, Dotson AR, Sackson A. Enhanced nasal cytokine production in human beings after in vivo challenge with diesel exhaust particles. J Allergy Clin Immunol 1996;98:114–123.
9. Takenaka H, Zhang K, Diaz-Sanchez D, Tsein A, Sackson A. Enhanced human IgE production results from exposure to the aromatic hydrocarbons from diesel exhaust: direct effects on B cell IgE production. J Allergy Clin Immunol 1995;95:103–115.
10. Ng MLS, Warlow RS, Chrishanthan N, Ellis C, Walls RS. Preliminary criteria for the definition of allergic rhinitis: a systematic evaluation of clinical parameters in a disease cohort (I and II). Clin Exper Allergy 2000;30:1314–1331, 1417–1422.
11. Gendo K, Larson EB. Evidence-based diagnostic strategies for evaluating suspected allergic rhinitis. Ann Intern Med 2004;140: 278–289.
12. Szeinbach SL, Barnes JH, Sullivan TJ, Williams PB. Precision and accuracy of commercial laboratories' ability to classify positive and/or negative allergen-specific IgE results. Ann Allergy Asthma Immunol 2001;86:373–381.
13. Sheikh A, Hurwitz B. House dust mite avoidance measures for perennial allergic rhinitis: a systematic review of efficacy. British J Gen Practice 2003;53:318–322.
14. McDonald LG, Tovey E. The role of water temperature and laundry procedures in reducing house dust mite populations and allergen content of bedding. J Allergy Clin Immunol 1992;90:599–608.
15. Ehnert B, Lau-Schadendorf S, Weber A, Buettner P, Schou C, Wahn U. Reducing domestic exposure to dust mite allergen reduces bronchial hyperreactivity in sensitive children with asthma. J Allergy Clin Immunol 1992;90:135–138.
16. Brunekreef B. On carpets, construction and covers. Clin Exp Allergy 1999;29:433–435.
17. Roberts JW, Clifford WS, Glass G, Hummer PG. Reducing dust, lead, dust mites, bacteria, and fungi in carpets by vacuuming. Arch Environ Contam Toxicol 1999;36:477–484.
18. Warner J, Frederick JM, Bryant TN, et al. Mechanical ventilation and high efficiency vacuum cleaning: a combined strategy of mite and mite allergen reduction in the control of mite sensitive asthma. J Allergy Clin Immunol 2000;105:75–82.
19. de-Blay F, Chapman MD, Platts-Mills TA. Airborne cat allergen (Fel d I). Environmental control with the cat in situ. Am Rev Respir Dis 1991;143:1334–1339.
20. Gergen PJ, Mortimer KM, Eggleston PA, et al. Results of the National Cooperative Inner-City Asthma Study (NCICAS) environmental intervention to reduce cockroach allergen exposure in inner-city homes. J Allergy Clin Immunol 1999;103:501–506.
21. Corren, J. Allergic rhinitis: treating the adult. J Allergy Clin Immunol 2000;105:S610–S615.
22. Borish L. Allergic rhinitis: systemic inflammation and implications for management. J Allergy Clin Immunol 2003;112:1021–1031.

23. Meltzer EO, Malmstrom K, Lu S, et al. Concomitant montelukast and loratadine as treatment for seasonal allergic rhinitis: a randomized, placebo-controlled clinical trial. J Allergy Clin Immunol 2000; 105:917–922.
24. Hadley JA. Cost-effective pharmacotherapy for inhalant allergic rhinitis. Otolaryngol Clin North Am 2003;36:825–836.
25. Nielsen LP, Dahl R. Comparison of intranasal corticosteroids and antihistamines in allergic rhinitis: a review of randomized, controlled trials. Am J Resp Med 2003;2: 55–65.
26. Weiner JM, Abramson MJ, Puy RM. Intranasal corticosteroids versus oral H1 receptor antagonists in allergic rhinitis: systematic review of randomised controlled trials. BMJ 1998;317:1624–1629.
27. Durham SR, Walker SM, Varga EM, et al. Long-term clinical efficacy of grass-pollen immunotherapy. N Engl J Med 1999;341:468–475.
28. Gendo K, Larson EB. Evidence-based diagnostic strategies for evaluating suspected allergic rhinitis. Ann Inter Med 2004;140:278–289.
29. Guerra S, Sherrill D, Martinez F, Barbee R. Rhinitis as an independent risk factor for adult-onset asthma. J Allergy Clin Immunol 2002;109:419–425.
30. Fuhlbrigge AL, Adams RJ. The effect of treatment of allergic rhinitis on asthma morbidity, including emergency department visits. Curr Opin Allergy Clin Immunol 2003;3: 29–32.
31. Smith H, White P, Annila I, et al. Randomized controlled trial of high-dose sublingual immunotherapy to treat seasonal allergic rhinitis. J Allergy Clin Immunol 2004;114: 512–516.
32. Novembre E, Galli E, Landi E, et al. Coseasonal sublingual immunotherapy reduces the development of asthma in children with allergic rhinoconjunctivitis. J Allergy Clin Immunol 2004;114:851–857.
33. Finn A, Gross G, Van Bavel J, et al. Omalizumab improves asthma-related quality of life in patients with severe allergic asthma. J Allergy Clin Immunol 2003;111:278–284.
34. Rolinck-Werninghaus C, Hamelmann E, Keil T, et al. The co-seasonal application of anti-IgE after preseasonal specific immunotherapy decreases ocular and nasal symptom scores and rescue medication use in grass pollen allergic children Allergy 2004;59:973–979.

5 Non-Allergic Rhinitis

Cardin Bell and Matthew L. Mintz

CONTENTS
>   CASE PRESENTATION
>   KEY CLINICAL QUESTIONS
>   LEARNING OBJECTIVES
>   EPIDEMIOLOGY
>   PATHOPHYSIOLOGY
>   DIFFERENTIAL DIAGNOSIS
>   DIAGNOSIS
>   TREATMENT
>   REFERRAL
>   FUTURE DIRECTIONS
>   REFERENCES

CASE PRESENTATION

A 23-year-old female college student presents to her primary care clinic complaining of persistent runny nose and nasal congestion for more than 10 months a year over the past several years. She does not remember exactly when her symptoms began, and states that they occur daily regardless of her location or the time of day. She denies any fever, chills, mucopurulent drainage, cough, dyspnea, headache, ocular or nasal pruritus, or ocular symptoms. Past medical history shows no evidence of allergies, asthma, recurrent upper respiratory tract infections, chronic sinusitis, nasal or head trauma, or nasal surgery or trauma. She takes no medications except an occasional acetaminophen for headache when studying for several hours. She works as a part-time legal aid in an office building downtown. Family history and review of systems are unremarkable. Physical exam shows enlarged nasal turbinates, clear nasal discharge, moist and clear oropharynx with no erythema or exudates, clear tympanic membranes, no tenderness to palpation over the maxillary and frontal sinuses, and no cervical lymphadenopathy.

KEY CLINICAL QUESTIONS

1. How is non-allergic rhinitis diagnosed and distinguished from allergic rhinitis with respect to symptoms, physical exam, and diagnostic testing, and what is the minimum diagnostic testing necessary?
2. Why is distinguishing between allergic rhinitis and non-allergic rhinitis important?
3. Are the treatments significantly different between allergic and non-allergic rhinitis, and if not, what is the need to distinguish between the two disorders?

LEARNING OBJECTIVES

1. Understand how to clinically diagnose non-allergic rhinitis and distinguish this from allergic rhinitis.
2. Recognize the common presenting types of non-allergic rhinitis.
3. Learn how to appropriately treat and manage non-allergic rhinitis.

EPIDEMIOLOGY

It is estimated that 17 million people in the United States are affected by non-allergic rhinitis, and only 2 to 4% of these people actually seek treatment for relief of their symptoms *(1,2)*. Approximately 50% of patients seeking treatment for rhinitis do not have allergic rhinitis, emphasizing the prevalence of non-allergic rhinitis, as well as mixed rhinitis *(3)*. Non-allergic rhinitis may contribute to the total number of patients with rhinitis more than previously estimated. A recent survey of nearly 1000 patients with rhinitis demonstrated that 43% of the patients had pure allergic rhinitis based on their symptoms and positive skin test and 23% had pure non-allergic rhinitis based on symptoms but negative skin tests *(4,5)*. A mixed rhinitis was diagnosed in 34% of the patients based on positive skin test but not complete accordance between the symptoms and skin test results, underscoring the importance of considering the mixed etiology of rhinitis and not only allergic and non-allergic etiologies in effectively managing the rhinitis in these individuals (Fig. 1).

PATHOPHYSIOLOGY

Unlike an allergic reaction, the immunopathological mechanisms involved in the inflammatory response of non-allergic rhinitis are not mediated by immunoglobulin (Ig)E, which is clinically proven by a negative allergy skin test. However, although IgE does not initiate the inflammatory response in non-allergic

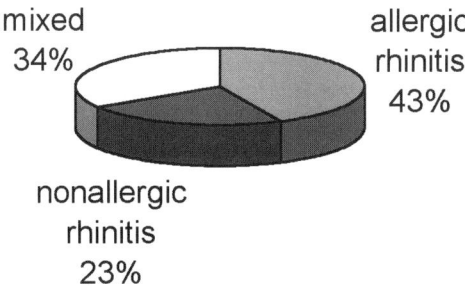

Fig. 1. Epidemiology of rhinitis.

rhinitis, many of the same inflammatory cells and mediators involved are the same as those present in allergic rhinitis. The term non-allergic rhinitis is actually a classification of rhinitis consisting of a broad group of heterogeneous syndromes that are commonly believed to have various distinct and unique etiologies, pathophysiologies, and cytological characteristics, in spite of their joint classification (6,7). Because of the wide degree of variance of opinion among researchers and clinicians on the classifications of the different forms of non-allergic rhinitis, the many mechanisms of action involved in the various types of non-allergic rhinitis remain generally unknown, and the diagnosis of non-allergic rhinitis is difficult; the various types of non-allergic rhinitis are described and diagnosed clinically.

Idiopathic Rhinitis

Idiopathic rhinitis is the most common form of non-allergic rhinitis affecting approximately 61% of patients with non-allergic rhinitis, and is characterized by persistent or sporadic perennial nasal symptoms for more than 9 months a year. Idiopathic rhinitis is commonly referred to as vasomotor rhinitis, and occasionally, non-allergic perennial rhinitis. These terms should not be used synonymously with non-allergic rhinitis. The exact etiology of idiopathic rhinitis is currently unknown. As with all types of non-allergic rhinitis, a specific test to diagnose idiopathic rhinitis does not currently exist. The diagnosis is one of exclusion by evidence of a negative allergy skin test, a lack of symptoms following allergen exposure, and exclusion of other possible types of non-allergic rhinitis (8). It is important that the clinician remember to consider the possibility of idiopathic rhinitis in a mixed rhinitis when administering allergy skin tests because idiopathic rhinitis is the most common and may be the most likely missed diagnosed type of non-allergic rhinitis, given that it has no specific or clearly detectable etiology.

Several different pathophysiological mechanisms for idiopathic rhinitis have been proposed. The most popular and dated of these is an imbalance of autonomic nervous input to the nasal mucosa. Although hyperactive parasympathetic innnervation and/or a hypoactive sympathetic innervation explain such an autonomic imbalance toward an excess in parasympathetic innervation, studies support that idiopathic rhinitis is more likely a result of a hypoactive sympathetic nervous system *(9,10)*. This autonomic imbalance in favor of parasympathetic innervation results in nasal edema from vasodilation of the nasal vasculature *(2)*. Autonomic dysfunction has also been demonstrated in patients with extra-esophageal manifestations of gastroesophageal reflux disease (GERD) and a significantly greater extent of autonomic dysfunction is observed in patients with both idiopathic rhinitis and GERD compared with patients with idiopathic rhinitis alone *(11)*. Further studies are needed to investigate a possible relationship between GERD and idiopathic rhinitis. Idiopathic rhinitis has also been described as a chronic complication of nonsurgical and surgical trauma. In approximately 80–90% of the nasal mucosa of patients with idiopathic rhinitis undergoing inferior turbinate reduction, microscopic and ultrasound studies have demonstrated microscopic abnormalities, such as reduced epithelial thickness, loss of goblet and ciliated cells, marked distension of intercellular spaces, absence of tight junctions, and ciliary loss *(12)*. Functional abnormality of sensory afferent nerves and/or C-fiber stimulation have also been suggested as a possible causes of idiopathic rhinitis *(13)*. Stimulation by noxious agent and pain stimulation of nasal sensory nerves eventually results in nasal congestion and pain sensation. Type C nocireceptive fibers are unmyelinated and unspecialized parts of the sensory neurons that originate from the ethmoidal and posterior nerves, and induce spreading of action potentials in peripheral branches of the sensory neurons and innervate the vessels, glands, and epithelium of the mucosa through the release of neuropeptides, such as calcitonin gene-related peptides and substance P (SP). Release of SP and calcitonin gene-related peptides result in localized increased vascular permeability, plasma extravasation, and glandular secretion. Local neuropeptide release may also lead to autonomic axon reflexes. This response is a protective reflex mechanism for clearing the nose under normal circumstances, but if altered, increased C-fiber activity may lead to nasal dysfunction in idiopathic rhinitis. Significantly elevated levels of vasoactive intestinal peptide neuropeptide tyrosine (NPY), and SP have also been identified in the nasal mucosa of patients with toxic rhinitis owing to chronic cigarette smoke exposure *(14)*. Ozone has been shown to induce release of SP, neurokinin A, and neuropeptides, which cause epithelial disruption and increased permeability, and may explain the increased responsiveness in patients with nasal hyperreactivity *(14,15)*. The free radical nitric oxide is cytostatic and cytotoxic to microbes and tumor cells, but also causes secondary decreased tissue viability and necrosis of normal tissue *(12,16)*. The resulting destruction of the epithelilium can lead to overexposure to the environment, causing hyperreactivity of afferent trigeminal fibers and recruitment of secretory and vascular reflexes *(17)*. The findings in one study of increased numbers of mast cells, IgE$^+$ cells, and eosinophils in the nasal mucosa of patients with idiopathic rhinitis compared with patients without rhinitis may suggest that inflammation in non-allergic rhinitis may be the result of localized IgE-mediated reactions not involving systemic Th$_2$ activity or atopy *(18)*.

Eosinophilic Types of Non-Allergic Rhinitis

Three types of non-allergic rhinitis resemble allergic rhinitis with a characteristic elevated level of eosinophils on nasal washings and blood smear. Like all non-allergic rhinitis types, these types are not IgE-mediated and display negative allergy skin tests. Eosinophilia is the distinguishing feature separating them from noneosinophilic types of non-allergic rhinitis, but intradermal tests show no difference between eosinophillic and non-eosinophillic types of non-allergic rhininits *(19)*.

NON-ALLERGIC RHINITIS WITH EOSINOPHILIA SYNDROME

Non-allergic rhinitis with eosinophilia syndrome (NARES) affects approximately 33% of patients with non-allergic rhinitis and exhibits high eosinophil counts in smears of nasal secretions. Cytological analysis of nasal secretions and epithelial scrapings from the inferior turbinate show more than 20% eosinophils *(3)*. Approximately 20% of the general population also demonstrates eosinophilia on nasal smear, but will not have an elevated eosinophil count equal to that of patients with NARES, nor the symptoms of rhinitis *(2)*. Patients with NARES will typically present with perennial symptoms of nasal congestion, sneezing, profuse rhinorrhea, nasal pruritis, and occasional hyposmia. Nasal polyps and asthma frequently develop later in life in patients with NARES *(20)*. The etiology and pathophysiology of NARES are not clearly understood. NARES is suspected by some researchers to be a precursor to the aspirin triad of intrinsic asthma, nasal polyposis, and aspirin intolerance. In approximately 50% of patients with NARES without a history of respiratory symptoms, bronchial responsiveness is associated with an increase in the number of eosinophils in sputum but not in nasal secretions *(21)*. Abnormal prostaglandin metabolism has also been suspected to cause NARES *(2)*.

BLOOD EOSINOPHILIA NON-ALLERGIC RHINITIS SYNDROME

Blood eosinophilia non-allergic rhinitis syndrome is similar to NARES, but eosinophilia is seen elevated in the blood levels rather than nasal smears. However, intense nasal symptoms, including perennial sneezing paroxysms, profuse watery nasal secretions, nasal itching, and loss of olfactory ability are observed in both syndromes.

NASAL POLYPS

Nasal polyps are also associated with eosinophilia. Clinical expression and symptoms vary among patients from those who are asymptomatic to those reporting considerable discomfort, sensation of fixed nasal obstruction, watery nasal secretions, continual sniffing because of an unfounded need to expel mucus, anosmia, absence of sneezing, and a nasal quality of the voice *(3,22)*. Polyps are usually bilateral, multiple, and painlessly manipulated on exam.

Drug-Induced Rhinitis

Drug-induced rhinitis may be separated into an unpredictable "aspirin hypersensitivity" subtype and predictable "pharmacological" subtype. Intolerance to aspirin and/or nonsteroidal anti-inflammatory drugs is unpredictable and typically results in rhinorrhea that may occur as part of a complex including nasal polyps, hyperplastic rhinosinusitis, and asthma, or it may occur independently *(3)*. Although a specific test to diagnose aspirin-induced rhinitis does not exists, it has been suggested that oral or nasal aspirin challenge may be useful to diagnose this condition, similar to provocation testing in diagnosing aspirin-induced asthma *(23)*. It has been suggested that increased numbers of eosinophils in both nasal secretions and blood may be seen in these patients for which corticosteroids may prove useful *(24)*. Vasoconstrictive intolerance to systemic drugs is infrequent. Systemic medications typically producing drug-induced rhinitis include penicillamine, oral contraceptives, exogenous estrogens, angiotensin-converting enzyme inhibitors, β-blockers, methyldopa, phentolamine, inhaled cocaine, and psychoactive drugs including reserpine, guanethidine, and gabapentin *(2)*. The term is typically used in reference to nasal congestion subsequent to prolonged use of topical decongestants for more than 5 to 7 days. Nasal congestion is commonly the primary complaint, with rhinorrhea, pruritis, and sneezing as accompanying symptoms. α-Receptors of the nasal vasculature become gradually desensitized to endogenous and exogenous stimulation, and adrenergic tone is eventually lost. Withdrawal of these drugs may also lead to a rebound nasal decongestion. Prolonged use of nasal sympathomimetics may result in rhinitis medicamentosa, a drug-induced rhinitis with nasal congestion, hypertrophy, and hyperactivity *(3,25)*. Patients with rhinitis medicamentosa complain of extensive nasal congestion and rhinorrhea, and can expect to see normal nasal function within 7–21 days after discontinuing decongestants.

Irritative-Toxic/Occupational Rhinitis

With irritative-toxic or occupational rhinitis, patients experience symptoms of rhinitis as a result of an inhaled irritant, such as wood dusts, glues, solvents, chemicals, grains, animal antigens, and cigarette smoke. Symptoms are experienced when exposed to precipitants, are decreased when precipitants are avoided in approximately 70% of patients, and include nasal pruritis, nasal obstruction, watery rhinorrhea, postnasal drip, and sneezing *(3,25,26)*. Irritative-toxic or occupational rhinitis is frequently associated with concurrent occupational asthma, bronchitis, sinusitis, and conjunctivitis. Although the specific mechanisms remain unknown, the reaction has been shown to not be immunological in nature. The disorder is believed to be the result of damage and/or stimulation of nasal epithelial cells and neurons inducing the synthesis of pro-inflammatory mediators and neuromediators that predispose the nasal mucosa to inflammation, infection, and subsequent rhinitis.

Hormonal Rhinitis

Hormonal rhinitis is commonly associated with hypothyroidism, puberty, oral contraceptive use, conjugated estrogen use, and acromegaly *(3,25)*. Rhinitis in pregnancy occurs in approximately 22% of pregnant women, and its incidence is markedly increased in pregnant women who were smokers, with a relative risk of 69% *(27)*. The hallmark of pregnancy rhinitis is nasal congestion that begins approximately in the second month and progressively increases over the course of pregnancy and subsides with parturition *(28)*. Some of these women may exhibit increased watery nasal secretions; sneezing and itching are less commonly experienced. Although the exact mechanism is still not precisely known, hormonal rhinitis is believed to be a result of physiological changes related to pregnancy; more particularly, the expanded blood volume and progesterone-induced vascular smooth muscle relaxation are believed to exacerbate a previously existing mild rhinitis condition *(22)*. Similar in its effect in the female genital tract, estrogen has also been shown to lead to vascular engorgement in the nose resulting in nasal obstruction and/or nasal hypersecretion *(24)*. Furthermore, progesterone and β-estradiol increase the expression of histamine H_1 receptors on nasal mucosal epithelium and microvascular endothelium, and induce eosinophil migration and/or degranulation *(29,30)*. These effects contrast those of testosterone in which eosinophilic activation and viability are consequently decreased.

Cholinergic Rhinitis

Within minutes to several hours of specific stimuli, vagally mediated nasal vasodilation results with profuse watery rhinorrheai. Gustatory rhinitis is a profuse watery rhinorrhea that occurs after ingestion of hot and spicy food, triggered by specific preservatives and dyes *(2)*. Similar profuse rhinorrhea is observed in certain individuals with hyperresponsiveness of sensory neurons to cold, dry air in what is commonly described jogger's or skier's nose.

Infectious Rhinitis

Infectious rhinitis is usually owing to an upper respiratory infection that is most commonly viral in origin and self-limiting within 7 to 10 days. Sore throat, fever, purulent nasal discharge, nasal congestion, sneezing, and the absence of associated allergy symptoms are suggestive of an infectious rhinitis *(28)*. These symptoms are generally self-limiting and respond to treatment with topical steroids. Persistent symptoms that present with mucopurulent nasal discharge, facial pain and pressure, change of sense of smell, and postnasal drainage with cough should be evaluated for chronic sinusitis and will generally require antibiotic administration.

DIFFERENTIAL DIAGNOSIS

Given that rhinitis is either allergic or non-allergic in nature, the differential diagnosis and diagnosis of non-allergic rhinitis are really one in the same. Rhinitis is quite often assumed to be allergic in nature without identification of the offending agents because there is uncertainty and doubt among many practitioners that differentiating allergic rhinitis from non-allergic rhinitis is cost-effective and appreciably changes management. Because of the similarity and overlap of symptoms that may be present in both types of rhinitis, distinguishing non-allergic rhinitis from allergic rhinitis by history alone may be difficult for the clinician. Nasal congestion, rhinorrhea, sneezing, postnasal drip, and nasal and pharyngeal pruritis may commonly be seen in both disorders. However, correctly distinguishing non-allergic rhinitis from allergic rhinitis is of clinical importance because the prognosis and pharmacotherapy for allergic rhinitis and non-allergic rhinitis differ substantially. It is important to consider that many patients may also present with a mixed rhinitis that comprises both allergic and non-allergic components, which may show symptoms of each disorder either simultaneously or separately at different times. Although a current categorical diagnosis for a mixed rhinitis does not exist, the concept is generally accepted. Unfortunately, mixed rhinitis and non-allergic rhinitis often go unrecognized or inadequately treated because rhinitis may be assumed by the clinician to be allergic in nature without identifying the cause, or the contribution of non-allergic rhinitis may be neglected in a patient with mixed rhinitis given a positive skin test. In the presence of a positive skin test, it is thus important for the clinician to not immediately exclude a comorbid non-allergic rhinitis in addition to the allergic rhinitis and consider the patient history for a possible mixed rhinitis.

In diagnosing non-allergic rhinitis or allergic rhinitis, infectious rhinitis must be initially excluded by the absence of purulent nasal discharge, sore throat, and fever because upper respiratory infections can be mistaken with either of these disorders *(28)*. A chronic rhinitis may also be consequent to chronic sinusitis, which is estimated to be prevalent in 13.5% of the general population and to occur concomitantly in 16% of patients with non-allergic rhinitis *(31)*. The familiar symptoms and signs of nasal congestion, discharge, headache, facial pain or pressure, and olfactory disturbances are generally sufficient for the practitioner in the clinical diagnosis of chronic sinusitis *(3,22,32)*. A rhinitis screening questionnaire in the initial patient visit, such as that in Fig. 2, may prove useful to the clinician in identifying critical information of the patient history to correctly differentiate between allergic rhinitis and non-allergic rhinitis or to appropriately diagnose a mixed rhinitis.

DIAGNOSIS

Non-allergic rhinitis is a diagnosis of exclusion. Because a specific diagnostic test for non-allergic rhinitis does not exist at present, diagnosis of non-allergic rhinitis is primarily based on clinical history, the absence of an identifiable allergy as evidenced by a negative skin test, and exacerbation of symptoms after exposure to nonimmunological stimuli.

History

Clinical history is the most important diagnostic tool of identifying non-allergic rhinitis because although a negative skin test may exclude the diagnosis of an allergic rhinitis in isolated non-allergic rhinitis, a positive allergy skin test does not rule out the presence of a non-allergic rhinitis, and the patient history will be critical to recognizing a mixed rhinitis. In the patent history, family history of allergy and early exposure to aeroallergens are the greatest risk factors for allergic rhinitis *(33)*. Atopic dermatitis and food allergies are usually observed during infancy and early childhood with subsequent asthma or allergic rhinitis seen in late childhood. The onset and progression of symptoms and age of the patient at presentation is of relative importance in diagnosing allergic rhinitis. The peak incidence of allergic rhinitis is observed between 12 and 15 years of age *(3)*. In the first several seasons in the onset of allergic rhinitis, patients describe symptoms that tend to worsen with each consecutive symptomatic season until the severity of the disease stabilizes, with usual improvement of symptoms in middle age. Allergic patients commonly suffer from eye irritation, pharyngeal pruritis, a sensation of fullness of the middle ear, popping of the eustachian tube. Although a positive family history, pollen-related seasonality, and sensitivity to animal dander or dust are more commonly associated with allergic rhinitis, the absence of nasal or ocular pruritis, nasal congestion and rhinorrhea with nonspecific irritants (e.g., odors, fumes), nasal polyps, changes in air temperature and humidity, certain medications, and food preservatives are more suggestive of non-allergic rhinitis. The effects of autonomic stimuli are much greater on patients with non-allergic rhinitis than patients with allergic rhinitis *(2)*. Approximately 64% of patients with allergic rhinitis have a first-degree relative with a history of allergy and are very likely to manifest with asthma and other allergic syndromes *(34,35)*.

PATIENT RHINITIS SCREEN Date: _____

This form will help determine the kind of rhinitis you have. Please check the box next to your symptoms.

Patient Name: _____

Patient Age: _____

Age when you first started having symptoms?

When do you have symptoms?

What symptoms do you have?	All Year?	Spring	Summer	Fall	Winter
Sneezing					
Stuffy nose/congestion					
Runny nose					
Postnasal drainage					
Itchy eyes/itchy nose					

What Medication[s] do you take for your symptoms? _____

Are your symptoms: ☐ completely controlled? ☐ somewhat controlled? ☐ uncontrolled?

Patient: Please check all the things that you think make your symptoms worse:

Allergens		Inhaled/Strong Odor Triggers	
Freshly mowed grass		Smoke (tobacco/burning items)	
Dead grass		Perfumes/colognes/fragrances	
Hay		Cosmetics	
Dead leaves		Cleaning products/detergents/soaps	
Pollen		Paint fumes or paint products	
Tree/Tree pollen		Hairspray	
Weeds (ragweed)		Outside dust	
Molds		Exhaust (cars/trucks/buses)	
House dust		Gasoline fumes	
Cats/cat hair			
Dogs/dog hair		**Weather Change Triggers**	
Feathers		Windy days	
		Cold days	
		Damp days	
		Humidity/temperature changes	
		Ingestant Triggers	
		Alcoholic beverages (beer, wine)	
		Spicy foods	
TOTAL		**TOTAL**	
Consider Allergic Rhinitis if ONLY boxes on this side are checked.		Consider Vasomotor (Nonallergic) Rinitis* if ONLY boxes on this side are checked.	

Consider "Mixed Rhinitis"
(or coexisting disease) if boxes on BOTH sides are checked.

*Vasomotor rhinitis is the major type of nonallergic rhinitis. Other types of nonallergic rhinitis include: infectous, hormonal-, exercise-, drug-, or reflex-induced etiologies, NARES and ciliary dyskinesia syndromes, and atrophic rhinitis. See guidelines by Dykewicz, et al for complete information *(Ann Allergy Asthma Immunol, 1998;81:478-518)*

Fig. 2. Rhinitis questionnaire. (Reproduced from ref. *35a* with permission.)

Physical Exam

The appearance of the nasal mucosa in non-allergic rhinitis shows a high degree of variability, often rendering the physical exam inconclusive. Consequently, visualization of the nasal mucosa should not be used as a basis for differentiation of non-allergic rhinitis from allergic rhinitis. Visible nasal anatomic abnormalities, such as septal deviation, polyps, and tumors, that can cause rhinitis may assist the clinician in diagnosing nasal polyp non-allergic rhinitis and idiopathic rhinitis secondary to trauma, and may also help rule out allergic rhinitis, especially with the absence of nasal pruritus, rhinorrhea, and sneezing *(34,36)*. The combination of pale, boggy, and cyanotic nasal mucosa is the classic description in patients with allergic rhinitis, but these patients may also present with normal appearing nasal mucosa *(34)*.

Clinical Testing

In consideration of the absence of studies undertaken to demonstrate adequate differentiation of these two disorders on the basis of clinical presentation, clinical testing is necessary to differentiate isolated non-allergic rhinitis from allergic rhinitis *(37)*. The minimum amount of diagnostic testing required to clinically differentiate these two conditions remains in question, yet clinical and ancillary testing remains the most definitive way to clinically exclude allergic rhinitis in patients with non-allergic rhinitis. Allergy skin testing is the current gold standard and necessary at present for distinguishing non-allergic rhinitis from allergic rhinitis. It is important to consider that irrelevant aeroallergens may occasionally result in a positive skin-prick test and may subsequently lead to a false diagnosis of allergic rhinitis *(22)*. Radioallergosorbent testing for allergen-specific IgE in serum may be as useful as specific allergy skin-prick test in confirming the diagnosis of allergic rhinitis. However, although radioallergosorbent testing for allergen-specific serum IgE provides roughly equivalent information for distinguishing non-allergic rhinitis from allergic rhinitis, it may be less sensitive, more expensive, and have a less favorable cost–reimbursement ratio *(38)*. Acoustic rhinometry, nasal peak flows, and anterior rhinomanometry may also be useful for clinical diagnosis.

TREATMENT

No studies have adequately addressed the question of the importance of differentiating allergic rhinitis from non-allergic rhinitis *(37)*. Differentiating non-allergic rhinitis from allergic rhinitis is clearly important if treatments are significantly different and if the outcomes of treatment, including prevention of complications, differ in response to those treatments. However, similar treatments are frequently employed in the two conditions, and differentiating non-allergic rhinitis from allergic rhinitis may not be necessary if nasal corticosteroids can be proven to significantly help treat most types of non-allergic rhinitis.

Avoidance of environmental factors or triggers is of primary therapeutic importance in treating non-allergic rhinitis. Nevertheless, because precipitants may not always be avoided or identified, pharmacotherapy is a mainstay in the treatment of non-allergic rhinitis. At present, pharmacotherapy modalities differ for the various types of non-allergic rhinitis; thus, the importance of correctly diagnosing the type of non-allergic rhinitis is underscored.

Antihistamines

Several studies have demonstrated that the second-generation antihistamine azelastine is highly efficacious in treating non-allergic rhinitis, in particular idiopathic rhinitis, for which the Food and Drug Administration (FDA) has approved its use in treatment *(39,40)*. One study showed that azelastine resulted in significant decreases in mean total scores of symptoms, including nasal congestion, rhinorrhea, postnasal drip, and sneezing when compared with placebo *(39)*. Because azelastine treats all four symptoms indiscriminately, it may prove to be highly effective in treating non-allergic rhinitis and particularly idiopathic rhinitis. In addition to its high efficacy, the 15- to 30-minute onset of action of topical azelastine with topical levocabastine is more rapid than that of other antihistamines currently in use *(41)*. As a second-generation antihistamine, azelastine is less lipophilic and has a decreased affinity for cholinergic and t-hydroxytryptaminergic receptors, leading to decreased central nervous system side effects, such as sedation, in comparison to first-generation antihistamines. Second-generation antihistamines also show an increased affinity for peripheral type 1 histamine receptors. Azelastine has anti-inflammatory effects that are also independent of type 1 histamine receptor inhibition, including decreased synthesis of leukotrienes, kinins, cytokines, prostaglandins, superoxide free radicals, decreased expression of intercellular adhesion molecules, decreased stimulation of irritant receptors, and reduced mucosal edema *(42)*. Some researchers suspect that the effectiveness of azelastine may also be a consequence of attenuation of the effects of neurokinins such as SP *(8)*.

Anticholinergics

Anticholinergics are most useful in treating patients with non-allergic rhinitis whose predominant symptom is rhinorrhea. The FDA has approved ipatropium bromide as the only intranasal anticholinergic for treatment of patients with non-allergic rhinitis whose predominant symptom is rhinorrhea. Ipatroprium bromide has been shown to reduce nasal blowing frequency, postnasal drip, and rhinorrhea, but has no activity against sneezing, itching, or nasal congestion. Consequently, it is the drug of choice for cholinergic syndromes of gustatory rhinitis and skier's or jogger's rhinitis. Nasal dryness, nasal irritation, epistaxis, pharyngitis, headache, and nausea occur in less than 10% of patients with the use of ipatroprium bromide.

Sympathomimetics/Decongestants

Oral decongestants, such as pseudoephedrine, are appropriate for short-term treatment of patients with non-allergic rhinitis whose predominant symptom is nasal congestion and with no comorbid contraindications to decongestants, such as severe cardiac disease and hypertension. Pseudoephedrine stimulates α-adrenergic receptors and augments the release of norepinephrine resulting in vasoconstriction and reduced nasal edema and airway obstruction. Pseudoephedrine also stimulates β-adrenergic receptors. If the patient is taking monoamine oxidase inhibitors, oral decongestions should not be taken concurrently and only started 2 weeks after their discontinuation. Oral decongestants may result in an arrhythmia when taken with epinephrine or isoproterenol and the sympathomimetic effect of decongestants may be potentiated by β-blockers. Caution must also be taken when used in patients with epilepsy, glaucoma, diabetes, urinary or gastrointestinal obstruction, and thyroid disease. Finally, patients may develop rhinitis medicamentosa if topical formulations are used for more than 5 to 10 days as a result of downregulation of adrenergic receptors subsequent to persistent stimulation.

Topical Corticosteroids

Topical steroids have been most useful in treating severe symptoms owing to an inflammatory pathogenesis. Three of the six topical corticosteroids, fluticasone propionate, budesonide, and beclomethasone, have been approved by the FDA for treatment of patients with non-allergic rhinitis. Inhaled corticosteroids are believed to permit local smooth muscle relaxation, reduce airway hyperresponsiveness, and reduce the quantity and activity of inflammatory mediators. Unfortunately, the efficacy of corticosteroids in non-allergic rhinitis has been inconsistent, and none have demonstrated significant improvement of all four major symptoms of nasal congestion, rhinorrhea, sneezing, and postnasal drip in idiopathic rhinitis. However, because of the variability and dual existence of symptoms of nasal congestion and rhinorrhea in patients with idiopathic rhinitis, a nonspecific "broad-based" therapy with topical steroids and topical antihistamines may be a more appropriate treatment.

Topical cortical steroid should be particularly effective in patients with in NARES, blood eosinophilia non-allergic rhinitis syndrome, and nasal polyps, in which response to treatment is adequately indicated by the change of eosinophils in nasal and blood smears *(22)*. Rhinitis in pregnancy has also shown responsiveness to topical corticosteroids, although safer therapies are available, such as steam inhalation and saline nasal sprays. As adjunctive therapy, topical steroids may also prove useful in treating the underlying condition of rhinitis medicamentosa and relieving the congestive symptoms while the decongestant spray is gradually discontinued. Because of a 1- to 2-week delayed onset of action with corticosteroids, administration requires a tapering course of oral glucocorticoids for 1 week while beginning topical corticosteroids on the third day *(22,34)*. Patient response will determine appropriate dosage for nasal corticosteroids, and continuous use is more effective than intermittent use as needed because of the delayed onset of action.

Antileukotrienes

Antileukotrienes may have a therapeutic role in the treatment of nasal polyposis, but further studies are needed to evaluate their efficacy in treating non-allergic rhinitis *(37,43)*.

Surgery

Surgical procedures of the inferior turbinates have been attempted in patients failing medical therapy, but the results have been mixed and believed to be the result of changes in the nasal valve *(44)*. Surgical treatments for intractable idiopathic rhinitis have included vidian neurectomy and sphenopalatine ganglion block *(45)*.

REFERRAL

Determining when it is appropriate to treat or refer a patient may be difficult in certain circumstances. The Joint Task Force on Practice Parameters in Allergy, Asthma and Immunology has given the following indications for referral to an allergist:

1. A prolonged history of rhinitis.
2. The presence of complications or of comorbid allergic or respiratory conditions.
3. Symptoms that significantly interfere with the patient's ability to function or that impair quality of life.
4. The need to further identify triggers of rhinitis.
5. Prior treatment that either is prolonged with multiple medications or is corticosteroid-based.
6. Current treatment that is either ineffective or produces adverse events.

FUTURE DIRECTIONS

In May 2002, the evidence-based practice program of the Agency for Healthcare Research and Quality released its review of 228 full-length articles on non-allergic rhinitis *(34)*. Their findings showed that few trials on non-allergic rhinitis have been performed and that these studies were generally small in size, funded by pharmaceutical companies with the intent to compare the pharmacotherapeutic efficacy of competing company drugs, and failed to address the optimal clinical management of patients. Many did not meet high standards for methodological quality despite being randomized controlled trials. No studies had attempted to distinguish non-allergic rhinitis from allergic rhinitis with respect to clinical symptoms, physical exam, or the existence of comorbid conditions, and none had attempted to determine the minimum level of diagnostic testing necessary to differentiate non-allergic rhinitis from allergic rhinitis. Additionally, no diagnostic test had been specifically developed to diagnose non-allergic rhinitis. The The Agency for Healthcare Research and Quality evidence-based practice program also determined that more research funded by nonproprietorial sources is needed to more adequately address these questions. Standardization of research variables and higher quality studies are also necessary for future research to reduce the heterogeneity of inclusion and exclusion criteria, diagnostic tests, outcome measures, and test circumstances among the studies on allergic and non-allergic rhinitis to allow more effective comparisons.

Regarding future diagnostic possibilities, several recent studies have shown that the concentration of certain proteins in nasal washes are elevated in both patient populations of allergic and non-allergic rhinitis, but with protein levels significantly greater in patients with allergic rhinitis than in patients with non-allergic rhinitis. Patients with non-allergic rhinitis have likewise been shown to have elevated serum concentrations of IgG subclasses 1 and 4 against IgE in comparison to placebo patients, and similar to the relative protein concentrations in nasal washings, elevated serum IgG levels in patients with allergic rhinitis are significantly higher than those found in non-allergic rhinitis patients. Concentrations of serum-soluble Fas, an inherent signal for cell death, are also elevated in patients with allergic rhinitis, whereas patients with non-allergic rhinitis do not show increased Fas serum levels. These findings may possibly allow for more expedient and practical clinical testing in the future to differentiate the two types of rhinitis.

REFERENCES

1. Settipane RA. Rhinitis: a dose of epidemiological reality. Allergy Asthma Proc 2003; 24:147–154.
2. Woodall BS, Meyers AD. Nonallergic rhinitis 2002. Available from: http://www.emedicine.com/ent/topic402.htm. Accessed January 15, 2005.
3. Dykewicz MS, Fineman S. Diagnosis and management of rhinitis: complete guidelines of the Joint Task Force on Practice Parameters in Allergy, Asthma, and Immunology. Ann Allergy Asthma Immunol 1998;81:478–518.
4. Settipane RA, Leiberman P. Update on nonallergic rhinitis. Ann Allergy Asthma Immunol 2001;86:494–508.
5. Kaliner MA, Lieberman P. Incidence of allergic, nonallergic and mixed rhinitis in clinical practice. Poster presented at the annual meeting of the American Academy of Otolaryngology-Head and Neck Surgery Foundation, September 24–27, 2000.
6. Togias AG, Naclerio RM, Proud DF, et al. Nasal challenge with cold, dry air results in release of inflammatory mediators. Possible mast cell involvement. J Clin Invest 1985;76:1375–1381.

7. Togias AG, Naclerio RM, Peters SP, et al. Local generation of sulfidopeptide leukotrienes upon nasal provocation with cold, dry air. Am Rev Respir Dis 1986;133:1133–1137.
8. Ciprandi G. Treatment of nonallergic perennial rhinitis. Allergy 2004;59,16–23.
9. Jaradeh SS, Smith TL, Torrico L, et al. Autonomic nervous system evaluation of patients with vasomotor rhinitis. Laryngoscope 2000;110:1828–1831.
10. Loehrl TA, Smith TL, Darling RJ, et al. Autonomic dysfunction, vasomotor rhinitis, and extraesophageal manifestations of gastroesophageal reflux. Otolaryngol Head Neck Surg 2002;126:382–387.
11. Loehrl TA, Smith TL, Darling RJ, et al. Autonomic dysfunction, vasomotor rhinitis, and extraesophageal manifestations of gastroesophageal reflux. Otolaryngol Head Neck Surg 2002;126:382–387.
12. Giannessi F, Fattori B, Ursino F, et al. Ultrastructural and ultracytochemical study of human nasal respiratory epithelium in vasomotor rhinitis. Acta Otolaryngol 2003;123:943–949.
13. Garay R. Mechanisms of vasomotor rhinitis. Allergy 2004;59:4–10.
14. Groneberg DA, Heppt, W, Cryer A, et al. Toxic rhinitis-induced changes of human nasal mucosa innervation. Toxicol Pathol 2003;31:326–331.
15. Schierhorn K, Hanf G, Fischer A, et al. Ozone-induced release of neuropeptides from human nasal mucosa cells. Int Archive Allergy Immunol 2002;129:145–151.
16. Ruffoli R, Fattori B, Giambelluca MA, et al. Ultracytochemical localization of the NADPH-d activity in the human nasal respiratory mucosa in vasomotor rhinitis. Laryngoscope 2000;110:1361–1365.
17. Lal D, Corey JP, Vasomotor rhinitis update. Allergy 2004;12:243–247.
18. Powe DG, Huskisson RS, Carney AS, Jenkins D, Jones NS. Evidence for an inflammatory pathophysiology in idiopathic rhinitis. Clin Exp Allergy 2001;31:864–872.
19. Milsevic D, Janosevic, L, Janosevic S, Invankovic Z, Dergenc R. Skin reactivity to vasomotor agents in non-eosinophilic and eosinophilic non-allergic rhinitis. J Laryngol Otol 2002;116:519–522.
20. Monoeret-Vautrin DA, Hsieh H, Wayoff M, Guyot JL, Mouton C, Maria Y. Non-allergic rhinitis with eosinophilia syndrome a precursor of the triad: nasal polyposis, intrinsic asthma, and intolerance to aspirin. Ann Allergy 1990;64:513–518.
21. Leone C, Teodoro C, Pelucchi A, et al. Bronchial responsiveness and airway inflammation in patients with nonallergic rhinitis with eosinophila syndrome. J Allergy Clin Immunol 1997;100:775–780.
22. Settipane RA, Lieberman P. Update on non-allergic rhinitis. Ann Allergy Asthma Immunol 2001;86:494–507.
23. Bush RK, Asbury DW. Aspirin-sensitive asthma. In: Busse WW, Holgate ST, eds. Asthma and Rhinitis, 2nd ed. Blackwell Science Ltd., Oxford, 2000;pp. 1315–1325.
24. Bachert C. Persistent rhinitis—allergic or nonallergic? Allergy 2004;59:11–15.
25. van Cauwenberge PB, Wang D-Y, Ingels KJAO, Bachert C. Rhinitis: the spectrum of the disease. In: Busse WW, Holgate ST, eds. Asthma and Rhinitis, 2nd ed. Blackwell Science Ltd., Oxford, 2000; pp. 6–13.
26. Tunnicliffe WS, O'Hickey SP, Fletcher TJ, Miles TF, Burge PS, Ayres JG. Pulmonary function and respiratory symptoms in a population of airport workers. Occup Environ Med 1999;56:118–123.
27. Ellegard E, Hellgren M, Toren K, Karlsson G. The incidence of pregnancy rhinitis. Gynecol Obstet Invest 2000;49:98–101.
28. Mastin T. Recognizing and treating non-infectious rhinitis. J Am Acad Nurse Pract 2003;15:398–409.

29. Hamano N, Terada N, Maesako K, et al. Expression of histamine receptors in nasal epithelial cells and endothelial cells—the effects of sex hormones. Int Arch Allergy Immunol 1998:115:220–227.
30. Hamano N, Terada N, Maesako K, Numata T, Konno A. Effect of sex hormones on eosinophilic inflammation in nasal mucosa. Allergy Asthma Proc 1998;19:263–269.
31. Settipane GA, Klein DE. Nonallergic rhinitis: demography of eosinophils in nasal smear, blood total eosinophil counts, and IgE levels. N Engl Reg Allergy Proc 1985;6:363–366.
32. Collins JG. Prevalence of selected chronic conditions, United States, 1983–1985. National Center for Health Statistics Advance Data 1988;155:1–16.
33. Bjorksten B. Risk factors in early childhood for the development of atopic disease. Allergy 1994;49:400–407.
34. Lieberman P. Rhinitis. In: Bone RC, ed. Current Practice of Medicine. Current Medicine, Philadelphia, PA, 1996, pp. 1756–1765.
35. Settipane GA. Rhinitis: introduction. In: Settipane GA, ed. Rhinitis. Oceanside: Providence, RI, 1991.
35a. Lieberman P, Rakel RE, Hedges HH III, et al. Quantifying the incidence of mixed rhinitis with a new patient screening tool. Today's Therapeutic Trends 2005;20:221–232.
36. Lieberman P. Rhinitis. In: Slavin RG, Reisman RE, eds. Expert Guide to Allergy and Immunology. Philadelphia: American College of Physicians: 1999, pp. 23–40.
37. Management of Allergic and Nonallergic Rhinitis. Summary, evidence report/technology assessment: No. 54, May 2002. Agency for Healthcare Research and Quality, Rockville, MD. Available from: http://www.ahrq.gov/clinic/epcsums/rhinsum.htm.
38. Lau J, Long A. Chronic rhinitis: allergic or non-allergic? Am Fam Physician 2003;67:705–706.
39. Banov CH, Lieberman P. Efficacy of azelastine nasal spray in the treatment of vasomotor (perennial non-allergic) rhinitis. Ann Allergy Asthma Immunol 2001;86:28–35.
40. Gehanno P, Deschamps E, Garay E, Baehre M, Garay RP. Vasomotor rhinitis: clinical efficacy of azelastine nasal spray in comparison with placebo. ORL J Otorhinolaryngol Relat Spec 2001;63:85–141.
41. Scadding GK. Clinical assessment of antihistamines in rhinitis. Clin Exp Allergy 1999;29:77–81.
42. Lieberman PL, Settipane RA. Azelastine nasal spray: a review of pharmacology and clinical efficacy in allergic and non-allergic rhinitis. Allergy Asthma Proc 2003;24:95–105.
43. Borish L. The role of leukotrienes in upper and lower airway inflammation and the implications for treatment. Ann Allergy Asthma Immunol 2002;88:16–22.
44. Prasanna A, Murthy PSN. Vasomotor rhinitis and sphenopalatine ganglion block. J Pain Symptom Manage 1997;13:332–338.
45. Hadley JA. Vasomotor rhinitis remains a true clinical problem. Arch Otolaryngol Head Neck Surg 2003;129:587–588.

6 Sinusitis

Neelam Gor and Matthew L. Mintz

CONTENTS
- CASE PRESENTATION
- KEY CLINICAL QUESTIONS
- LEARNING OBJECTIVES
- EPIDEMIOLOGY
- PATHOPHYSIOLOGY
- DIFFERENTIAL DIAGNOSIS
- DIAGNOSIS
- TREATMENT
- FUTURE DIRECTIONS
- SOURCES

CASE PRESENTATION

A 27-year-old female is seen at her primary care physician's office for a second visit for re-evaluation of her symptoms. She was previously seen 2 weeks ago with symptoms of elevated temperature, rhinorrhea, and productive cough. Her symptoms improved after 3 days of treatment with first-generation antihistamine and ibuprofen. At this time, the patient's symptoms have worsened to include a fever, purulent cough, nasal congestion, mild facial pressure, and headache. Her past medical history is only remarkable for seasonal allergic rhinitis for which she takes an over-the-counter antihistamine as needed. Her family and social history are noncontributory.

KEY CLINICAL QUESTIONS

1. What factors have led this patient's symptoms to worsen?
2. What is the double sickening effect?
3. What complications in this patient would you most worry about?
4. What is the most effective treatment for sinusitis?

From: *Current Clinical Practice: Disorders of the Respiratory Tract:
Common Challenges in Primary Care*
By: M. L. Mintz © Humana Press, Totowa, NJ

LEARNING OBJECTIVES

1. Identify the patient with clinical signs and symptoms consistent with acute, chronic, and allergic sinusitis.
2. Formulate a management plan based on the pathophysiology of sinusitis.
3. Recognize that sinusitis is a problem that without prompt, effective treatment may lead to potentially debilitating complications.
4. Use a protocol for first-line medical management of acute and chronic sinusitis.
5. Identify patients who might benefit from appropriate referral for specialized care.

EPIDEMIOLOGY

According to the National Center for Disease Statistics, sinusitis has become the number one chronic illness for all age groups in the United States. Approximately one in eight persons are affected by the condition at least once in their lifetime and an estimated 35 million Americans suffer each year. Most patients with sinusitis are treated medically by their primary care physicians, accounting for almost 25 million physician office visits in the United States per year. Therefore, it is important for primary care physicians to recognize and properly diagnose acute, subacute, and chronic sinusitis. In most cases, treatment eliminates causative factors and controls the inflammatory and infectious components of the disease without leading to significantly debilitating complications.

PATHOPHYSIOLOGY

Sinusitis refers to the inflammation of the mucosal lining of the nose and paranasal sinuses. Often, it is referred to as rhinosinusitis in more modern texts named for its appropriate pathophysiology. Care in diagnosing the condition must be given in differentiating the various classes of sinusitis and appropriately treating the underlying factors contributing to the disease process. To understand the modality of treatment, it is important to define the illness and understand sinus anatomy, function, pathophysiology, and microbiology.

The functions of the four paired paranasal sinuses are not completely understood. Theories proposed include regulation of intranasal pressure, olfaction, humidification and warming of inspired air, lightening of the skull, improvement of voice resonance, shock absorption during trauma, and secretion of mucus to moisten the nasal passages. The normal physiology of the paranasal sinuses depends on normal sinus secretions, functioning cilia, and draining sinus ostia. These three components allow continuous clearance of sinus secretions. If any of these components of sinus physiology is altered, then the patient is predisposed to developing sinusitis.

Chapter 6 / Sinusitis

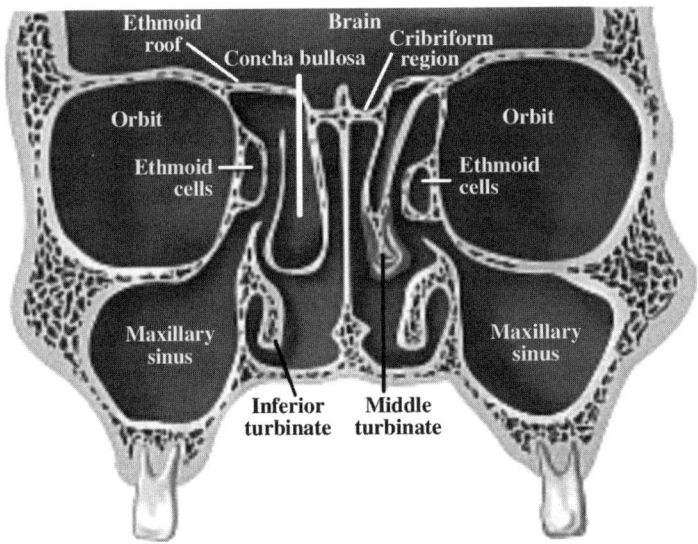

Fig. 1. Sinuses. (Courtesy of Dr. Daniel Becker, www.sinustreatmentcenter.com.)

The four paired paranasal sinuses are the ethmoid, frontal, maxillary, and sphenoid, named after the cranial bones that house them (Fig. 1). They have developed as outpouchings of the nasal mucosa and connect to the nasal cavity by a narrow ostium. The sinuses are normally lined by ciliated, pseudostratified columnar epithelium, interspersed with mucus-secreting cells. The air and fluid that accumulate within these spaces drain into the nasal cavity. The ostia of the frontal, maxillary, and anterior ethmoid sinuses lead into the osteomeatal complex (OMC) (Fig. 2), a key anatomic area in the pathophysiology of sinusitis. It is bound medially by the middle turbinate, posteriorly by the basal lamella, and laterally by the lamina papyracea, a paper thin bone that separates the orbit from the ethmoid sinus.

The cycle of events that leads to sinusitis begins with blockage of the OMC. Many factors contribute to the obstruction, including failure of normal mucus transport, mucosal edema, bacterial or viral infections, allergic rhinitis, anatomic variations, such as deviated septum (Fig. 3) and turbinate hypertrophy, barotraumas, dental infections, hormone factors, immunodeficiency states, irritants, mechanical ventilation, nasal dryness, and nasotracheal/nasogastric tubes. During the development of the OMC obstruction, mucosal congestion or anatomic obstruction blocks airflow and drainage. The secretions become stagnant and thicken within the sinus cavities. The pH and lowered oxygen tension create a

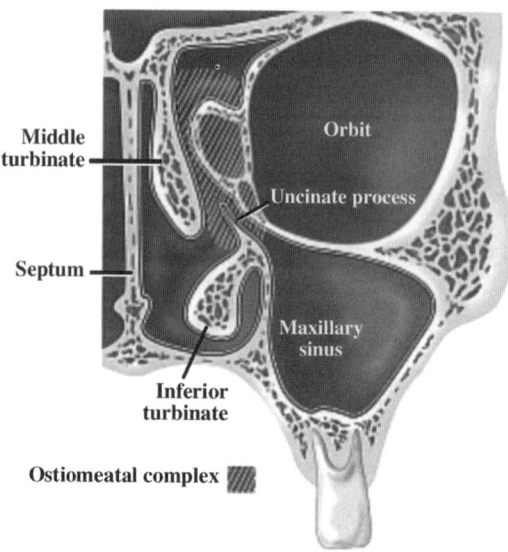

Fig. 2. Osteomeatal complex. (Courtesy of Dr. Daniel Becker, www.sinustreatment center.com.)

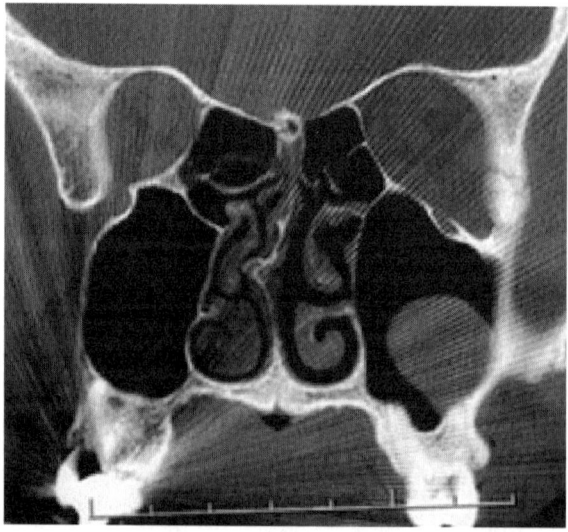

Fig. 3. Deviated septum causing nasal obstruction. (Courtesy of Dr. Daniel Becker, www.sinustreatmentcenter.com.)

medium for bacterial colonization and initiation of mucosal gas metabolism changes. The cilia, that normally clear mucous and air toward the OMC ostia, become damaged. Retained secretions also cause tissue inflammation and bacterial infection can develop in the sinus cavity. Sinusitis occurs because of a vicious cycle that leads to further mucosal thickening and edema, creating further blockage.

Microbiology

The most common factor that predisposes one to bacterial sinusitis is viral upper respiratory infections. Rhinovirus, parainfluenza, and influenza viruses are among the notable culprits. Approximately 2% of viral rhinosinusitus develops into bacterial sinusitis. Another small percentage of bacterial rhinosinusitis results from extension of dental root infection into the sinus cavity. Bacterial sinusitis can be divided into community-acquired and nosocomial infections. Seventy percent of cases of community-acquired sinusitis in adults and children are caused by *Streptococcus pneumoniae* and *Haemophilus influenzae*. One-fourth of pediatric acute sinus infections are caused by *Moraxella catarrhalis*. Other species that have been documented in sinusitis include other streptococcal species such as *Staphylococcus aureus*, *Neisseria* species, anaerobes, and Gram-negative rods, especially in hospitalized patient with nasogastric tubes. Polymicrobial infections have also been noted in this setting. Fungi are part of the normal flora, however, they can become pathological in immunocompromised and diabetic patients.

DIFFERENTIAL DIAGNOSIS

The differential diagnosis of acute bacterial sinusitis includes viral upper respiratory infection, dental infection, nasal foreign body, migraine/cluster headache, temporal arteritis, tension headache, allergic rhinitis, and temporomandibular joint disorders. History and physical exam can reveal the underlying causes of sinusitis, as mentioned previously. Among the signs and symptoms used to increase the likelihood of accurate diagnosis of acute sinusitis is the concept of double sickening that often occurs in sinusitis. Double sickening is a phenomenon in which a patient presents with a biphasic illness. After an initial presentation of a cold, the patient begins to recover for a brief period of time until worsening symptoms return. It is very easy to confuse the common cold for acute sinusitis especially during the first week of presentation of symptoms.

DIAGNOSIS

Sinusitis encompasses a basic classification system based on chronology and etiology. Patients with acute sinusitis present with symptoms of frontal headache or facial pain, tooth pain, fever higher than 100°F, and purulent nasal discharge for less than 4 weeks duration. Most cases of acute sinusitis present after an upper respiratory tract infection. The most common cause of acute bacterial sinusitis is a viral upper respiratory infection. Patients with symptoms present for 4 to 12 weeks can be classified as having subacute sinusitis. These cases have a more likely suspicion of bacterial etiology. When patients present with symptoms for longer than 12 weeks, they have chronic sinusitis with a pathophysiology that differs from that of acute sinusitis. Often it presents as an ongoing inflammation characterized by eosinophilia. Repeated insults to the sinus mucosa cause loss of the normal function of mucociliary clearance. This holds true, especially in pediatric cases. In contrast to acute sinusitis, the role of bacterial infection in subacute and chronic sinusitis is less certain. Fungus may also contribute in these cases.

The diagnosis of sinusitis is often presumptive and treatment is empirical, which presents further challenges to primary care clinicians. Certain diagnostic tools may be helpful to differentiate a common cold from sinusitis, especially in the case of bacterial sinusitis. One-half to two-thirds of patients with sinus symptoms who visit their clinicians are unlikely to have bacterial sinusitis. Studies performed in primary care settings have shown that there is no single symptom or sign that is both sensitive and specific for diagnosing acute sinusitis. In cases of acute sinusitis, the predictive power is improved by combining signs and symptoms into a clinical impression.

Diagnosing sinusitis is made on the basis of the signs, symptoms, and findings. These findings can be grouped into major and minor criteria (Table 1). The major criteria of sinusitis include facial pain/pressure, nasal congestion, facial fullness, purulent nasal discharge, hyposmia/anosmia, and fever (in the case of acute sinusitis). The minor criteria include headache, fever (in the cases of subacute and chronic sinusitis), halitosis, fatigue, cough, dental pain, and ear pressure. The accuracy rate of combining major and minor signs and symptoms is more than 55%. The Rhinosinusitis Task Force Committee of the American Academy of Otolaryngology-Head and Neck Surgery have developed diagnostic criteria that can be used to assess a potential patient with sinusitis based on signs and symptoms. A history that strongly supports the diagnosis of sinusitis is indicated by the presence of two major criteria or one major and two minor criteria.

On physical examination, palpation and percussion of the involved sinus may elicit tenderness or increased pressure. Areas that should be palpated include the palate (to evaluate the maxillary floor), cheek (to evaluate the anterior maxillary wall), medial canthus (to evaluate the lateral ethmoid wall), roof of the orbit (to evaluate the frontal sinus floor), and supraorbital skull (to evaluate the anterior frontal wall). There is a lack of correlation with transillumination methods when assessing the sinuses. Although transillumination is commonly used, it has poor reproducibility among patients.

Table 1
Diagnosis of Sinusitis

Major criteria

Facial pain/pressure
Nasal congestion
Facial fullness
Purulent nasal discharge
Hyposmia/anosmia
Fever (for acute sinusitis)

Minor criteria

Headache
Halitosis
Fatigue
Cough
Dental pain
Ear pressure
Fever (for subacute and chronic sinusitis)

- A history that strongly supports the diagnosis of sinusitis is indicated by the presence of two major criteria or one major and two minor criteria.

Computed tomography (CT) studies may reveal thick nasal walls, engorged turbinates, and occluded maxillary ostia. Imaging may also be helpful in determining the presence of air–fluid levels in the sinus spaces; however, these studies are not cost-effective in the initial assessment and treatment of patients with clinical findings. Radiographs have been suggested to help in uncertain or recurrent cases. A normal sinus X-ray has a negative predictive value of more than 90%. Signs and symptoms that may suggest a more thorough evaluation or hospitalization include those recently discharged from the hospital in which an intubation, feeding, or suction device was in the nasal cavity, immunocompromised states, severe headache or mental status changes, severe facial pain, or orbital involvement.

If an episode of acute sinusitis prolongs to beyond 4 weeks, the patient should be evaluated for subacute sinusitis. Such cases present after failure of treatment or no treatment of acute sinusitis. Symptoms are usually less severe with fever excluded from the major criteria for diagnosis. When a patient has been symptomatic for sinusitis for a period longer than 12 weeks, an evaluation by an otolaryngologist should be considered. Physiologically, patients with chronic sinusitis suffer from irreversible mucosal damage. Despite appropriate medical management, often these patients may find a definitive cure only after surgery. There are several factors involved in diagnosing chronic sinusitis. Patient history is critically important, and after combined with the physical exam, medical treatment can be initiated. The diagnostic criteria based on signs and symptoms are the same for chronic sinusitis as they are for acute sinusitis, except the presence of fever is classified as a minor criterion. Chronic sinusitis is determined by the duration of sinus symptoms. Most patients at this stage of the disease present with mucopurulent discharge and mild nasal congestion, whereas systemic symptoms are generally absent.

It is important to fully recognize the disease at this stage because of the debilitating complications that may result. The physical exam includes examination of orbits, extraocular motility, pupillary response, vision, cranial nerve function, and palpation for sinus pressure/tenderness. Careful skin examination that reveals erythema with periorbital swelling may indicate ethmoid sinusitis. Use of an otoscope with a nasal speculum provides better visualization of the inferior turbinate and anterior nasal septum, whereas a nasal endoscope is ideal for evaluating the entire nasal cavity. Common findings in patients with chronic sinusitis include deviated septum, nasal polyps, mucous crusts, and turbinate edema or hypertrophy. Plain X-ray films have been replaced by CT technology to evaluate patients who do not improve with medical therapy. A standard sinus CT without contrast injection is the radiographic study of choice because it can define the extent and location of disease. This imaging modality is used to confirm and stage the disease and to evaluate the anatomy before possible surgical intervention. Endoscopically guided cultures taken from the middle meatus may provide useful information for medical management of patients who fail to respond to empiric therapy.

TREATMENT

Once sinusitis is diagnosed, medical management is initiated. Underlying causes will affect the treatment modality. These include medical management of seasonal or perennial allergies, eosinophilic nonallergic rhinitis, vasomotor rhinitis, aspirin intolerance and nasal polyps, tumors, atrophic rhinitis, immunodeficiency states, anatomic causes, and so on. These underlying conditions must be kept in mind when starting treatment on any patient with acute or chronic sinusitis. The treatment of acute bacterial sinusitis includes antibiotics, decongestants, nasal lavage or saline spray, and an optional topical nasal corticosteroid. Adjuvant therapies are designed to promote ciliary function and decrease edema to improve drainage through the ostia. Decongestants constrict the sinusoids in the nasal mucosa, which are regulated by both $\alpha 1$- and $\alpha 2$-adrenoreceptor agonists. When choosing decongestants, studies have shown that $\alpha 2$-agonists may interfere with the healing of maxillary sinusitis. Using an $\alpha 1$-agonist, such as phenylephrine or oxymetazoline (i.e., Afrin™), is the preferred topical decongestant. Because of the risk of rebound rhinitis with topical nasal decongestants, it is important to restrict use to 5 days. Oral decongestants have also been implicated for symptomatic relief, but side effects should be regarded before prescribing to patients with hypertension. There is no rationale for using antihistamines in the case of acute sinusitis. Antihistamines further dry the mucous membranes, inspisate secretions, and may contribute to further obstruction of the OMC.

The incidence of the bacterial species causing acute sinusitis has not changed for many decades; however, the prevalence of antimicrobial resistant organisms continues to increase each year and it is difficult to predict emerging resistance patterns. The overuse of antibiotics, inappropriate dosing, and the use of broad-spectrum antibiotics as a first-line treatment have contributed to increasing numbers of resistant organisms. Although 40% of patients will recover spontaneously, antibiotics are indicated in the treatment of correctly diagnosed acute sinusitis, especially to hasten recovery. Hueston et al. noted that three of four randomized trials support the use of antibiotics in cases of acute sinusitis. Appropriate use of antibiotics may decrease the rate of orbital or intracranial complications and prevent the progression of an acute process to a chronic disease, in which mucosal damage can become irreversible. The Joint Task Force on Practice Parameters for Allergy and Immunology recommends antibiotic therapy for acute sinusitis if the symptoms have persisted for more than 7 days. The initial choice of antibiotic should begin with amoxicillin or trimethoprin–sulphamethoxazole for 10 to 14 days that target community-acquired organisms such as *S. pneumoniae* and *H. influenzae*. Second-line antibiotics depend on clinical efficacy, resistance patterns, dosing schedules, adverse events, compliance, patient allergies, and clinician experience. Penicillin, erythromycin, cephalexin, tetracycline, and cefixime are not recommended antibiotics for treatment because of inadequacy of their spectrum of activity.

The treatment for chronic sinusitis is similar to that of acute sinusitis with some minor differences. The medical management includes antibiotics, a topical nasal corticosteroid, an oral decongestant, nasal lavage or saline spray, humidification, and a mucolytic. Antibiotic treatment in chronic sinusitis is recommended for 3 to 4 weeks and nasal corticosteroids are prescribed on a long-term basis. In addition to the community-acquired pathogens associated with acute sinusitis, *S. aureus* and anaerobic species should be considered for chronic disease. Therefore, broad-spectrum coverage is required. Few studies focus on the choice of antibiotics for chronic disease. Amoxicillin is not considered a first-line treatment for chronic sinusitis. Recommendations include cefuroxime and amoxicillin-clavulanate as first-line agents. Patients with penicillin allergies may be treated with clindamycin or a quinolone. The treatment of patients with chronic sinusitis may require otolaryngology consultation. CT imaging of the sinuses followed by functional endoscopic sinus surgery often restores function and drainage in approximately 80 to 90% of patients.

It is important to know when to refer patients with severe or chronic disease to an otolaryngologist for further evaluation. Improperly treated sinus infections may spread through anastomosing veins or direct extension. Referral is appropriate when there are recurrent or chronic symptoms, nasal polyposis, asthma, and concomitant allergies. Complications that require a referral include deteriorating conditions, treatment failure, immunocompromised states, or development of a nosocomial infection. Referral to an otolaryngologist should be considered in a patient who has required more than three courses of antibiotic therapy for chronic sinusitis over a 12-month period. Otolaryngologists are able to perform aspiration of the maxillary sinuses to obtain cultures, diagnose and address contributing factors, and provide surgical intervention when necessary. Surgery should be considered only when all medical options are exhausted and patients present with refractory disease or anatomic abnormalities.

In addition, a patient with a normal sinus CT scan may benefit from an allergy consultation. The incidence of environmental allergy in patients who present for sinus surgery ranges from 15 to 60%. Other complications that may result from untreated or inappropriately treated sinusitis include meningitis, orbital cellulites/abscess, and osteitis of the sinus bones.

FUTURE DIRECTIONS

In the era of antibiotic therapy and adequate access to primary care, most patients do not experience serious complications from sinusitis. However, with increasing office visits and annual expenditures on prescription medications, especially antibiotics, sinusitis has been shown to have a significant effect on the patient's quality of life. Knowing how to appropriately manage this disease can relieve the financial and lifestyle burdens for a large portion of patients that are seen in primary care clinics. Although the literature is full of clinical studies and articles on management of sinusitis, the optimal management of the disease remains controversial. Future research is needed into the most cost-effective and efficient protocols for primary care physicians to follow. Although recommendations do exist, validated guidelines would be beneficial. In addition, newer antibiotics and other agents (inhaled nasal steroids, decongestants) continue to be developed for other reasons that will ultimately improve the treatment of sinusitis.

SOURCES

Benninger MS, Ferguson BJ, Hadley JA, et al. Adult chronic rhinosinusitis: definitions, diagnosis, epidemiology, and pathophysiology. Otolaryngol Head Neck Surg 2003;129:S1–S32.

Brook I, Gooch III WM, Jenkins SG, Pichichero ME. Medical management of acute bacterial sinusitis. Recommendations of a clinical advisory committee on pediatric and adult sinusitis. Ann Otol Rhinol Laryngol 2000;109:2–20.

Conde MV, Williams JW, Witsell DL, Piccirillo JF. Management of a 35-year-old man with acute nasal and sinus complaints. JCOM 1998;5:63–76.
Druce HM. Diagnosis of sinusitis in adults: history, physical examination, nasal cytology, echo, and rhinoscope. J Allergy Clin Immunol 1992;90:436–441.
Evans KL. Recognition and management of sinusitis. Drugs 1998;56:59–71
Fagnan LJ. Acute sinusitis: a cost effective approach to diagnosis and treatment. Am Fam Physician 1998;58:1795–1802, 1805–1806.
Gliklich RE, Metson R. The health impact of chronic sinusitis in patients seeking otolaryngologic care. Otolaryngol Head Neck Surg 1995;113:104–109.
Gooch WM III. Antibacterial management of acute and chronic sinusistis. Managed Care Interface 1999(February);92–94.
Gwaltney JM Jr. Acute community-acquired sinusitis. Clin Infect Dis 1996;23:1209–1223.
Gwaltney JM Jr, Hendley JO, Phillips CD, et al. Nose blowing propels nasal fluid into the paranasal sinuses. Clin Infect Dis 2000;30:387–391.
Gwaltney JM Jr, Scheld WM, Sande MA, Sydnor A. The microbial etiology and antimicrobial therapy of adults with acute community-acquired sinusitis: a fifteen-year experience at the University of Virginia and review of other selected studies. J Allergy Clin Immunol 1992;90:457–461; discussion 462.
Gwaltney, JM Jr, Wiesinger, BA, Patrie, JT. Acute community-acquired bacterial sinusitis: the value of antimicrobial treatment and the natural history. Clin Infect Dis 2004;38:227–233.
Hueston WJ, Eberlein C, Johnson D, Mainous AGIII. Criteria used by clinicians to differentiate sinusitis from viral upper respiratory tract infection. J Fam Pract 1998;46:487–492.
Kaliner MA, Osguthorpe JD, Fireman P, et al. Sinusitis: bench to bedside. Current findings, future directions. J Allergy Clin Immunol 1997;99;S829–S848.
Le J, Lipsky MS. Management of bacterial rhinosinusitis. Fam Pract Recert 2004;3–8.
McCaig LF, Hughes JM. Trends in antimicrobial drug prescribing among office-based physicians in the United States. JAMA 1995;273:214–219.
Metson R, Sindwani R. Chronic Sinusitis. Available from: www.uptodate.com. Accessed March 13, 2005.
National Institutes of Health. Data book 1990. US Department of Health and Human Services, Bethesda, MA, 1990; table 44, publication 90-1261.
Pankey GA, Gross CW, Mendelsohn MG. Classification. In: Contemporary Diagnosis and Management of Sinusitis. Handbooks in Health Care, Newton, PA, 1997, pp. 31–35.
Pankey GA, Gross CW, Mendelsohn MG. Diagnosis. In: Contemporary Diagnosis and Management of Sinusitis. Handbooks in Health Care, Newton, PA, 1997, pp. 36–47.
Pankey GA, Gross CW, Mendelsohn MG. Antimicrobial therapy. In: Contemporary Diagnosis and Management of Sinusitis. Handbooks in Health Care, Newton, PA, 1997, pp. 81–90.
Poole MD. A focus on acute sinusitis in adults: changes in disease management. Am J Med 1999;106:38S–47S.
Spector SL, Bernstein IL. Parameters for the diagnosis and management of sinusitis. J Allergy Clin Immunol 1998;102:S107–S144.
Su WY, Liu C, Hung SY, Tsai WF. Bacteriological study in chronic maxillary sinusitis. Laryngoscope 1983;93:931–934.
United States Department of Health and Human Services. National health survey. Prevalence of selected chronic conditions, United States, 1983–85. US Department of Health and Human Services, Hyattsville, MD, 1987.
Wald ER. Microbiology of acute and chronic sinusitis in children and adults. Am J Med Sci 1998;316:13–20.

Williams JW Jr, Simel DL. Does this patient have sinusitis? Diagnosing acute sinusitis by history and physical examination. JAMA 1993;270:1242–1246.

Yonkers AJ. Sinusitis—inspecting the causes and treatment. Ear Nose Throat J 1992;71:258–262.

7
Pharyngitis

David Jager and Matthew L. Mintz

CONTENTS

>   CASE PRESENTATION
>   KEY CLINICAL QUESTIONS
>   LEARNING OBJECTIVES
>   EPIDEMIOLOGY
>   PATHOPHYSIOLOGY
>   DIFFERENTIAL DIAGNOSIS
>   DIAGNOSIS
>   TREATMENT
>   FUTURE DIRECTIONS
>   REFERENCES

CASE PRESENTATION

A 40-year-old woman presents to her primary care physician complaining of fever, malaise, and sore throat for the last 3 days. The patient has a past medical history significant for hypothyroidism. She takes only levothyroxine pills and recent thyroid tests have been normal. The patient denied nausea, vomiting, diarrhea, cough, chest pain, and shortness of breath. She is a nursery school teacher who reports having taken care of multiple children with "colds" in the recent week. She drinks one glass of wine every week and denied smoking or other drug use. The patient is married and lives with her husband, who has not been sick.

Physical examination reveals a normal pulse and blood pressure, but a temperature of 101°F. She has no acute distress. Her turbinates are nonerythematous and her tympanic membranes appear normal. Her throat has erythematous tonsils bilaterally with white exudates and her neck reveals palpable anterior cervical adenopathy bilaterally. Her lungs are clear to auscultation bilaterally, with no wheezing, rales, or rhonchi. The remainder of her exam is normal.

> From: *Current Clinical Practice: Disorders of the Respiratory Tract:
> Common Challenges in Primary Care*
> By: M. L. Mintz © Humana Press, Totowa, NJ

KEY CLINICAL QUESTIONS

1. Can we make the diagnosis of group A streptococcus (GAS) pharyngitis on a clinical basis alone?
2. What is the differential diagnosis for pharyngitis?
3. Are there laboratory tests used to diagnose GAS?
4. What treatment modalities are available for pharyngitis?

LEARNING OBJECTIVES

1. Understand the proposed theories of how pharyngitis causes the symptoms of a "sore throat."
2. Be familiar with the laboratory tests and clinical findings used to diagnose GAS pharyngitis.
3. List the differential diagnosis of viral, bacterial, and fungal causes of pharyngitis.
4. Know the different treatment options available for GAS pharyngitis as well as other causes of pharyngitis.

EPIDEMIOLOGY

Pharyngitis is an inflammatory process of the pharynx, hypopharynx, uvula, and tonsils. Acute pharyngitis is one of the most common causes of physician visits, accounting for 2% of ambulatory visits in the United States every year *(1)*. In adults, GAS is found in only 10% of patients who seek medical attention. Although the majority of causes of pharyngitis do not require treatment with antibiotics, the majority of patients nonetheless receive them. According to the National Ambulatory Medical Care Survey, 18 million patients sought care for a sore throat in the United States during 1996 *(2)*. Therefore, because approximately 75% of patients who see physicians for pharyngitis receive antibiotics *(3)*, the treatment of pharyngitis is a major cause of excess antibiotic use in the United States. In addition to side effects from medications, the consequences of unnecessary antibiotic use have led to more resistant bacterial organisms.

Upper respiratory infections are the most common cause of illness. During the 1990s, an average of 6.5 million adults presented as outpatients with the chief complaint of sore throat in the United States *(4)*. Children are affected more often than the adult population. GAS (*Streptococcus pyogenes*) accounts for 15–36% of pediatric cases of pharyngitis. It has been estimated that children between the ages of 6 months and 2 years who are in day care have an upper respiratory infection approximately every 3 weeks *(5)*. A large portion of these infections are pharyngitis.

PATHOPHYSIOLOGY

Pharyngitis is frequently found in the setting of a viral upper respiratory infection. The pathogenesis of pharyngitis is not well-understood, but many theories have been offered. When a group of volunteers were given rhinoviral infections, bradykinin and lysylbradykinin were produced. These are known inflammatory mediators that can excite nerve endings in the pharynx, resulting in pain *(5)*. Other research done with laboratory animals found that viral infections produced an inflammatory response by invading pharyngeal cells *(4)*. Adenovirus and Epstein-Barr virus produce lymphoid hyperplasia and tonsilar exudates *(4)*. Herpes simplex virus causes oral mucosa ulcerations that are frequently found in the anterior portion of the mouth. In contrast, coxsackievirus causes oral ulcers located in the posterior mouth and pharynx. Pharyngitis caused by streptococcus B produces inflammation of the posterior pharynx. In patients with Epstein-Barr virus, as many as 10% of patients will have a GAS superinfection *(4)*. In some patients with *Corynebacterium diphtheriae* pharyngitis, a gray membrane can be seen over the posterior pharynx.

GAS (*S. pyogenes*) is transmitted through inhalation or contact with secretions *(6)*. Studies have shown that if a person is colonized with *S. pyogenes*, then 10% of family members will become colonized *(7)*. If that person has symptomatic pharyngitis, the percentage of family members who will become colonized increases to 25% *(8)*. Research has shown that school-age children are most likely the initial carriers of streptococcus into the family unit *(6)*. In patients who are colonized, 40% will develop streptococcal pharyngitis *(7)*. Differentiating streptococcal pharyngitis from other causes is important because GAS is the only major organism to which antibiotic therapy should be directed.

GAS infection also has associated infections regarded as complications. These complications include acute rheumatic fever, toxic shock syndrome, and acute glomerulonephritis. Acute rheumatic fever occurs after a latent period of 2 to 3 weeks after the pharyngitis begins. Symptoms of acute rheumatic fever include carditis, arthritis, chorea, erythema marginatum, and subcutaneous nodules. During World War II, the incidence of rheumatic fever among US army personnel reached 388 cases per 100,000 at its apex *(9)*. Secondary to improved antibiotics, increased access to health care, and decreased crowding, the incidence fell to 0.23 to 1.14 cases per 100,000 school-aged children during the 1970s and 1980s *(10)*. The current annual incidence of rheumatic fever is approximately one case per 1 million people *(10)*.

Streptococcal toxic shock syndrome is rarely associated with pharyngitis. The site of initial infection is commonly localized to skin, vagina, pharynx, and mucosa but in 45% of cases, no portal of entry can be determined *(11)*.

Timely therapeutic intervention to treat GAS pharyngitis does not prevent acute poststreptococcal glomerulonephritis (APG), the most common cause of postinfectious glomerulonephritis *(12)*. APG is a common cause of acute and chronic renal failure in children *(13)*. APG is most commonly found between the ages of 2 and 12 *(12)*. Although commonly found in the pediatric population, 5 to 10% of APG is found in patients ages 49 and older *(14)*. There is a male-to-female ratio of 2:1 in APG *(13)*. The glomerulonephritis develops 10 days after pharyngitis *(15)*. Some patients present with nephritic syndrome, whereas others present with hematuria. In more than 90% of patients with APG, the presentation is that of acute nephritic syndrome *(16)*. The average risk of developing APG following GAS infection is 15%, but during epidemics that risk can increase to 25% *(14)*. APG is an acute inflammatory disorder of the glomerulus initiated by GAS *(12)*. The development of APG is likely dependent on the virulence of the bacterial strain and the immune response created by the patient.

DIFFERENTIAL DIAGNOSIS

Sore throat is one of the most common complaints of adults in the outpatient setting. The differential diagnosis includes thyroiditis, gastroesophageal reflux, oropharyngeal/laryngeal tumor, pharyngitis, peristonsillar abscess, epiglottitis, retropharyngeal abscess, and Ludwig angina. However, the majority of patients with a "sore throat" will have pharyngitis.

The differential diagnosis for causative agents of pharyngitis is extremely diverse as shown in Table 1.

Viruses are estimated to cause roughly 30% of pharyngitis cases *(17)*. Rhinovirus is the most common viral cause. The other common viral causes in descending order are coronavirus, adenovirus, parainfluenza, and influenza virus *(18)*. Viral infections are more common during the winter months with the exception of adenoviruses, which occur year round. Patients with influenza can be diagnosed secondary to other cases in the community. The differential includes acute retroviral syndrome, which may be difficult to differentiate from mononucleosis. In patients in which HIV is in the differential diagnosis, risk factors for HIV must be explored by the physician. The symptoms may develop from 6 days to 3–5 weeks depending on the length of incubation. The symptoms of acute retroviral syndrome include pharyngitis, lymphadenopathy, fever, myalgia, and lethargy *(19)*. Herpes virus type I has been noted to cause a pharyngitis, as well as herpes virus type 2 if oral–genital contact has occurred.

Infectious mononucleosis is another viral infection that can cause pharyngitis. The majority of cases of mononucleosis are caused by Epstein-Barr virus with the remainder of cases caused by cytomegalovirus. Pharyngitis and tonsillar exudates in addition to lymphadenopathy, fatigue, and splenomegally point to a diagnosis of mononucleosis. Viral pharyngitis is spread through similar mecha-

Table 1
Causes of Pharyngitis

Bacteria	*Arcanobacterium haemolyticum*
	Corynebacterium diptheriae
Corynebacterium other spp.	
	Haemophilus influenzae
	Legionella pneumophilia
	Neisseria gonorrhoeae
	Neisseria meningitides
	Streptococcus pyogenes
	(group A b- hemolytic)
	Streptococcus spp.
	(groups B, C, and G)
	Treponema palidum
	Yersinia enterolitica
Fungal/rickettsial/intracellular organisms	*Candida* spp.
	Mycoplasma pneumoniae
	Coxiella burnettii
	Chlamydia pneumoniae
Viruses	Adenovirus
	Coronavirus
	Coxsackie A virus
	Cytomegalovirus
	Epstein-Barr virus
	Herpes simplex virus
	Human immunodeficiency virus-1
	Influenza A and B
Parainfluenza	Measles
	Reovirus
	Respiratory syncytial virus

nisms as other viral infections. Hand-to-mouth contact, contact with oral secretions, and sharing common utensils all contribute to viral spread. Prevention of the spreading of disease is based on frequent hand washing and avoidance of aerosolized secretions. Mycoplasma and chlaymdia typically cause pharyngitis in young patients with acute bronchitis.

Streptococci groups C and G are responsible for food- and water-borne pharyngitis outbreaks *(19)*. These bacteria have also been documented to cause a less severe form of pharyngitis that mimics GAS. These organisms commonly colonize the respiratory tract, therefore, differentiating this state from acute infection is often difficult. *Arcanobacterium haemolyticum* produces a pharyngitis that is difficult to distinguish from GAS pharyngitis *(19)*. *A. haemolyticum* infection should be suspected in adolescents and young adults with a clinical presentation consistent with GAS but with a negative culture.

Diphtheria was once a more common cause of pharyngitis in the United States, but is now rare. One probable case was reported to the Centers for Disease Control and Prevention (CDC) in 1998 *(19)*. With the advent of immunization, diphtheria cases are now rare in industrialized nations. Pharyngeal infection with *C. diphtheriae* produces a grayish-brown membrane on the pharynx, uvula, and larynx. Diagnosis is usually made based on clinical and epidemiological factors.

DIAGNOSIS

The majority of cases of viral pharyngitis are associated with an upper respiratory infection. An upper respiratory infection commonly begins with malaise, fever, headache, myalgias, and then coryza and sore throat. In assessing patients with pharyngitis, there is great importance in differentiating GAS from all other causes. Research has showed that physicians are poor predictors of which patients will have positive throat cultures for GAS pharyngitis. The sensitivity and specificity range from 55 to 74% and 58 to 76%, respectively *(1)*. The Centor criteria were created to aid physicians in diagnosing GAS. The four criteria are tonsillar exudates, history of fever, absence of cough, and tender anterior cervical adenopathy. If three or four criteria are met, the positive predictive value is 40 to 60% *(20)*. The negative predictive value of less than three criteria is 80% *(20)*. The sensitivity and specificity are both increased to approximately 75% when the criteria are implemented according to some studies *(21)*. Clinical features that are consistent with GAS pharyngitis include sore throat, sudden onset of symptoms, fever, and headache. Clinical symptoms consistent with a viral etiology include conjunctivitis, coryza, cough, and diarrhea.

The CDC has released principles to govern diagnosing and treating patients with GAS. The CDC recommends that all adult patients with pharyngitis should be screened with the Centor criteria. If patients have none or one criterion, these patients shouldn't be tested or treated because they are unlikely to have GAS *(22)*. When patients have two, three, or four criteria, a rapid antigen test (RAT) should be performed. If the RAT is positive, then antibiotic therapy should be started. The algorithm that we recommend is to test patients with two or three criteria with an RAT, and treat those with a positive test and those with four criteria. The final option is to not use diagnostic tests and use antibiotics to treat patients with three or four criteria *(22)*. The guidelines do not apply to immunocompromised patients and patients with a history of rheumatic fever, valvular heart disease, sore throats not caused by acute pharyngitis, and patients that have recurrent or chronic pharyngitis *(22)*. The guidelines do not apply during outbreaks of GAS.

The diagnosis of acute GAS pharyngitis in children should be similarly based on clinical grounds and then verified by RAT or throat culture. There is great debate as to what clinical guidelines should be implemented. We recommend using the Centor criteria (fever, tonsillar exudates, absence of cough, cervical lymphadenopathy) as well as including seasonal risk factors (November to May) and personal or family contact history of rheumatic fever. If a patient has one or less of these criteria, GAS is less likely, so no further testing or treatment is needed. For two or more criteria, we recommend either RAT or throat culture. The Infectious Disease Society of America recommends that if a child has a negative RAT, it must be confirmed by a throat culture. If either the RAT or throat culture are positive, then treatment must be started *(23)*.

The gold standard for diagnosis of GAS is the throat culture. The drawbacks of traditional throat cultures have been the 24 to 48 hours required for growth. This duration of time makes decisions about whether to start antibiotics difficult. Other criticisms include the insensitivity of the test secondary to variations in specimen collection and laboratory processing *(24)*. Another drawback of throat cultures is the false-positives secondary to 5% carrier rate for GAS *(25)*. Plating of the specimen is to occur under direct visualization of the specimen with immediate plating onto sheep's blood agar with low dextrose content. With proper technique, sensitivity and specificity in adults are at least 90%, but in clinical practice, sensitivity and specificity are significantly lower. The delay in information provided by standard throat cultures makes their usefulness of question.

The advent of the RAT has provided faster results that can be given at the bedsides and done quickly in office labs. Most rapid streptococcus tests detect the surface carbohydrate that designates a streptococcus as a member of Lancefield group A. The early tests used latex agglutination methods, whereas the second-generation tests employed enzyme immunoassays. Modern tests use DNA probes and optical immunoassays *(26)*. Recent studies have showed sensitivity of 80 to 90% and specificity of 90 to 100% *(27)*. The American Academy of Pediatrics has guidelines that consider a positive RAT to be considered definitive evidence of streptococcal pharyngitis *(28)*. If the RAT is negative, but there is strong clinical suspicion, then a standard throat culture should be performed.

Serological testing is of little use in the diagnosis of streptococcal pharyngitis. In the picture of acute streptococcal pharyngitis, a fourfold rise in antistreptolysin or anti-deoxyribonuclease B may be seen. The titers will rise during acute infection and will peak within 2 weeks. The serological results are not present when treatment decisions must be made.

TREATMENT

There are numerous factors that influence selecting an antibiotic treatment for streptococcal pharyngitis. These factors include bacteriological and clinical efficacy, patient allergies, compliance concerns, and frequency of drug administration, palatability, cost, spectrum of activity, and side effects *(9)*. Table 2 lists some of the potential antibiotic choices.

Table 2
Antibiotic Treatment for Group A β-hemolytic Streptococcal Pharyngitis

Penicillin V
Penicillin G benzathine
Amoxicillin
Erythromycin ethylsuccinate
Erythromycin estolate
Azithromycin
Amoxicillin-clavulanate potassium
Cefadroxil
Cephalexin

Penicillin has been the drug of choice for streptococcal pharyngitis in both adults and children. Initially, GAS pharyngitis was treated with a single injection of penicillin G benzathine. Studies conducted in the 1960s and 1970s have shown that oral and intramuscular penicillin were equally effective treatment regimens *(9)*. Based on this information, oral penicillin V has been the treatment of choice since the 1980s *(29)*. Drawbacks to penicillin use are allergic reactions and compliance with four times daily dosing regimen. Studies have shown that clinical failure rates range from 5 to 15% and bacteriological failure rates range from 10 to 30% *(30)*. Adults with GAS pharyngitis should be given penicillin V 500 mg orally two or three times daily for 10 days or one intramuscular injection of penicillin. Children should receive penicillin V 250 mg orally two or three times daily for 10 days.

Amoxicillin has benefit over penicillin of having longer half-life and improved palatability. Skin rashes and gastrointestinal side effects are more common with amoxicillin *(9)*. The first-line alternative for patients with a penicillin allergy is erythromycin. The gastrointestinal side effects cause 15 to 20% of patients to be unable to tolerate erythromycin therapy *(31)*. Azithromycin is an alternative treatment with fewer side effects than erythromycin, but is much more expensive.

Cephalosporins have been found to be superior to penicillin V in a meta-analysis of 19 trials. The bacteriological cure rate for cephalosporins was 92% compared with 84% for penicillin *(32)*. The first-generation cephalosporins are preferred over the second- or third-generation antibiotics. The cost and penicillin crossreactivity make cephalosporins less desirable for first-line treatment of streptococcal pharyngitis. The broadest spectrum antibiotic choice is amoxicillin-clavulanate potassium, which is expensive and has diarrhea as a side effect. Amoxicillin-clavulanate is typically used to treat recurrent streptococcal pharyngitis *(33)*.

A chart review study found that recurrent group A β-hemolytic streptococcal infections were more common in the 1990s than in previous decades *(34)*. It is unclear whether patients have a relapse of the initial infection or are becoming re-infected. Numerous theories have been created to explain these findings, which include lack of compliance, repeat exposure, eradication of protective pharyngeal microflora, penicillin resistance, and antibiotic suppression of immunity *(30)*. In patients with continued infection, other reservoirs of infection must be examined. Group A β-hemolytic streptococci can persist for up to 15 days on unrinsed toothbrushes and orthodontic appliances *(35)*. Thorough rinsing of these items may decrease spread of infection and help to prevent re-infection.

There is no need to repeat throat cultures following treatment. If a patient has a positive posttreatment culture, it means that the patient is a chronic carrier and is of little concern to spread infection. Chronic carriers will only be treated if they are associated with treatment failure in a close contact *(9)*. The CDC recommends that throat cultures should not be used for screening adults with pharyngitis or used for confirmation of negative rapid tests when the test sensitivity exceeds 80% *(22)*. Another treatment recommendation is that all patients with pharyngitis should be offered analgesics, antipyretics, and other supportive care.

FUTURE DIRECTIONS

The future of diagnosis of GAS pharyngitis involves the development of more rapid tests using optical immunoassay and chemiluminescent DNA *(9)*. These tests will increase the accuracy of diagnosis, but will likely be more costly. Research is currently underway to create a vaccine to prevent the disease. The target for the vaccine is the streptococcal M protein, but this research will take many years to potentially reach the market *(36)*. Future research may also need to be directed into recurrences of infection and changing drug sensitivities.

REFERENCES

1. Cooper RJ, Hoffman JR, Bartlett JG, et al. Principles of appropriate antibiotic use for acute pharyngitis in adults: background. Ann Intern Med 2001,134.509–517.
2. Schappert SM. Ambulatory care visits to physician's offices, hospital outpatient departments, and emergency departments: United States, 1996. Vital Health Stat Series 13 1998; 134:1–37
3. Gonzales R, Steiner JF, Sande MA. Antibiotic prescribing for adults with colds, upper respiratory infections, and bronchitis by ambulatory care physicians. JAMA 1997;278:901–904.
4. Clements DA. Pharyngitis, laryngitis, and epiglottis. In: Cohen J, Powedeny WG, eds. Infectious Diseases, 2nd ed. Elsevier, New York, 2004, pp. 341–348.
5. Proud D, Reynolds CJ, Lacapra S, et al. Kinins are generated in nasal secretions during natural rhinovirus colds. J Infect Dis 1990;161:120–123.
6. Wannamaker LW. The epidemiology of streptococcal infections. In: McCarty M, ed. Streptococcal infections. Columbia University Press, New York, 1954; pp. 157–175.

7. Dingle JH, Badger GF, Jordan WS Jr. Illness in the home: a study of 25,000 illnesses in a group of Cleveland families. Western Reserve University Press, Cleveland, 1964.
8. Hamburger M Jr, Green MJ, Hamburger VG. The problem of the "dangerous carrier" of hemolytic streptococci. Number of hemolytic streptococci expelled by carriers with positive and negative nose cultures. J Infect Dis 1945;77:68–81.
9. Hayes CS, Willaimson H. Management of group A beta-hemolytic streptococcal pharyngitis. Am Fam Physician 2001;63:1557–1564.
10. Bronze MS, Dale JB. The reemergenceof serious group A streptococcal infections and acute rheumatic fever. Am J Med Sci 1996;311:41–54.
11. Stevens DL, Tanner MH, Winship J, et al. Reappearance of scarlet fever toxin A among streptococci in the Rocky Mountain West: Severe group A streptococcal infections associated with a toxic shock-like syndrome. N Engl J Med 1989;321:1–7.
12. Lang MM, Toers C. Identifying poststreptococcal glomerulonephritis. Nurse Pract 2001;26:34,37,38,40–42,44,47.
13. Berry PL, Brewer ED. Glomerulonephritis and nephrotic syndrome. In: Long SS, Pickering LK, Prober CG, eds. Principles and Practice of Pediatrics, 2nd ed. J.B. Lippincott Co., Philadelphia, 1994, pp. 1785–1788.
14. Rodriguez-Iturbe B. Acute endocapillary glomerulonephritis. In: Davison AM, Cameron JS, Grunfeld J-P, Ponticelli C Winearls CG, VanYpersele C, eds. Oxford Textbook of Clinical Nephrology, 2nd ed. Oxford University Press, New York, 1998 pp. 613–622.
15. Brady HR, O'Meara YM, Brenner BM. The major glomerulopathies. In: Kasper DL, Braunwald E, Fauci AS, et al., eds. Harrison's Principles of Internal Medicine, 14th ed. McGraw-Hill, New York, 1998; pp. 1536–1545.
16. Rodriguez-Iturbe B. Postinfectious glomerulonephritis. Am J Kidney Dis 2000;35:xlvi–xlviii.
17. Mandell GL, Bennett JE, Dolin R. Principles and Practices of Infectious Diseases, 5th ed. Churchill Livingstone, Philadelphia, 2000.
18. Bisno AL, Gerber MA, Gwaltney JM, et al. Diagnosis and management of group A streptococcal pharyngitis: a practice guideline. Clin Infect Dis 1997;25:574–583.
19. Bisno AL. Primary care: acute pharyngitis. New Engl J Med 2001;344:205–211.
20. Centor RM, Witherspoon JM, Dalton HP, et al. The diagnosis of strep throat in adults in the emergency room. Med Decis Making 1981;1:239–246.
21. Zwart S, Sachs AP, Ruijs GJ, et al. Penicillin for acute sore throat: randomized double blind trial of seven days versus three days treatment or placebo in adults. BMJ 2000;320:150–154.
22. Cooper RJ, Hoffman JR, Bartlett JG, et al. Principles of appropriate antibiotic use for acute pharyngitis in adults: background. Ann Emerg Med June 2001;37:711–719.
23. Bisno AL, Peter GS, Kaplan EL. Practice guidelines for the diagnosis and management of group A streptococcal pharyngitis. Clin Infect Dis 2002;35:126–129.
24. Krober MS, Bass JW, Michels GN. Streptococcal pharyngitis: placebo-controlled double-blind evaluation of clinical response to penicillin therapy. JAMA 1985;253:1271–1274.
25. Kellogg JA, Manzella JP. Detection of group A streptococci in the laboratory or physician's office. Culture vs antibody methods. JAMA 1986;255:2638–2642.
26. Corneli HM. Rapid strep tests in the emergency department: an evidence-based approach. Ped Emerg Care 2001;17:272–278.
27. Gieseker KE, Mackenzie T, Roe MH, Todd JK. Comparison of two rapid Streptococcus pyogenes diagnostic tests with a rigorous culture standard. Pediatr Infect Dis J 2002;21:922–927.
28. American Academy of Pediatrics. Group A streptococcal infectuions. In: Pickering LK, ed. 2000 Red Book: Report of the Committee on Infectious Diseases, 25th ed. American Academy of Pediatrics, Elk Grove Village, IL, 2000; pp. 526–536.

29. Bass JW. Treatment of streptococcal pharyngitis revisited. JAMA 1986;256:740–743.
30. Pichichero ME. Streptococcal pharyngitis: is penicillin still the right choice? Compr Ther 1996;22:782–787.
31. Feder HM, Gerber MA, Randolph MF, Stelmach PS, Kaplan EL. Once-daily therapy for streptococcal pharyngitis with amoxicillin. Pediatrics 1999;103:47–51.
32. Pichichero ME, Margolis PA. A comparison of cephalosporins and penicillins in the treatment of group A beta-hemolytic streptococcal pharyngitis. Pediatr Infect Dis J 1991;10:275–281.
33. Brook I. Treatment of patients with acute recurrent tonsillitis due to group A beta-hemolytic streptococci: a prospective randomized study comparing penicillin and amoxycillin/clavulanate potassium. J Antimicrob Chemother 1989;24:227–233.
34. Pichichero ME, Green JL, Francis AB, et al. Recurrent group A streptococcal tonsillopharyngitis. Pediatr Infect Dis J 1998;17:809–815.
35. Brook I, Gober AE. Persistence of group A beta-hemolytic streptococci in toothbrushes and removable orthodontic appliances following treatment of pharyngotonsillitis. Arch Otolaryngol Head Neck Surg 1998;124:993–995.
36. Markowitz M. Pioneers and modern ideas. Rheumatic fever—a half century perspective. Pediatrics 1998;102:272–274.

8 Laryngitis and Hoarseness

Matthew Chandler and Matthew L. Mintz

CONTENTS

> CASE PRESENTATION
> KEY CLINICAL QUESTIONS
> LEARNING OBJECTIVES
> EPIDEMIOLOGY
> PATHOPHYSIOLOGY
> DIFFERENTIAL DIAGNOSIS
> DIAGNOSIS
> TREATMENT
> CONCLUSIONS/CASE WRAP-UP
> REFERENCES

CASE PRESENTATION

A 42-year-old female jazz singer presents with a 3-day history of hoarseness. She had the onset of symptoms 3 days after a concert at a local club where she performs as a soloist in a jazz trio. Four days before her performance she complained of a cold with symptoms that included nasal congestion and sore throat. She was previously healthy with no history of systemic diseases. She occasionally drinks alcohol, but denies history of smoking.

On physical exam, she is a healthy-appearing individual who speaks with a hoarse voice. Her weight is 105 pounds, unchanged from baseline. Her blood pressure is 108/72. Head and neck exams are normal without oropharyngeal erythema or exudates. The remainder of the physical exam is normal.

KEY CLINICAL QUESTIONS

1. What is the cause of this woman's hoarseness?
2. At what point should clinicians work this patient up for something more serious?
3. What would be the most appropriate treatment for this patient?

LEARNING OBJECTIVES

1. Recall the common causes of laryngitis and hoarseness.
2. Understand the anatomy and physiology of the pharnyx to appreciate the complexity of voice production.
3. List the various pharmacological treatments of hoarseness and laryngitis.
4. Differentiate between acute and chronic hoarseness and the appropriate approach to the patient.

EPIDEMIOLOGY

Hoarseness is a common complaint of patients presenting to their primary care physicians (1). This clinical symptom has a variety of etiologies and can present in all patients at different stages of their lives. For this reason, data on all causes is difficult. However, the incidence is high, particularly in children, with one study suggesting that up to one-fourth of childhood patients have chronic laryngitis. Although the character or quality of hoarseness may be helpful in identifying the underlying cause, the evaluation of the patient with a thorough history of the onset of symptoms and associated complaints in addition to a directed physical exam is essential in making a diagnosis. It is crucial that patients presenting with longer than 2 weeks history of hoarseness be referred for evaluation by a specialist because of the potential for malignancy as the underlying cause for the symptom (2).

PATHOPHYSIOLOGY

Understanding the anatomy and histology of the larynx and vocal folds can broaden one's understanding of voice production and the mechanisms of hoarseness. The larynx is positioned along the airway below the glottis and is comprised of the thyroid, cricoid, and arytenoids cartilages. Within this structure, intrinsic laryngeal muscles are involved in the altering the shape, tension, and position of the vocal cords. Extrinsic muscles attach to the cartilaginous structures of the larynx connecting it with surrounding tissues. The larynx is primarily innervated by two branches of the vagus nerve. The superficial laryngeal nerve enters the larynx after branching from the vagus nerve within the neck and primarily innervates the epiglottis, the false vocal folds, and the cricothyroid muscle. The recurrent laryngeal nerve branches from the vagus nerve within the mediastinum, loops around the arch of the aorta on the left, and the subclavian artery on the right, and migrates upward through the tracheoesophageal groove into the inferior portion of the larynx. The recurrent laryngeal nerve primarily innervates the intrinsic muscles of the larynx *(3)*.

Voice production involves passing air across the true focal folds producing vibratory waves. The true vocal folds, like most epithelial tissue is comprised of an outer mucosal cover of stratified squamous epithelium and a deeper lamina propria. The lamina propria, or vocal ligament, is comprised of three distinct layers. The outer layer, also known as Rienke's space, is made of loose, gelatinous material. The second and third layers are comprised of elastic and collagenous material, respectively. Below the lamina propria is the vocalis muscle, which alters the overlying mucosal cover as it vibrates *(2)*. Voice production involves three distinct processes: air production, vibration, and resonance. Air originating in the lungs will flow through the larynx toward the mouth during expiration. This flow of air will generate a vibration along the vocal folds. The character of the vibration will be enhanced by adduction of the vocal folds and approximation of the mucosal elements. The production of the mucosal wave along the vocal folds will result in sound generation. The oropharynx and nasopharynx form a resonance chamber augmenting sound into speech as it travels upward and out through the mouth. Altering any of the three components of voice production is likely to distort the quality and/or volume of the speech produced.

Hoarseness occurs as a result of disruption of normal air production, vibration of the vocal folds, and resonation in the oropharynx and nasopharynx. Causes can be distinguished as acute or chronic by the length of symptoms. There is some overlap of the causes of acute and chronic hoarseness. A thoughtful consideration of the causes of hoarseness (Table 1) promotes a more orderly approach to the evaluation of a hoarse patient. Hoarseness lasting for longer than 2 weeks should be evaluated by a specialist.

Acute hoarseness presents with symptoms occurring less than 2 weeks in duration, occurs abruptly, and is often self-limiting *(2)*. Most causes of acute hoarseness are the result of acute inflammation of the vocal folds by infection or irritation. Acute infectious laryngitis is the most common cause of hoarseness *(4)*. Typically, laryngitis occurs in association with a viral upper respiratory tract infection and may present with cough and coryza. The most common viruses implemented in laryngitis are rhinovirus, adenovirus, and respiratory syncytial virus. In most cases, these viral infections are self-limiting. Secondary bacterial infections may occur and should be considered if symptoms persist. Organisms to consider as likely causes are *Moraxella catarrhalis*, *Haemophilus influenzae*, pneumococcus, streptococcus, staphylococcus, and mycoplasma. *Moraxella* is the most common bacterial infection occurring in 50% of cases *(4)*. Other rare infectious causes include tuberculosis, diphtheria, and mycotic infections.

Table 1
Causes of Laryngitis

Infectious	Upper respiratory tract infection
	Rhinovirus, adenovirus, and respiratory syncytial
	Bacterial infection (usually secondary)
	Moraxella catarrhalis, *Haemophilus influenzae*, pneumococcus, streptococcus, and staphylococcus
Noninfectious	Postnasal drip
	Gastroesophageal reflux disease
	Tobacco
	Alcohol use
Other benign causes	Polyps
	Nodules and cysts of the vocal fold
	Functional dysphonia

Noninfectious causes of acute laryngitis primarily result from exposure of the vocal folds to irritants. Laryngeal irritants include postnasal drip, gastroesophageal reflux disease (GERD), and tobacco and alcohol use, all of which can progress to chronic laryngitis if left untreated. Postnasal drip may present with associated cough and frequent throat clearing in patients with a previous history of allergies or sinusitis. Laryngitis is an atypical presentation of GERD, and will rarely be associated with symptom of heartburn, or a bitter taste in back of the throat *(4)*. Tobacco smoke and alcohol are direct irritants of the vocal folds and may result in hoarseness in an acute setting. Prolonged use by patients who present with hoarseness should also prompt an investigation of head and neck or other malignancies. Finally, acute hoarseness may be the result of functional dysphonia. In this setting, hoarseness presents as a result of abnormal contraction of the muscles while speaking, such as abnormal supraglottic contraction. Functional dysphonia may occur with abnormal compensation of laryngeal dysfunction that results from infectious or irritant laryngitis. Other causes include voice overuse and abuse, which may result in benign inflammation of the vocal cords. Symptoms occur as a result of speaking too long, too much, and too loud.

Chronic hoarseness requires a thorough head and neck evaluation to look for a cause, especially malignancy. Hoarseness lasting longer than 2 weeks should be evaluated by a specialist in head and neck diseases *(2)*. Although chronic hoarseness may be related to exposure to irritants, it is often a symptom of head and neck malignancy, especially glottic and vocal cord cancers. Because early detection results in favorable prognosis, suspicious lesions should be referred to a head and neck surgeon for further evaluation and possible biopsy or removal *(4)*.

Prolonged exposure to irritants and inflammation can progress to chronic laryngitis. Postnasal drip, GERD, and tobacco and alcohol use should be considered in patients with known exposures. GERD may present with isolated hoarseness as stomach acid refluxes up the esophagus and comes in contact with the larynx. This reflux laryngitis presents without typical symptoms of heartburn and bitterness in the back of the throat. Other symptoms include nocturnal coughing, throat clearing, and a sensation of having a lump in the throat, called "globus hystericus" *(5)*. Patients with reflux laryngitis have posterior laryngeal inflammation resulting in erythema, mucosal thickening, granuloma formation, and ulcers in the mucosal overlying the arytenoids. Bullemia may also present with laryngitis both from laryngeal reflux disease as well as small focal hemorrhages of the vocal folds.

Other benign causes of chronic laryngitis are polyps, nodules, and cysts of the vocal fold. These lesions occur as a result of prolonged use or abuse of the voice, and may be aggravated by upper respiratory infections, sinusitis, smoke, and alcohol. Nodules and polyps interfere with normal voice production by preventing closure and disrupting vibration along the vocal fold. Nodules commonly form bilaterally along the anterior and middle third of the vocal fold along the vibrating edge of the fold. Polyps are unilateral lesions that form along the vibrating edge of the vocal folds as a result of vocal misuse or prolonged exposure to inflammatory irritants. Polyps occur more commonly in men and appear as smooth, soft, broad-based, pedunculated masses. Cysts are submucosal lesions that more greatly interfere with the vibratory motion on the vocal folds. The etiology of cysts is unknown, but is likely the result of voice overuse or irritant exposure. Other cystic lesions that may present with hoarseness include retention cysts, laryngoceles, and ventricular prolapse. Retention cysts generally occur at the epiglottis, the false cords, ventricle, and the artyepiglottic fold, all areas in which mucous glands are present. Laryngoceles are air-filled sacs of the appendix of the laryngeal ventricle, and may present with hoarseness, cough, a foreign body sensation, or a neck mass. Ventricular prolapse occurs when the ventricle protrudes into the larynx, which occurs as a result of chronic inflammation producing an inflammatory infiltration and hypertrophy of the ventricular wall *(2)*.

DIFFERENTIAL DIAGNOSIS

Laryngitis is a disease entity causing the symptom of hoarseness. We have discussed infectious and noninfectious laryngitis, both acute and chronic, as well as functional dysphonia. However, many diseases affect the anatomy and/or physiology of the larynx and cause hoarseness as a secondary effect (Table 2).

Vocal cord paralysis occurs as a result of a number of causes but may often be idiopathic. Paralysis may involve one or both cords and will present with inadequate closure or approximation of the vocal cords. Patients will present with breathy voices because air passes open vocal folds *(2)*. With unilateral paralysis, patients may have subtle changes in voice quality because they may have com-

Table 2
Differential Diagnosis of Hoarseness

Vocal cord paralysis
Presbylaryngeus
Cardiopulmonary disease
Neuromuscular disorders
Infiltrative disease
Hormone level fluctuation
Collagen vascular disease
Psychological disorders
Malignancy

pensation by the normally functioning vocal cord. Vocal cord paralysis occurs with injury or damage to the nerves involved with normal function of the vocal cords. In patients with recent neck surgery, injury to the recurrent laryngeal nerve should be suspected. Surgical procedures of the thyroid gland, spinal cord, and carotid arteries may result in injury or damage of the laryngeal nerves, especially the recurrent laryngeal nerves. Without a history of recent surgery, a thorough investigation for tumors or lesions along the path of the nerves of the larynx must be completed. Viruses and autoimmune diseases may result in paralysis of the focal folds because of damage or irritation of the nerves innervating the larynx. The recurrent laryngeal nerve may also be compressed by intrathoracic masses, especially on the left as it wraps around the arch of the aorta. Head and neck cancers may infiltrate the laryngeal nerves and present with vocal cord paralysis. Apical lung masses as well as left atrial enlargement have been implemented in some cases. Bilateral paralysis of the vocal cords may be a result of a central process and a thorough evaluation and imaging of the brain may be useful (2).

The most common cause of the hoarseness in the elderly is presbylaryngeus (2). As an individual ages, the larynx undergoes changes affecting voice quality. There is loss of tone of the abdominal and laryngeal muscles decreasing the effort of voice production. Other changes include thickening of mucus secretions, laryngeal cartilage ossification, and arthritis in joints. On exam, the vocal folds may appear bowed when adducted as a result of the loss of tone in the vocalis muscles. Presbylaryngeus occurs more commonly in women and may be related to postmenopausal decreases in circulating estrogens. In the past, the onset has been delayed in women with postmenopausal hormonal therapy, but current understanding of postmenopausal estrogen use is likely to limit its use specifically in this case. Medialization thyroplasty may be used as a surgical correction for this problem.

Patients with cardiopulmonary disease may present with changes in their voice because of the loss of adequate air production. Patients with intrinsic pulmonary disease or neuromuscular disorders affecting respiration and ventilation may complain of decreased voice volume and hoarseness related to limited air movement across the vocal folds. Individuals using chronic oxygen therapy are at risk for drying and irritation of the vocal cords resulting in hoarseness.

Patients with obstructive/reactive lung disease who use inhaled medications may also present with complaints of hoarseness. Theses medications may cause laryngeal edema or may result in thrush. Changing medications or the use of "spacer" may decrease the frequency or improve hoarseness *(4)*.

Some neurological and systemic diseases may also present with hoarseness. Parkinson's disease is a disorder of motor neuron functioning and may result in abnormal voice production described as weak and monotone, which may be difficult to understand because of the lack of articulation. Essential tremors of the head and neck may also present with hoarseness. Strokes and multiple sclerosis should also be considered in the differential for neurological causes of hoarseness. A much less common neurological cause of hoarseness is spasmodic dysphonia, or vocal stuttering *(4)*. It results from hyperfunctioning of the vocal folds resulting in abnormally tight closure producing a strangulated voice. It may be associated with facial tics and grimacing. Normal vocal production may be achieved by temporarily paralyzing one of the vocal cords with botulinum toxin.

Infiltrative disease may result in changes in the larynx or nerves involved with voice production, such as sarcoidosis and amyloidosis. Wegener's granulomatosis results in granuloma formation and destruction of normal tissue along all parts of the airway. Hypothyroidism may present with diffuse myxedema of the vocal folds. Patients presenting with obesity, cold intolerance, and menstrual irregularities should raise the awareness of hypothyroidism as a possible cause.

Hoarseness may also be associated with changes in hormone levels is some women. It may occur as a result of fluctuating levels in the menstrual cycle, pregnancy, or with menopause *(4)*.

Other systemic diseases that should be considered include systemic lupus erythematous and rheumatoid arthritis. Systemic diseases should be considered when no other obvious cause for hoarseness can be identified.

Psychological disorders may also present with hoarseness. Anxiety, depression, and hypochondriasis are a few examples. Professional voice users are particularly susceptible to psychological causes because of the pressures of relying on their voice as a way of life. Special consideration should be taken when evaluating these individuals. Substance abuse may present as either a psychological cause or as a result of direct irritation by substances used. Alcohol and tobacco smoke are direct irritants. Cocaine may cause hoarseness through several mechanisms, including vasoconstriction and rebound vasodilation of the respiratory mucosa, disruption of fine motor control of the larynx, and direct laryngeal irritation *(4)*.

Patients presenting with more than 2 weeks of hoarseness should alert the practitioner to the possibility of malignant laryngeal lesions and should prompt referral to a specialist *(2)*. Ninety to 95% of malignant lesions of the larynx are squamous cell carcinomas *(5)*. Because 75% of these malignancies are in the glottic region involving the vocal cords, patients will present early in the clinical course with a complaint of hoarseness *(5)*. Symptoms associated with glottic carcinomas include dysphagia, odynophagia, otalgia, and hemoptysis in addition to hoarseness. Malignant lesions have been associated with tobacco and alcohol use, history of ionizing radiation, human papilloma virus, and herpes virus. Early carcinomas *in situ* will appear as hyperkeratotic lesions on exam. This cancer rarely metastasizes because of the relatively small blood and lympthatic supply. Under the guidance of a specialist, the tumor should be staged using the tumor, node, metastasis (TNM) strategy. Based on the stage, the tumor may be amenable to vocal cord microexcision or surgical excision, laser therapy, radiation therapy, and/or chemotherapy. Early detection and treatment may result in a more than 90% 5-year survival rate and preservation of phonation *(4)*.

DIAGNOSIS

As with any clinical problem, a thorough history is important in the evaluation of hoarseness. Patients presenting with longer than 2 weeks of symptoms should be referred to a specialist for further evaluation *(2)*. At presentation, a physician should collect information about the onset of symptoms. The quality and character of hoarseness may be useful in elucidating the underlying cause. Historical information should include vocal patterns of the patient, including recent use or abuse and recent speaking environments, such as noisy and smoky environments. Careful attention to these details may be important, because patients may undervalue these issues. In the case of professional singers, it is important to know level of training, type of music performed, and environment of concerts. The jazz singer with no formal training performing in a smoky environment is more likely to present with a complaint of hoarseness. Recent upper respiratory infection may predispose to infectious laryngitis, postnasal drip, and frequent throat clearing. It is important to know if patients smoke or consume alcohol because both of these are common laryngeal irritants. A history of smoking and alcohol use should also prompt an investigation for head and neck or other cancers. Important associated symptoms should include pain, otalgia, cough, shortness of breath, dysphagia, and acid taste in the mouth, although reflux laryngitis does not commonly present with typical symptoms of GERD. Nausea, vomiting, and weight loss may suggest a diagnosis of bullemia predisposing to irritant laryngitis.

In the primary care setting, a thorough head and neck evaluation is crucial. This should include careful inspection of the ears, nose, mouth, and throat with particular attention to the mucosa, looking for signs of inflammation and/or unusual masses. Careful palpation of the neck for masses and adenopathy should be performed. The examination should include careful assessment of cranial nerve function. A thoughtful consideration of the signs of other systemic diseases including hypothyroidism and neurological diseases, such as tremor, Parkinson's disease, and multiple sclerosis is also important. For presentations of hoarseness that are not obvious on routine examination, further work-up should include routine labs, chest X-ray, and referral to an ear, nose, and throat specialist for direct laryngoscopy and further evaluation.

TREATMENT

After careful consideration of the patient's presentation, specific therapy may be prescribed to address the underlying problem. Most cases of acute laryngitis are self-limiting *(2)*. Treatment options are directed towards symptomatic complaints and preventing complications. Patients should be taught vocal hygiene to expedite recovery and prevent future episodes of acute laryngitis. Patients should avoid excessive and loud talking, including whispering, which results in excess strain on the inflamed larynx.

In cases of infectious laryngitis, hoarseness will resolve as the upper respiratory tract infection improves. Decongestants and antihistamines should be avoided if possible because of the anticholinergic effects of drying the mouth and throat. Instead, voice rest and adequate hydration should be preserved, whereas caffeine, smoking, and other irritants should be avoided. Adequate hydration keeps the vocal folds well-lubricated and free of irritating mucous. A mucolytic agent also may be helpful to minimize mucus from irritating the vocal cords. Aspirin and non-steroidal anti-inflammatory drugs should be avoided because their use in this setting may increase the risk of vocal cord hemorrhage *(4)*. Antibiotics should only be considered if the practitioner is suspicious of the presence of a secondary bacterial infection.

For non-infectious acute laryngitis, treatment should be targeted at eliminating or minimizing exposure to the causative irritants to the vocal folds. Acid suppressors can be useful in GERD-associated laryngitis. Allergen avoidance, antihistamines, and intranasal steroids may be appropriate medical therapies to minimize symptoms caused by laryngitis from postnasal drip. Rarely, sinus surgery may be considered when conservative medical therapies have failed.

Chronic laryngitis may respond to good vocal hygiene and irritant avoidance, but may require more sophisticated therapy, which should be directed at the underlying cause. Nodules are reversible lesions that improve with vocal hygiene and speech therapy. Polyps and cysts are less commonly reversible and often require surgical excision. Oral steroid therapy and speech therapy may be beneficial before surgical interventions. Vocal therapy after surgery is expected to improve voice quality postoperatively *(2)*.

Patients with functional dysphonia should be reassured of the benign, reversible nature of their condition and referred for speech therapy. The goals of voice therapy are to correct maladaptive vocal behaviors and produce appropriate speaking mechanics. With the assistance of a therapist and voice analysis, patients learn appropriate behaviors related to pitch, loudness, and voice quality. Patients are taught posture coordination, as well as ventilation control. Whispering and whistling should be avoided because these potentially further damage the vocal folds. If left untreated, voice overuse may result in chronic inflammation. Therapy may be conducted over a 6- to 8-week period *(3)*.

Patients with hoarseness lasting for longer than 2 weeks should be referred to a specialist for a work-up of possible malignancy *(2)*. Part of the evaluation should include visualization of the larynx. Flexible nasolaryngoscopy allows direct visualization of the larynx and the opportunity to identify pathology. Strobovideolaryngoscopy may be used to visualize the vibrating vocal cords. This allows the examiner to evaluate the high-speed vibrations of the vocal cords. Using this technique, small lesions of the vocal cord mucosa can be detected as the possible source of the patient's hoarseness *(3)*.

Glottic carcinomas are managed according to their TNM stage. Early detection of squamous carcinomas often results in a good prognosis, owing to their tendency to metastasize late in their clinical course. Local T1N0M0 lesions are either endoscopically excised or treated with primary radiation. This modality minimizes resection of healthy tissue and preserves voice production. More advanced tumors may require laryngectomy *(2)*.

In the case of bilateral vocal cord paralysis, a temporary tracheostomy may be indicated if return of function is expected. Unilateral arytenoidectomy may allow decanulation from a tracheostomy should the condition become permanent. For unilateral paralysis, re-approximation may be achieved with injection of gelfoam or autologous fat into the affected vocal cord. This may improve voice production and minimize aspiration with improved glottic closure. Medialization thyropolasy may also be indicated in some cases *(2)*.

CONCLUSIONS/CASE WRAP-UP

Hoarseness is a relatively common complaint of patients presenting to a primary care provider *(1)*. Although most cases are acute in nature and self-limiting, a careful history and thorough evaluation of the patient is important *(2)*. Hoarseness lasting longer than 2 weeks should prompt the clinician to consider malignant causes for the patient's complaint and arrange referral to a specialist for a more complete evaluation *(2)*.

In the case presented here, the patient is most likely presenting with hoarseness secondary to an acute viral infection. Although her symptoms are expected to be self-limiting, she should be encouraged to avoid other irritants. She could be at risk for functional dysphonia, given her profession. In addition to reassurance, the patient should be referred to a voice therapist for treatment and education about vocal hygiene.

REFERENCES

1. Banfield G, Tandon P, Solomons N. Hoarse voice: an early symptom of many conditions. Practitioner. 2001;244:267–271.
2. Garret CG, Ossoff RH. Hoarseness: contemporary diagnosis and management. Comp Ther 1995;21:705–710.
3. Rosen CA, Anderson D, Murray T. Evaluating hoarseness: keeping your patient's voice healthy. Am Fam Physician 1998;57:2775–2782.
4. Hausfeld JN. Hoarseness: current concepts on etiologies and treatment alternatives. Md Med 1998:47:59–63.
5. Berke GS, Kevorkian KF. The diagnosis and management of hoarseness. Comp Ther 1996;22:251–255.

III DISORDERS OF THE LOWER AIRWAY

9 Croup

Jeremy Spencer and Matthew L. Mintz

CONTENTS
> CASE PRESENTATION
> KEY CLINICAL QUESTIONS
> LEARNING OBJECTIVES
> DEFINITION
> EPIDEMIOLOGY
> ETIOLOGY
> DIFFERENTIAL DIAGNOSIS
> PATHOPHYSIOLOGY
> DIAGNOSIS
> TREATMENT
> FUTURE DIRECTIONS
> REFERENCES

CASE PRESENTATION

Case 1

A 20-month-old boy is brought to his family practitioner by his mother. The boy has a 12-hour history of a loud cough, slight fever to 101°F, and a hoarse voice. The mother reports that the child had a difficult time sleeping the previous night because of the harsh cough. On examination, the boy is playful and smiling with a temperature of 99°F. It is noticed that he has a seal-like barking cough and subtle evidence of audible stridor. His chest is clear on auscultation with a normal respiratory rate. No chest wall recession is noted. The rest of the exam is unremarkable. The patient is sent home with a suspected upper respiratory infection. Later that evening, the family practitioner receives a phone call from the emergency department informing him that the patient has had worsening respiratory difficulty with visible signs of inspiratory stridor and is being admitted to the hospital for further observation.

From: *Current Clinical Practice: Disorders of the Respiratory Tract:
Common Challenges in Primary Care*
By: M. L. Mintz © Humana Press, Totowa, NJ

Case 2

A 25-year-old woman presents to her primary care physician with a 3-day history of sore throat now with dysphagia, hoarseness, and shortness of breath. The patient was noted to have a low-grade fever of 101°F and an oxygen saturation of 95% on room air. Suspected of having an upper respiratory infection, the patient was sent home with a prescription for antibiotics. Later that evening, the primary care doctor receives a phone call from the emergency department informing the physician that the patient has been admitted to the hospital for further observation. In the emergency department, the patient was found to have an oxygen saturation of 85% with improvement after receiving 35% oxygen via facemask. A white blood cell count of 8.7×10^9/L was obtained with a predominance of lymphocytes. The patient's symptoms improved over the next 8 hours. There was no bacterial growth from throat cultures and the patient was discharged on the seventh day after admission.

KEY CLINICAL QUESTIONS

1. What signs and symptoms in these patients help establish the diagnosis?
2. What might have warned the physicians that these patients would become worse?
3. Could any intervention have been done in the outpatient setting to prevent the emergency room visits?

LEARNING OBJECTIVES

1. What is the typical presentation of a patient with croup and why would you suspect this diagnosis?
2. What are the etiological agents of croup?
3. What is the clinical course and complications of croup?
4. What is the pathophysiology of croup and how is it treated?

DEFINITION

Croup is a term used to describe a syndrome that is caused by a variety of respiratory illnesses that involve the larynx, trachea, and bronchi. These illnesses include laryngotaheitis, laryngotracheobronchitis, laryngotracheobronchopneumonitis, and spasmodic croup. The various forms of croup all involve upper airway obstruction causing a seal-like barking cough, inspiratory stridor, hoarseness, and varying degrees of respiratory distress. Croup is most often a self-limiting illness but can result in severe airway obstruction with respiratory failure and death.

EPIDEMIOLOGY

Croup affects children from 6 months to 12 years old. Most cases occur at 2 years old and there is a significant decrease in its incidence after 6 years of age.

It affects boys more often than girls in a ratio of 2:1 *(1)*. Annually, it has an incidence of 50 new cases per 1000 children aged 2 *(1)*. Croup can occur any time during the year but is seen most often in the fall and winter with a recurrence rate of 5% *(1)*.

More rarely, acute laryngotracheitis can occur in adults causing a community-acquired adult croup. This entity was first identified in 1990 by Deeb and Einhorn *(2)* and only 10 cases have been reported since 1996 *(3)*, although the incidence is probably much higher owing to the lack of accurate diagnoses. Because of the relative rarity of adult croup, it has not been extensively studied and cases of the entity have only been examined retrospectively.

ETIOLOGY

Croup is usually a viral illness most frequently caused by the parainfluenza virus type I. Other pathogens known to cause croup include parainfluenza virus types II and III. Combined with type I, these viruses account for 75% of the cases of croup annually *(4)*. Less common causes of croup include parainfluenza type IV, influenza types A and B, adenovirus, respiratory syncytial virus, herpes simplex virus, measles, rhinovirus, coxsackievirus A and B, and echovirus. *Mycoplasma pneumoniae* is an extremely rare cause of croup. Other bacterial causes of tracheitis causing a croup-like syndrome include *Staphylococcus aureus, Haemophilus influenzae, Corynebacterium diphtheriae, Streptococcus pneumoniae,* and *Moraxella catarrhalis.* Non-infectious causes of croup include spasmodic croup but this form is often difficult to distinguish from infectious croup.

The adult form of croup is also caused by various viral and bacterial pathogens as well as a fungal cause. The viral causes of adult croup include herpes simplex, cytomegalovirus, and influenza type B. The bacterial causes include *S. aureus* and *H. influenzae.* The fungal cause of adult croup is Aspergillus. Table 1 highlights the more common causes of croup in children and adults. The reason for the difference between adults and children is a result of viral-specific memory T-helper cells and B-lymphocytes in adults.

DIFFERENTIAL DIAGNOSIS

The differential diagnosis of croup is extensive and includes any etiology causing stridor in young children. In addition to the viral causes of croup, the differential diagnosis includes the bacterial pathogens causing tracheitis. One of the most important, and often overlooked, causes of a croup-like presentation in children is foreign body aspiration. In contrast to croup, foreign body aspiration would not present with a seal-like barking cough and a history of aspiration or choking can be obtained in 90% of cases *(5)*. Table 2 lists some other disease entities causing stridor in children.

Table 1
Causes of Croup in Children and Adults

Organism	Adults	Children
Viral	Herpes simplex	Parainfluenza virus
	Cytomegalovirus	Influenza type A, B
	Influenza type B	Respiratory syncytial virus
		Adenoviruses
		Rhinovirus
		Varicella-Zoster
		Measles
		Echovirus
		Coxsackievirus
		Corona virus
		Enterovirus
Bacterial	*Staphylococcus aureus*	*Mycoplasma pneumoniae*
	Haemophilus influenzae	*Corynebacterium diptheriae*
		Streptococcus pneumoniae
Fungal	Aspergillus	

Table 2
Differential Diagnosis of Stridor in Children

Acute laryngeal fracture	Angioneurotic edema	Arnold-Chiari deformity
Burns or thermal injury	Dandy-Walker syndrome	Diphtheria
Epiglottitis	Inhalation injury	Laryngeal papillomatosis
Laryngomalacia	Measles	Neoplasm
Peritonsillar abscess	Retropharyngeal abscess	Subglottic stenosis
Vascular ring	Vocal cord paralysis	

Epiglottitis used to be a major cause of stridor in children. However, with the use of the *H. influenzae* vaccine, this entity is much less common. It can be distinguished from croup by a sudden onset, high fever, inflammation of the supraglottic region, dysphagia, lack of cough, and a thumb sign on radiography. Another common cause of stridor in children is a peritonsillar abscess. In contrast to croup, the child with a peritonsillar abscess will often have difficulty opening the mouth and visualization of the tonsils will reveal erythema, swelling, and tonsillar exudates.

Although many entities may present with stridor, history and clinical course remain the most important means of making an accurate diagnosis.

PATHOPHYSIOLOGY

Various viruses that are transmitted via the respiratory route cause croup. The virus enters through the nose and begins replication in the nasopharyngeal respiratory epithelium causing coryza as the first symptom. The infection spreads distally causing laryngeal and tracheal erythema and edema with diffuse inflammation of the airway walls. Because of this inflammation, the airways secrete a fibrinous exudate causing partial obstruction of the tracheal lumen. The infection also involves the vocal cords and subglottic larynx. Inflammation of the vocal cords causes vocal cord immobility and hoarseness. In the subglottic region where the airway lumen is the narrowest because of a ring of cartilage surrounding the area, a small amount of edema restricts airflow leading to audible inspiratory stridor and the seal-like barking cough. In younger children, the infection and inflammation can cause significant airway obstruction as a result of the smaller circumference of the lumen. This can result in mild to severe hypoxemia.

Spasmodic croup is a variant of the syndrome that may occur without an infectious agent. This entity is often indistinguishable from viral croup in that up to 40% of children will have features of both spasmodic (multiple recurrences, atopy) and viral croup (fever, upper respiratory infection symptoms) *(6)*. This variant is often triggered by allergy and occurs at night with noninflammatory edema of the airway structures and possible spasm of the glottis resulting in stridor and the seal-like barking cough owing to the same mechanisms described previously. This variant of croup is short-lived and responds well to humidify air with recurrence of symptoms limited to the first few days after the initial episode. Spasmodic croup should be suspected in a child who has had multiple bouts of croup with sudden onset at night and has a history of allergy or gastroesophageal reflux.

In croup caused by bacterial tracheitis, the inflammation can result in necrosis of the mucosa of the airway wall with ulceration and microabscess formation. A loosely attached pseudomembrane may form over areas of necrosis and ulceration and can result in worsening airway obstruction if it becomes detached.

DIAGNOSIS

Viral croup usually begins with a mild, nonspecific prodrome of 12 to 72 hours. During the prodrome period, the patient may experience a low-grade fever and coryza as the virus replicates in the nasopharyngeal mucosa. Other symptoms during this period include nasal congestion, sore throat, and a mild cough. As the illness progresses, the child will begin to develop a harsh, seal-like barking cough, and a hoarse voice. The cough often wakes the child from sleep and is frightening to the parents. With further airway obstruction, the child may develop inspiratory stridor, which is usually the first clue that the illness is not a common cold. The symptoms of croup tend to be worse at night, especially in the first and second days of the illness. Crying tends to worsen the symptoms and children with croup prefer to be in an elevated position. The symptoms are usually self-limited and resolve within 1 week.

Findings on the physical exam are usually minimal because the child is usually in less distress during the day than at night. Mild to severe respiratory distress may be apparent. The chest exam is often normal, but sometimes reveals expiratory wheezes. Inspiratory stridor may be evident on observation of the child. In more severe forms of the illness, expiratory stridor may also be present with nasal flaring as well as suprasternal and intercostal retractions. Lethargy and agitation may result from hypoxemia. With severe respiratory distress, tachycardia and tachypnea may be present that appears out of proportion to the rest of the clinical exam ultimately developing into cyanosis. Dehydration may be seen if the child has had difficulty maintaining adequate oral intake. In contrast to epiglottitis, drooling and dysphagia are absent in croup as well as rapid deterioration to toxicity. In bacterial tracheitis, the child will worsen after a few days of illness when the viral illness would be resolving. A child with bacterial tracheitis will often develop high fever, toxicity, and worsening respiratory distress.

A research tool developed by Westley and associates *(3)* is helpful in assessing the severity of croup and monitoring response to treatment. Table 3 outlines this severity scoring.

Adult croup presents with a prodromal upper respiratory tract illness lasting 2 to 4 days and includes cough, sore throat, and malaise. Fever may be low grade or absent and a white blood cell count is usually not elevated with a lymphocyte predominance. Following the prodromal period, there is a rapid deterioration with respiratory compromise and obstruction. Recovery is almost always complete in cases of adult croup with no evidence of complications.

The diagnosis of croup is usually made in the clinical setting. Monitoring the course of the illness is best done by frequent follow-up visits and physical exams, keeping in mind the typical clinical course previously outlined. This technique is the best method for obtaining a good outcome and avoiding preventable complications. Some studies and imaging may be beneficial in aiding the physician in the diagnosis of croup if the presentation is atypical or another cause for the child's condition is suspected.

Radiologic studies include plain films of the soft tissues of the neck that may show the classic "steeple sign." The "steeple sign" is seen on a posteroanterior plain film as a narrow column of air in the subglottic region. On lateral plain film, the "steeple sign" is represented by an overdistended hypopharynx. These findings are found in only 50% of the cases of croup with many children having radiologic plain films with normal findings *(4)*. Because radiography does not correlate well with a diagnosis of croup, radiographic studies should be reserved

Table 3
Severity Scoring for Croup

Level of consciousness	
Normal or sleeping	0
Disoriented	5
Cyanosis	
None	0
With agitation	1
At rest	2
Stridor	
None	0
With agitation	1
At rest	2
Air entry	
Normal	0
Decreased	1
Markedly decreased	2
Retractions	
None	0
Mild	1
Moderate	2
Severe	3

Adapted from ref. 3.

if the clinical presentation is atypical for croup or suspicious for another etiology, such as epiglottitis or foreign body aspiration, in which radiography may be diagnostic. A more sensitive, and likely more useful, imaging study in the diagnosis of airway obstruction and stridor is rapid computed tomographic scanning of the neck.

Sometimes pulse oximetry is useful in measuring the degree of hypoxia in a child with croup. However, croup is a disease of the larger upper airways with pulse oximetry being normal except in the most severe cases of obstruction and respiratory distress caused by the illness. Pulse oximetry may be useful in differentiating croup from bronchospasm, in which the oxygen saturation is lower than expected.

Direct visualization of the laryngeal area and intubation is rarely required in the setting of croup. Laryngoscopy may be necessary if epiglottitis is suspected or the child has a rapidly deteriorating course. Intubation may be required if the illness appears to be deteriorating to complete airway obstruction. Direct visualization may also be useful if foreign body aspiration is suspected. Other uses of direct visualization include a child whose illness does not resolve, continues to have frequently recurring bouts of croup, or was intubated during the illness and now may have subglottic stenosis.

Laboratory studies are rarely helpful as the white blood cell count is usually normal except for possible lymphocytosis or leukopenia. Arterial blood gases are also usually normal except in severe disease when hypoxia and hypercarbia may be present. If bacterial traheitis is suspected, it can be useful to obtain blood cultures to direct treatment.

TREATMENT

Complications are rare following an episode of croup. The most common complication is airway obstruction with respiratory distress. If a child begins developing hypoxemia, tachycardia, and tachypnea, endotracheal intubation may be required. Pneumothorax, pneumomediastinum, and subglottic stenosis may be complications of endotracheal intubation. Dehydration may result from inability of the child to maintain adequate oral intake. Other complications include lymphadermatitis and otitis media. The viral type of croup may result in bacterial superinfection resulting in bacterial tracheitis. Pneumonia is a rare complication associated with bacterial traheitis and toxic shock syndrome has been seen in bacterial tracheitis owing to *S. aureus*. Death from croup is exceedingly rare if an appropriate airway is maintained.

Adult croup has not been associated with complications. The initial therapeutic approach to a child with suspected croup is general evaluation of the degree of respiratory distress and maintenance of an adequate airway for effective oxygenation and ventilation. This can be accomplished by monitoring the heart rate, respiratory rate, and pulse oximetry. In the setting of severe respiratiory distress and hypoxia, it may be necessary to provide 100% oxygen via a bag–valve–mask device. If this is unsuccessful and the child's oxygenation does not improve, it may be necessary to maintain an airway with endotracheal intubation. Any patient requiring supplemental oxygen to maintain adequate oxygenation should be admitted and monitored as an inpatient. This determination is made more accurately by observing the clinical picture and degree of distress and stridor rather than by pulse oximetry alone. Most children do not present with severe stridor and respiratory distress and do not require either technique to maintain an adequate airway. These children can typically be managed on an outpatient basis. It is important to avoid stressful situations in the treatment of children with croup because agitation and crying can aggravate the symptoms and worsen the respiratory distress. Another important initial aspect in the treatment of a child with croup is the evaluation of volume status. A child should be provided oral rehydration if tolerated, but it may be necessary to administer intravenous fluids if oral intake is not adequate.

Humidity has been used for hundreds of years to alleviate the symptoms of croup. Also known as mist therapy, it is believed to be beneficial by providing cooler inhaled air with moisture to cause vasoconstriction and alleviation of the mucosal edema. In addition to this effect, it is believed to decrease the viscosity of mucous secretions facilitating removal from the airway. The cool moisture also provides a soothing relief to the inflamed mucosa of the airway walls. Despite its extensive use, humidified air has not been shown in studies to be beneficial in improving the outcome of croup and despite its use being abandoned in many hospitals, no observable differences have occurred in the number of hospitalizations or complications incurred in cases of croup *(6)*. It is still argued, however, that the use of humidified air may be beneficial as a placebo effect, especially in the home, by reducing anxiety in both the child and the parent. Devices used to provide humidity include croup tents, croupettes, masks, and blow-by oxygen.

The use of corticosteroids in the management of croup remains controversial. However, corticosteroids are routinely used by physicians in the management of croup. Use of corticosteroids in the inpatient setting has been shown to be of benefit in the first 6 to 12 hours *(7)*. Its use has been shown to improve croup scores and shorten hospital stays with less requirement of treatment by other pharmacological agents *(7)*. The method of administration of the steroid has also been studied and has shown no difference between nebulized budesonide and oral dexamethasone as evidenced by equal decrease in croup scores *(7)*. In the outpatient setting, studies have also focused on the best method of administration of steroids in the treatment of croup. It has been shown that there is no significant difference between oral administration of dexamethasone versus intramuscular dexamethasone in the improvement of symptoms caused by croup *(7)*. Further studies have shown benefit in the use of 0.15 mg/kg oral dexamethasone over placebo and higher doses of steroid *(7)*. These studies have provided convincing evidence for the use of corticosteroids in the treatment of croup in both the inpatient and outpatient setting. It also appears that the use of oral corticosteroids in a low dose can provide an equal benefit to any other method of administration.

Racemic epinephrine in nebulized form is also used in the treatment of severe croup. Epinephrine acts to stimulate the α-adrenergic receptors causing capillary constriction and reduction of laryngeal mucous. This allows for a larger airway diameter and reduces respiratory difficulty and inspiratory stridor. The effects of epinephrine are short-lived, lasting for 2 hours. Patients should not be discharged for at least 3 to 4 hours after the administration of epinephrine, given the possibility of return of symptoms after the effects of the therapy have worn off. The use of epinephrine in the treatment of croup should be reserved for those patients who are seriously ill or have had a poor response to other treatment modalities, including mist therapy and analgesics.

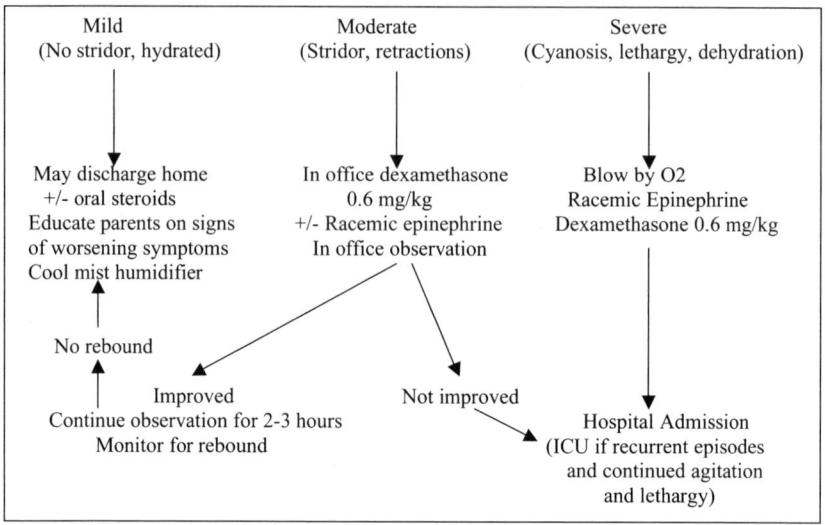

Fig. 1. Algorithm for the management of croup *(9,10)*.

For more than 20 years, the use of a mixture of helium and oxygen called heliox has been used in the treatment of severe croup. This mixture improves laminar gas flow in the airway decreasing the work of breathing. Blood oxygenation is improved over using oxygen alone when this treatment modality is used. Heliox is also beneficial when used with other treatments such as epinephrine and corticosteroids by extending the time in which these drugs have action on the laryngeal airway.

Treatment of adult croup is empiric and aimed at early recognition and airway stabilization. Use of the flexible fiberoptic laryngoscope has been used to assess the degree of airway obstruction *(8)*. Intubation may be necessary with severe respiratory compromise. Adjuvant therapy may also be employed with use of oxygen, humidification, steroids, and nebulized epinephrine, similar to the treatment used for croup in children.

Figure 1 illustrates an algorithm, based on the severity of the illness at presentation, used in the management of croup. The decision to hospitalize is based on the response to initial treatment in all cases.

FUTURE DIRECTIONS

Because the absolute treatment of croup remains controversial, further studies will continue to look at the benefits of modalities such as humidified air and steroids in the management of the illness. Also, children hospitalized for treatment of croup may be at a higher risk of subsequent bronchial hyperresponsiveness and asthma as well as being more prone to cutaneous hypersensitivity reactions. However, these correlations are still under investigation.

REFERENCES

1. Muniz A. Croup. eMedicine Journal. 2003. Available from www.emedicine.com/emedclass/topic510.htm. Accessed September 15, 2004.
2. Deeb ZE, Einhorn KH. Infectious adult croup. Laryngoscope 1990;100:455–457.
3. Westley CR, Cotton EK, Brooks JG. Nebulized racemic epinephrine by IPPB for the treatment of croup: a double-blind study. Am J Dis Child 1978;132:484–487.
4. Knutson D, Aring A. Viral croup. Am Fam Physician 2004;69:535–542.
5. Leung A, Cho H. Diagnosis of stridor in children. Am Fam Physician 1999;60:2289–2296.
6. Macdonald W, Geelhoed GC. Management of childhood croup. Thorax 1997;52:757–759.
7. Russell K, Wiebe N, Saenz A, et al. Glucocorticoids for croup. Cochrane Acute Respiratory Infections Group, The Cochrane Database of Systematic Reviews 2005;4.
8. Rosekrans JA. Viral croup: current diagnosis and treatment. Mayo Clin Proc 1998;73:1102–1107.
9. Alberta Clinical Practice Guideline Working Group. Guideline for the diagnosis and management of croup. 2003. Available from www.albertadoctors.org. Accessed January 25, 2005.
10. Dern M. UCSD Medical Group, Croup (Laryngotracheobronchitis). 1998. Available from http://gort.ucsd.edu/chaynes/Ncroup.pdf. Accessed January 25, 2005.

10 Pediatric Asthma

Katrina Dafnis and Matthew L. Mintz

CONTENTS

    CASE PRESENTATION
    KEY CLINICAL QUESTIONS
    LEARNING OBJECTIVES
    EPIDEMIOLOGY OF ASTHMA
    PATHOPHYSIOLOGY OF ASTHMA
    CLINICAL PRESENTATION
    DIFFERENTIAL DIAGNOSIS
    DIAGNOSIS
    TREATMENT
    FUTURE DIRECTIONS
    REFERENCES

CASE PRESENTATION

A 6-year-old male is brought to his pediatrician by his mother for an unrelenting cough. The patient is an otherwise healthy child except for some allergies to dust and pollen that he has experienced for the past 2 to 3 years. His cough is intermittent and dry in nature. He has had no fevers, mucus production, or sore throat, and denies any other symptoms. The cough is worse at night and often keeps him up for 30 to 60 minutes before he can get back to sleep. The boy's mother has tried over-the-counter cough suppressants but they have only shown minimal effect. He is beginning to become very sleepy during the day and is having trouble focusing in school secondary to being overly tired.

From: *Current Clinical Practice: Disorders of the Respiratory Tract:
Common Challenges in Primary Care*
By: M. L. Mintz © Humana Press, Totowa, NJ

KEY CLINICAL QUESTIONS

1. What factors predispose a child to developing asthma, and which children recover and which children go on to suffer from adult asthma?
2. How can you make the diagnosis of asthma in this patient?
3. How would you initiate treatment for this patient?

LEARNING OBJECTIVES

1. Understand the pathophysiology of asthma in children and how that may impact future disease status.
2. Understand the difficulties associated with diagnosing pediatric asthma, and identify the components of an accurate diagnosis
3. Become familiar with the most current recommendations for treatment of asthma in children, and understand the evidence behind these recommendations.

EPIDEMIOLOGY OF ASTHMA

Asthma is a growing health problem among our nation's children. Between 1980 and 1996, the number of children diagnosed with asthma rose from 36 per 1000 children to 62 per 1000 *(1)*. Roughly 6.1 million children were estimated to currently have asthma in 2004 *(2)*. Asthma is the number one cause for emergency department visits and missed school days among the pediatric population *(3)*. In 2002 alone, 14.6 million school days were lost to asthma *(2)*. Sadly, despite increased awareness and continued research, the mortality due to asthma increased annually between 1980 and 1998 *(1)*.

According to the National Health Interview Survey in 2002, boys are roughly 1.5 times more likely to develop asthma than girls *(4)*. The gender difference is most profound earlier in childhood. As children approach puberty, the rate of asthma among girls increases and by age 16, males and females show a similar prevalence. An interesting finding in the Tuscon Children's Respiratory Study relates to the role obesity plays in the prevalence of asthma among boys and girls. This study showed that girls who were obese or overweight just before puberty were 7.1 times more likely to develop new asthma symptoms between ages 11 and 13 than the girls who were normal weight. Remarkably, obesity during childhood did not have an effect on the rate of asthma among boys *(5)*.

Asthma studies throughout the years show that African-American children are affected more frequently than Caucasian children. In 2000, the ratio of prevalence was almost 2:1 and the ratio of hospitalization rates was (and continues to be) 3 to 4:1 *(1)*. African-American children also continue to have the highest death rates *(3)*. Investigators have not been able to completely explain the reasons behind increased prevalence of asthma in African Americans. Contributing factors may include lack of access to health care and high exposure to allergens, such as dust mites and molds often found in urban settings. Other factors that may play a role include lack of education regarding the disease and treatment options *(1)*. It is known that people who live in urban settings have higher rates of asthma, but whether this explains the racial differences among asthma prevalence is yet to be fully determined *(6)*.

A variety of factors may influence the onset of asthma in children and its persistence in later life. A large study was performed in Tuscon by Martinez et al. that followed 1200 infants through their childhood and tracked their respiratory symptoms. Martinez et al. separated wheezing children into three different categories: transient early wheezers (wheezing before age 3), late-onset wheezers (after age 3), and persistent wheezers (still wheezing at age 6). They studied risk factors for each group and found that maternal smoking was the number one predictor of transient early wheezing. Late-onset wheezing was most prevalent in children whose mothers had asthma and in male children. Finally, persistent wheezing was highly associated with maternal asthma, eczema, and rhinitis in the absence of cold symptoms. In addition, both late-onset and persistent wheezing were found to be associated with increased levels of immunoglobulin (Ig)E. When these children were followed into their teens, the factors were most associated with continued asthma symptoms were personal history of eczema or a parental history of asthma *(7)*. This evidence goes to show both the strong genetic and atopic association in asthma. Allergy plays a significant role in the persistence of asthma into adulthood. Roughly 60% of children who are diagnosed with asthma have resolution by adulthood, most often during adolescence. Of the 40% who go on to suffer from asthma as adults, most have at least one type of atopic disorder.

Despite the high prevelance of asthma, a good understanding of the disease, and efficacious therapuetic options, the mortality rate has not improved in the last 20 years *(1)*. The patients at the highest risk for a fatal asthma attack are those who have had life-threatening attacks in the past and those who require chronic oral steroids to control their symptoms (Table 1).

PATHOPHYSIOLOGY OF ASTHMA

The main factors underlying asthma in children are the same that define asthma in the adult population: airway inflammation and edema, airway hyperresonsiveness, and mucus plug formation. These elements cause airflow limitation that by definition in asthma is reversible. However, over time airway remodeling may occur, causing the airflow obstruction to become only partially reversible.

Airway inflammation is the first step in the pathophysiological mechanism that leads to asthma (Fig. 1). In the case of the asthmatic child, atopy is often involved. The airways of an atopic child have been sensitized to various antigens in the environment. For an unknown reason, these airways have an increased

Table 1
Risk Factors for Asthma Deaths

- Past history of sudden severe exacerbations
- Prior intubation and mechanical ventilation for asthma
- Prior asthma admission to the intensive care unit
- Two or more asthma hospitalizations in the last year
- Three or more emergency department visits for asthma in the last year
- Hospitalization or emergency department visit in the last month
- Use of more than two canisters of short-acting bronchodilators per month
- Current use of systemic steroids or recent withdrawal from steroids
- Difficulty perceiving airflow obstruction and its severity
- Comorbidity that may affect cardiopulmonary status (e.g., heart disease)
- Serious psychiatric disease or psychosocial problems
- Low socioeconomic status and urban residence
- Illicit drug use
- Sensitivity to *Alternaria*

Adapted from ref. 9.

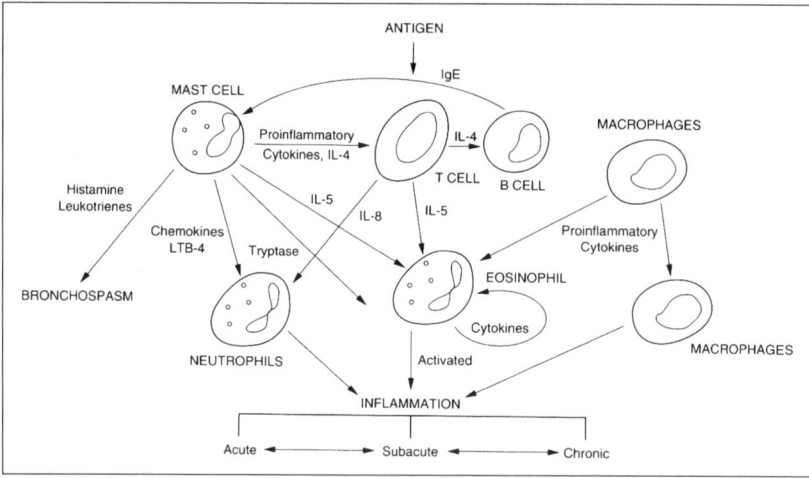

Fig. 1. Cellular mechanisms involved in airway inflammation and the interaction of multiple cell types and mediators in airway inflammation. IL, interleukin; Ig, immunoglobulin; LTB, leukotriene B. (From ref. 9.)

number of inflammatory cells, such as mast cells, eosinophils, and activated T-helper cells *(6)*. After re-exposure to an allergen, IgE antibodies on mast cells bind the allergen and become crosslinked in the process. The mast cells are located in the airways and crosslinking of the IgE molecules causes a release of inflammatory mediators that opens the junctions between the epithelial cells that line the airway. Mast cells release interleukin -4 and other pro-inflammatory cytokines, which stimulates proliferation of T-cells. They also release interleukin-5, which leads to further recruitment of eosinophils, cells that play a major role in asthma pathogenesis *(8)*. Chemokines released by mast cells stimulate the recruitment of neutrophils, which aid in the inflammation of and damage to the airways. Lastly, mast cells also release histamine and leukotrienes, which lead to the bronchospasm observed during an asthma episode *(9)*. The allergen is then able to enter into the mucosa where it can activate more mast cells and eosinophils. The further activation leads to increased release of vasoactive and inflammatory mediators. In addition to stimulating mediator release, the antigen is able to directly stimulate receptors on the vagal nerve, leading to more bronchoconstriction. The process described in this paragraph constitutes the acute phase of the asthma attack and usually lasts 15 to 30 minutes. The end result includes airway edema, bronchoconstriction, mucus production, and increased vascular permeability *(10)*.

The late phase of the asthma reaction begins hours after the initial insult and may persist for a day or more. The chemokines and cytokines released during the acute phase lead to an influx of leukocytes, namely neutrophils, basophils, and eosinophils, which release their own mediators. These mediators result in further bronchoconstriction and airway edema, thus prolonging the asthmatic event *(6)*.

Over time, asthma can lead to permanent airway remodeling, especially when the asthma is not well-controlled. One aspect of the remodeling response is thickening of the airway wall. The clinical consequences of this are not completely understood, but several studies have linked increased airway thickness with increased severity of disease. It has also been shown that increased wall thickness increases the narrowing of the airways that already occurs with asthma, thus causing increased bronchospasm. Subepithelial fibrosis is another aspect observed in airway remodeling that has shown correlation with disease severity. Fibrosis has also been linked in reports to a decrease in forced expiratory value in 1 second (FEV_1) as well as increase in frequency and duration of asthma symptoms. Mucus hypersecretion and mucus gland metaplasia are a third way that airway remodeling occurs. As a result, over time, asthmatic airways are more obstructed and more prone to mucus plugging, thus making it more difficult to recover from each exacerbation *(11)*. The exact pathophysiology behind airway remodeling and its regulation are not well-established. However, the remodeling process likely relates to the chronicity of asthma and the reason for many cases of treatment failure *(8)*.

CLINCAL PRESENTATION

The clinical presentation of asthma can be quite variable. The most common presenting symptoms are dry cough, wheezing, chest tightness, and dyspnea *(6)*.

A young child may be unable to explicate the sensation of chest tightness, but may instead complain of generalized chest pain *(12)*. Respiratory symptoms, especially cough, tend to be worst at night when airway inflammation is at its peak *(6)*. Signs of allergic rhinitis or chronic sinusitis may also be clues to the diagnosis of asthma in certain patients. In the case of acutely ill patients, they may be using accessory muscles to breathe and may not be able to speak in complete sentences. In the most severe cases, patients can appear cyanotic and may in fact have a "silent chest" because of either minimal or absent air exchange *(3)*. Asthmatic episodes often begin with exposure to certain triggers. Different patients are susceptible to different triggers and it is important for the physician to identify those triggers to help educate his patients (Table 2).

DIFFERENTIAL DIAGNOSIS

The differential diagnosis for asthma in children is wide, and complicated by the fact that diagnosis is often difficult (Table 3). Furthermore, certain conditions that can present like asthma may also co-exist with asthma, such allergic rhinitis. Practitioners should be suspicious of other causes when the diagnosis is uncertain, when patients have other unrelated findings, or when there is a failure to respond to treatment. In these cases, specialty referral may be necessary.

DIAGNOSIS

Although asthma is a common disease in our society, the diagnosis is often difficult to establish, especially in a child. Asthma is a disease of chronic, intermittent symptoms, so the history is an important tool in yielding a diagnosis. Screening questions regarding episodes of wheezing or dry cough over the last year are very important during regular clinic visits. Physicians should also ask about symptoms related to allergic rhinitis and eczema *(8)*. Children not currently experiencing an exacerbation will not usually reveal any physical signs. During an exacerbation, expiratory wheezing accompanied by a long expiratory phase can be heard on auscultation. Auscultation may also demonstrate decreased breath sounds if atelectasis has occurred. Crackles or rhonchi may also be heard because of increased mucus production in the airways. This may make the differentiation between pneumonia and asthma difficult to determine. As mentioned in discussing the physical exam, the child may be using accessory muscles to breathe and the physician can sometimes visualize nasal faring as well as suprasternal and intercostals retractions *(6)*.

The National Asthma Education and Prevention Program (NAEPP) provides guidelines for asthma diagnosis, classification, and treatment. The most recent guidelines were published in 2002. Although treatment recommendations have changed, the diagnosis and classification criteria remain the same. The diagnosis of asthma relies on three criteria: episodic symptoms of airflow obstruction,

Table 2
Common Asthma Triggers

- Exercise
- Weather changes
- Cold air
- Allergens (dust, mold, animal dander, pollen)
- Air pollution
- Environmental changes
- Tobacco smoke exposure
- Irritants
- Acid reflux
- Viral respiratory infections

Table 3
Differential Diagnosis of Coughing and Wheezing (Infants and Children)

Allergic rhinosinusitis
Cystic fibrosis
Enlarged lymph nodes
Foreign body
Heart disease
Tumor
Viral bronchiolitis
Vocal cord dysfunction
Laryngotracheomalacia

From ref. 9.

partial to full reversibility of airflow obstruction, and exclusion of alternative diagnoses (Table 4) *(8)*. Pulmonary function testing can be challenging in children younger than 7 years old and is almost impossible in children younger than 4 years of age, thus making the diagnosis difficult in this age group *(13)*. When children can perform spirometry, peak expiratory flow (PEF), FEV_1, and forced vital capacity (FVC) are analyzed. An asthmatic will show decreased PEF, FEV_1, and FEV_1:FVC ratio during pulmonary function testing. In children who are wheezing but cannot perform spirometry, it is reasonable to begin treatment and monitor them closely.

In certain cases, additional testing may be needed to confirm the diagnosis of asthma. In fact, unlike adults, most children with asthma have normal pulmonary function. In these circumstance, if the diagnosis is in question, the practioner may consider bronchoprovocation testing or may choose to follow the daily variation in PEF for 1 to 2 weeks. Chest X-ray should be consider if the situation is compli-

Table 4
Diagnosis of Asthma in Children and Adults

Episodic symptoms of airflow obstruction
- Difficulty breathing
- Chest tightness
- Cough (worse at night)
- Symptoms occurring or worsening at night, awakening the patient
- Symptoms occurring or worsening with exercise, viral infections, changes in weather, strong emotions, or menses; or in the presence of animals, dust mites, mold, smoke, pollen, or chemicals

Airflow obstruction at least partially reversible
- Diurnal variation in PEF of more than 20% for 1 to 2 weeks
- Increase in at least 12% and 200 mL in FEV_1 after bronchodilator use (indicates reversibility)
- Reduced FEV_1 (<80% predicted) and FEV_1:FVC (<65%) ratio using spirometry (indicates obstruction)

Alternatve diagnoses excluded (*see* Table 3)

From ref. 9.
FEV, forced expiratory value; PEF, peak expiratory flow.

---

cated by comorbid conditions such as infection, heart disease, or foreign body ingestion. Lastly, children with asthma often have the atopic form and exhibit other conditions, such as allergic rhinitis and atopic dermatitis. In the cases in which the diagnosis may be confusing, allergy testing and nasal examinations may help the physician build a case for the diagnosis of asthma *(8)*.

Once a child is diagnosed with asthma, it is then necessary to classify them according to severity because this will be used to determine an appropriate treatment regimen. There are four different classifications based on daytime and nighttime symptoms as well as on pulmonary function testing results: mild intermittent, mild persistent, moderate persistent, and severe persistent (Table 5).

The diagnosis of asthma is not always easy or straightforward, especially in children. The important thing to remember is to screen carefully during well-child visits for history of episodic wheezing or dry cough and when suspicious, refer for pulmonary function testing. Also, when in doubt, treat. A firm diagnosis of asthma is not required to begin treatment in a wheezing child.

TREATMENT

Treatment of asthma involves both pharmacotherapy as well as patient and family education. Treatment is directed by the severity of asthma at the time of diagnosis and by the response to initial treatment *(1)*. The guidelines (*see* Table 6)

Table 5
Asthma Classification System

Class	Symptoms	Night symptoms	Spirometry
Mild intermittent	Two or less times per week	Two or less times per month	FEV_1 or PEF ≥80% predicted
			PEF variability <20%
Mild persistent	Less than two times per week, but less than once a day	More than twice a month	FEV_1 or PEF ≥80% predicted
	Exacerbations may affect activity		PEF variability 20–30%
Moderate persistent	Daily use of short-acting β2 agonists	More than once a week	FEV_1 or PEF ≥60% but <80% predicted
	Exacerbations two or more times a week affect activity		PEF variability >30%
Severe persistent	Continuous symptoms Frequent exacerbations; limited activity	Frequent	FEV_1 or PEF <60% predicted
			PEF variability >30%

From ref. 9.
FEV, forced expiratory value; PEF, peak expiratory flow.

are set by the NAEPP and were most recently updated in 2002 *(9)*. The only patients for whom no daily treatment is recommended are patients with mild intermittent disease.

One of the major changes in the updated guidelines was the recommendation that inhaled corticosteroids now be considered first-line treatment in children of all ages with mild persistent disease. The previous guidelines recognized the utility and efficacy of corticosteroids in treating asthma, but using steroids in children and in mild disease was considered controversial *(14)*. The NAEPP expert panel reviewed clinical trials that showed conclusive evidence that inhaled corticosteroids provided better control of asthma than short-acting β2 agonists do. This was evidenced by decreased symptom frequency, higher FEV_1 measurements, decreased bronchospasm, fewer hospitalizations and clinic visits, and less need for oral corticosteroids. Although there have not been many studies in children under 5 years because of the difficulty of diagnosis in this age group, the NAEPP panel still recommends inhaled steroids in this age group based on the evidence. Head-to-head studies between inhaled corticosteroids and other long-term medications (cromolyn, nedocromil, leukotriene modifiers, theophylline) are limited in young children, but the available evidence consistently demon-

Table 6
Asthma Treatment Guidelines for Children

Asthma classification	Treatments in infants and children younger than 5 years of age	Treatment in children older than 5 years of age (and adults)
Mild intermittent	No daily medication necessary	No daily medication necessary
Mild persistent	**Preferred:** Low-dose inhaled corticosteroid (with nebulizer or metered-dose inhaler with holding chamber) **Alternative:** Cromolyn or leukotriene receptor antagonist	**Preferred:** Low-dose inhaled corticosteroid **Alternative:** Cromolyn, leukotriene modifier, nedocromil or sustained-release theophylline
Moderate persistent	**Preferred:** Low-dose inhaled corticosteroid and long-acting inhaled β2 agonist or medium-dose inhaled corticosteroid **Alternative:** Low- to medium-dose inhaled corticosteroid and either leukotriene modifier or theophylline	**Preferred:** Low- to medium-dose inhaled corticosteroid and long-acting inhaled β2 agonist **Alternative:** Increase steroid dose within medium-dose range or inhaled corticosteroid and either leukotriene modifier or theophylline
Severe persistent	High-dose inhaled corticosteroid and long-acting inhaled β2 agonist plus systemic steroids if needed	High-dose inhaled corticosteroid and long-acting inhaled β2 agonist plus systemic steroids if needed

From ref. 8.

strates superiority of inhaled corticosteroids, and the current guidelines recommend that any other medications be used as alternatives. Cromolyn and nedocromil decrease inflammation in asthma by blocking chloride channels on mast cells. This prevents the release of many inflammatory mediators that trigger the cascade of events in an asthma event. Leukotriene modifiers block the release of leukotrienes, which ordinarily cause bronchoconstriction. Theophylline is a phosphodiesterase inhibitor and leads to increased bronchodilation. For mild persistent disease in children younger than 5 years of age, alternative treatments are restricted to cromolyn and leukotriene modifiers. In children older than 5 years, all four aforementioned alternative treatments are options *(9)*.

The reason inhaled steroids were not recommended as first-line treatment in children in the 1997 guidelines were a result of controversy over the potential side effect of growth restriction. In reviewing several clinical trials, the 2002 NAEPP panel found steroids to be safe for use in children. The major study that led the panel to this conclusion was performed by the Childhood Asthma Management Program. This study followed more than 1000 children who either took inhaled steroids, nedocromil, or placebo. After 1 year, the children on corticosteroids showed a small difference in rate of growth velocity (roughly 1 cm), but by the end of the trial (mean 4.5 years) there was no difference in target adult height. In addition, the children on inhaled steroids had improved asthma control compared with the other groups *(9)*.

Treatment guidelines for children with moderate disease have changed as well. Guidelines now recommend that children older than 5 years take combination therapy involving low- to medium-dose inhaled steroids and a long-acting β2 agonist. This change is based on overwhelming clinical evidence that combined treatments lead to decreased symptoms and improved lung function *(9)*. A systematic review performed by Shrewsbury et al. demonstrated the efficacy of combining inhaled steroids and long-acting β2 agonists over increasing the steroid dose *(15)*. This study reviewed nine trials with 3685 patients. In addition, other studies have shown the superiority of combinaed inhaled steroid and long acting β2 agonist compared with inhaled steroid combined with a leukotriene modifier *(16)*. In children under 5 years old, the evidence is less clear, although studies are still ongoing. There are currently two options for first-line treatment in children under five: low-dose inhaled corticosteroid with an inhaled long acting β2 agonist, or a medium-dose inhaled corticosteroids alone. Addition of leukotriene modifiers or theophylline are again considered alternatives *(9)*.

The guidelines for severe persistent disease were not changed in the 2002 NAEPP updated guidelines. Children of all ages with severe disease are recommended to take high-dose inhaled corticosteroids along with a long-acting β2 agonist. Also, systemic steroids are indicated when exacerbations occur *(9)*. Although there is no evidence to support the use of leukotriene modifiers in this group of patients, they are often used in an attempt to avert the need for oral steroids *(17)*.

There are several medications that are used in the emergency room to treat asthma exacerbations. Some are standard treatments, some are more controversial because of conflicting evidence regarding their efficacy. Mild asthma exacerbations (defined as a decrease in peak flow to 50 to 80% of predicted value) are most often treated successfully with a short-acting inhaled β2 agonist, such as albuterol. All patients should have this medication on hand at home in the event of an asthma attack. Most often albuterol alone is enough to control mild exacerbations *(17)*.

Moderate to severe exacerbations require more than a β2 agonist, although albuterol or its isomer levalbuterol are standard treatments in asthma exacerbations of all severities. In the cases that come to the emergency room, 2.5 to 5.0 mg of albuterol is usually given via a nebulizer every 20 minutes for a total of three treatments *(18)*. The albuterol treatments will help to dilate the airways, but steroids are needed to treat the inflammatory component of the exacerbation. Studies have proven that systemic corticosteroids given within 1 hour of arrival to the emergency department decreases the rate of hospitalizations as well as the number of relapses after discharge *(19)*. The route of steroid administration has not been shown to play any role in the efficacy of the treatment. The steroids may be given orally, intramuscularly, or intravenously, as long as they are given as soon as possible. After discharge from the hospital, children should be sent with a burst of oral steroids consisting of 1 to 2 mg per kg per day for 5 to 10 days *(18)*.

Anticholinergic medications exert their effect by blocking stimulation of the postganglionic parasympathetic vagal fibers that normally promote bronchoconstriction. Ipratropium bromide is the most widely used of the anticholinergics and helps to dilate the central airways. There is strong evidence demonstrating that when anticholinergics are combined with short-acting β2 agonists, peak expiratory flow rate increases by 31.5 L per minute more than patients who are treated with β2 agonists alone. There are some studies that have shown no benefit in the addition of ipatropium, however, based on the majority of studies showing added benefit and the low side-effect profile of these medications, the NAEPP has recommended the addition of anticholinergics in cases in which the PEF rate or FEV_1 drops to less than 80% predicted *(18)*.

There are several medications that are sometimes used in acute asthma exacerbations despite conflicting evidence. One of these is magnesium. The exact mechanism of action is unknown, but it is hypothesized that magnesium blocks calcium channels in airway smooth muscle and therefore leads to bronchodilation. The effect is seen within 2 to 5 minutes of infusion, but rapidly wears off once the infusion is stopped. There is conflicting evidence regarding whether magnesium actually is of benefit in the acute setting, but if a physician decides to use it, the patient must be monitored closely. Magnesium can cause hypotension, cardiac arrhythmias, and neurological abnormalities. Heliox is another treatment that is considered controversial. This mix of helium and oxygen is thought to decrease both the work of breathing and airway resistance. Heliox has shown benefit in severe exacerbations, but because it has not shown benefit in mild or moderate exacerbations, it is not recommended as standard treatment *(18)*.

The NAEPP 2002 panel also addressed the question of whether using antibiotics in acute exacerbations would improve outcomes. After reviewing the literature, the panel maintained its position that antibiotic therapy is not warranted in the treatment of acute asthmatic episodes unless there is clear evidence of a bacterial infection *(9)*.

Once a patient is diagnosed, classified, and started on treatment it is important to ensure that the patient, parent, and physician are all involved in monitoring the progress of the disease. Newly diagnosed patients should be seen approximately every 3 months for the first year, then every 6 to 12 months after that. Patients with severe disease should be seen more frequently. Interval monitoring, including pulmonary function testing once or twice a year, is appropriate for all patients who have persistent asthma *(17)*. The updated asthma guidelines addressed two issues regarding monitoring of disease severity: written asthma plans compared with medical management alone and peak flow-based versus symptom-based written action plans. Written action plans help patients control their asthma by instructing them on which environmental triggers to avoid and how to adjust their medications on normal days and during attacks *(20)*. The data regarding written action plans was inconclusive; however, the panel continues to recommend their use as part of the self-management of asthma *(9)*. In 2004, a Cochrane review of 25 studies showed that written action plans lead to less emergency room visits, decreased hospitalizations, and better lung function *(21)*. The 2002 panel also found evidence regarding use of peak-flow monitoring to be inconclusive. Results are especially inconclusive in children because it is more difficult for children to perform the technique *(9)*. In fact, several studies, including the Childhood Asthma Management Program study, have found that children with significant deterioration in FEV_1 and symptoms actually showed similar peak-flow values *(22)*. Despite inconclusive evidence, the NAEPP panel continues to recommend peak-flow monitoring in patients with moderate to severe disease. It is thought to increase caregiver awareness as well as patient–physician communication *(9)*.

One of the most important issues in ensuring adequate control is to educate the child and the caregiver about the disease. The physician and the patient need to establish a common goal and definition for what it means to have the asthma under control. Often times the parent and the physician have different perceptions of what constitutes good control, which can be detrimental to the child's health. Clarifying treatment goals and the reasons behind the need for treatment can enhance compliance significantly. It is difficult with a disease in which objective measures are not always available, but the more educated the patient and the family are about the disease and the more they feel comfortable communicating with their physician, the more likely it is for their asthma to remain under control *(23)*.

FUTURE DIRECTIONS

Despite extensive research in asthma, new therapies, and updated guidelines, many questions still exist regarding pediatric asthma. First, there are not nearly enough studies in younger children, especially under 2 years old. This is obviously a difficult population to study. Techniques to measure pulmonary function and airway inflammation that can be used in infants and young children are in currently in development. These techniques will enable us to determine the best treatment options for young children as well as better understand which children will progress to severe disease, thus requiring more aggressive therapy. Retrospective claims analysis *(25)* have shown that the infants and children that are younger than two have far fewer exacerbations when initiated directly on nebulized inhaled steroids compared with oral steroids and other agents, but prospective studies are needed.

Newer therapies are also on the horizon. Inhaled corticosteriods with better safety profiles and additional combination therapies will come to market soon, which may have an impact on how asthma is treated. Monoclonal antibodies have been used successfully in allergic asthma, but they are costly and difficult to use. Better formulations of these types of medications may prove to have significant benefits, particularly in children.

Etiology of asthma is also a critical area of investigations. Researchers have established a clear correlation between viruses early in life, but have not been able to clarify the pathogenetic mechanism by which viruses may lead to long-term wheezing. Protective benefits of early exposure to upper respiratory infections as well as animals have been observed, but further investigation should provide a better understanding of asthma etiology.

REFERENCES

1. Guill, MF. Asthma update: epidemiology and pathophysiology. Pediatr Rev 2004;25:299–305.
2. American Lung Association. Asthma and children fact sheet. Available from: http://www.lungusa.org/site/pp.asp?c=dvLUK9O0E&b=44352. Accessed January 2, 2005.
3. Steyer TE, Mallin R, Blair M. Pediatric asthma. Clin Fam Pract 2003;5:343.
4. Akinbami LJ, Schoendorf KC. Trends in childhood asthma: prevalence, health care utilization, and mortatlity. Pediatrics 2002;110:315–322.
5. Taussig LM, Wright AL, Holberg CT, Hanonen M, Morgan WJ, Martinez FD. Tucson children's respiratory study: 1980 to present. J Allergy Clin Immunol 2003;111:661–675.

6. Behrman R, Kliegman RM, Jenson HB. Nelson Textbook of Pediatrics, 17th ed. Elsevier, Philadelphia, 2004; pp. 760–774.
7. Martinez FD, Wright AL, Taussig LM, et al. Asthma and wheezing in the first six years of life. New Engl J Med 1995;332:133–138.
8. National Asthma Education and Prevention Program. Guidelines for the diagnosis and management of asthma: update on selected topics—2002. US Department of Health and Human Services, Public Health Service, National Institutes of Health, National Heart, Lung, and Blood Institute, Bethesda, MD, 2003; NIH publication no. 02-5074.
9. National Asthma Education and Prevention Program. Guidelines for the diagnosis and management of asthma: expert panel report 2. US Department of Health and Human Services, Public Health Service, National Institutes of Health, National Heart, Lung, and Blood Institute, Bethesda, MD, 2003; NIH publication no. 97-4051.
10. Kumar V, Abbas AK, Fausto N. Robbins and Cotran Pathologic Basis of Disease, 7th ed. Elsevier, Philadelphia, 2005; pp. 723–727.
11. Zhu Z, Chupp G, Homer RJ. Airway Remodeling in Asthma. J Clin Invest 1999;104:1001–1006.
12. Burkhart PV, Ward HJ. Children's self-reports of characteristics of their asthma episodes. J Asthma 2003;40:909–916.
13. Michael MA. Scope and impact of pediatric asthma. Nurse Pract 2002;27:3–6.
14. Mintz M. Asthma update: part II. Medical management. Am Fam Physician 2004;70:1061–1066.
15. Shrewsbury S, Pyke S, Britton M. Meta-analysis of increased dose of inhaled steroid or addition of salmeterol in symptomatic asthma. BMJ 2000;320:1368–1373.
17. Nelson HS, Busse WW, Kerwin E, et al. Fluticasone propionate/salmeterol combination provides more effective asthma control than low-dose inhaled corticosteroid plus montelukast. J Allergy Clin Immunol 2000;106:1088–1095.
17. Guill MF. Asthma update: clinical aspects and management. Pediatr Rev 2004;25:335–344.
18. Adams BK, Cydulka RK. Asthma evaluation and management. Emerg Med Clin North Am 2003;21:315–330.
19. Rowe BH, Spooner CH, Ducharme FM, et al. Early emergency department treatment of acute asthma with systemic corticosteroids. Cochrane Database Sys Rev 2001;1:CD000195.
20. Mintz M. Asthma update part I: diagnosis, monitoring and prevention of disease progression. Am Fam Physician 2004;70:893–898.
21. Gibson PG, Powell H, Coughlan J, et al. Self-management education and regular practitioner review for adults with asthma. Cochrane Database Syst Rev 2004;(1):CD001117.
22. Kelly HW. The assessment of childhood asthma. Pediatr Clin North Am 2003;50:593–608.
23. Becker, A.B. Challenges to treatment goals and outcomes in pediatric asthma. J Allergy Immunol 2002;109:1–11.
24. Abbott A. Beta-blocker goes on trial as asthma therapy. Nature. 2003. Available from: http://www.nature.com/news/2004/041101/pf/432007a_pf.html. Accessed January 3, 2005.
25. Murphy KR, Bukstein DA, Katz LM, et al. Earlier use of nebulized inhaled corticosteroids is associated with fewer asthma exacerbations in young children. J Allergy Clin Immunol 2005;115: S1.

11 Adult Asthma

Dharti Patel and Matthew L. Mintz

CONTENTS

>CASE PRESENTATION
>KEY CLINICAL QUESTIONS
>LEARNING OBJECTIVES
>EPIDEMIOLOGY
>PATHOGENESIS
>DIFFERENTIAL DIAGNOSIS
>DIAGNOSIS
>MONITORING
>TREATMENT
>FUTURE DIRECTIONS
>REFERENCES

CASE PRESENTATION

A 23-year-old male with a childhood history of mild persistent asthma presents to his primary care physician for an albuterol prescription refill earlier than expected. On further questioning, the patient reveals progressively worsening episodic shortness of breath following his evening runs as well as nighttime awakenings once or twice a week. His current medication regimen includes albuterol for acute attacks and a low dose of fluticasone proprionate for long-term control. The patient is worried about chronic steroid use because of side effects. Physical findings are unremarkable except for a slightly elevated respiratory rate of 25 and scattered wheezes.

KEY CLINICAL QUESTIONS

1. What factors determine asthma classification of severity?
2. What is triggering acute exacerbations in this patient?

>From: *Current Clinical Practice: Disorders of the Respiratory Tract:
>Common Challenges in Primary Care*
>By: M. L. Mintz © Humana Press, Totowa, NJ

3. Is the patient overusing his albuterol inhaler? What changes, if any, would you make to his medication regimen to assure control as well as compliance?
4. Is the patient's concern about chronic corticosteroid use appropriate?
5. What recommendations would you make for monitoring and follow-up?

LEARNING OBJECTIVES

1. Understand the pathophysiology of asthma.
2. Learn how to diagnose, classify, and monitor asthma.
3. Be familiar with the updated evidence-based treatment recommendations.
4. Understand the importance of patient–provider communication in the management of asthma and learn tools for improvement.

EPIDEMIOLOGY

Asthma continues to be a growing burden in the United States despite the advent of multiple medications and an increased understanding of asthma pathophysiology. There are nearly 2 million emergency department (ED) visits and more than 10 million physician office visits each year. Females, children aged 14 or younger, and blacks as compared with whites have higher rates of office visits. Blacks also share higher rates of asthma-related ED visits, hospitalizations, and deaths. The numeric increase over the years in numbers and rates of office and ED visits can largely be accounted for by an increase in prevalence. The lifetime prevalence of asthma in the United States is estimated at nearly 26.7 million people and a 12-month attack prevalence (persons with one or more attacks) estimated at nearly 11.1 million. Despite increased treatment options, the morbidity and mortality associated with asthma remains high. Asthma accounts for nearly 500,000 hospitalizations and 5000 deaths each year *(1)*. Even patients with mild intermittent and persistent asthma were often identified in a review of asthma-related deaths during sports, underscoring the seriousness of asthma and suggesting possible undertreatment *(2)*. In an effort to address such disparity between the availability of asthma treatment options and an increase in morbidity, the National Asthma Education and Prevention Program (NAEPP) updated clinical guidelines in 2002 to define a new standard of care *(3)*.

PATHOGENESIS

Asthma is an obstructive airway disease characterized by episodic airway narrowing that resolves either spontaneously or with treatment. Two major factors that contribute to such narrowing are (1) airway hyperresponsiveness to stimuli, which otherwise elicit minimal to no bronchoconstrictor response in nonasthmatics, and (2) chronic inflammation, which over time can lead to airway remodeling and thus partial irreversibility in severe cases. Stimuli vary from individual to individual and may include various allergens, respiratory viruses, exercise, cold air, stress, and/or occupational exposures.

The inflammation triggered in asthmatics is a complex multicellular process that leads to marked airway edema, mucus plug formation, increase in hyperresponsiveness, and airway remodeling, all of which contribute to airflow limitation. Acute airway obstruction results in paroxysms of wheezing, dyspnea, chest tightness, and cough, usually lasting minutes to hours. Symptoms are often worse at night and in the early morning. In rare cases, acute episodes can persist for days or weeks either with mild obstructive symptoms with or without superimposed exacerbations or, in status asthmaticus, with continual severe obstructive symptoms. During acute exacerbations, asthma can be potentially fatal.

Asthma develops more often in childhood than in adulthood. Atopy, a genetic predisposition to an immunoglobulin (Ig)E-mediated response to environmental stimuli, is a major risk factor for the development of asthma in childhood. The relationship between atopy and asthma is complex. For example, studies indicate that the link between asthma and rhinitis may go beyond shared risk factors, including genetic predisposition, because they failed to fully explain the strong association between the two. Patients with rhinitis were at a significantly increased risk for asthma and bronchial hypersensitivity than those without asthma, even after adjusting for total IgE, parental history of asthma, and allergen sensitization *(4)*. Allergy and a family history of allergy also play an important role in adult-onset asthma. Adult-onset asthma can also be triggered by occupational exposures, for which symptoms can persist even after the elimination of exposure. Although the mechanisms of the non-allergic, or intrinsic, form of adult-onset asthma are still unclear, it shares a similar inflammatory process to that of atopic asthma.

Inflammation is a key contributor to the onset and persistence of asthma, in which the Th2 lymphocytic cytokine profile including interleukin-4 and -5 plays a significant role. Primary players in the inflammatory process include mast cells, eosinophils, macrophages, T-lymphocytes, and epithelial cells. The release of inflammatory mediators from these cells following contact of the bronchial epithelium with stimuli serves to recruit more cells and potentiate the pathological response of airway narrowing. They affect airway tone, neural stimulation, mucus secretion, microvascular permeability and leakage, and over time, can affect the structural integrity of the tracheobronchial tree (Table 1). Long-standing inflammation can lead to collagen deposition in the basement membrane and fibrosis of subbasement membrane tissues, which contributes to airway rigidity and persistent abnormalities in pulmonary function unresponsive to treatment. Hence, early anti-inflammatory treatment is significant in that it may halt or slow the development of such airway remodeling and modify the disease process. It is further important to diagnose and treat asthma early because studies have

Table 1
Components of Airway Wall Remodeling That Lead to Permanent Air-Flow Limitation

Airway smooth muscle hypertrophy
Angiogenesis
Epithelial cell destruction
Increased submucosal vascularity
Subepithelial collagen deposition
Thickening of the basement membrane

shown that active asthma can serve as a significant risk factor for the future development of chronic bronchitis, emphysema, and chronic obstructive pulmonary disease (COPD) *(5)*.

The component of bronchial hyperresponsiveness is present apart from as well as potentiated by the inflammatory process. Bronchoconstriction contributes significantly to the symptoms of wheezing and dyspnea and the degree of constriction correlates closely with clinical severity. Acute bronchoconstriction following allergen exposure results from IgE-dependent mast cell degranulation of mediators, such as histamine, tryptase, leukotrienes, and prostaglandins, whereas aspirin-induced bronchoconstriction results from non-IgE-dependent mediator release. The mechanism of airflow obstruction is less well understood for other stimuli, such as exercise, cold air, irritants, and stress.

DIFFERENTIAL DIAGNOSIS

Although asthma often presents with recurrent coughing and wheezing, there are multiple other diagnoses that can present with similar symptoms and some may require more urgent intervention (Table 2). It is important to entertain the differential diagnostic possibilities of asthma not only for patients with new onset of coughing and wheezing, but also for patients for whom the diagnosis of asthma has already been established. Some diagnoses to consider are congestive heart failure, pulmonary embolism, laryngeal or vocal cord dysfunction, pulmonary infiltration, mechanical obstruction with tumors, as well as medications such as angiotensin-converting enyzyme inhibitors. COPD (chronic bronchitis or emphysema), for which asthma is a significant risk factor, is also among the differential. Whether asthma and COPD are distinct entities or a spectrum remains to be determined, but primary care physicians should consider COPD in their patients with a history of asthma *(5)*.

Table 2
Differential Diagnosis of Asthma in Adults

Chronic obstructive pulmonary disease
Congestive heart failure
Pulmonary embolism
Laryngeal dysfunction
Mechanical obstruction of the airways (benign or malignant)
Pulmonary infiltration with eosinophilia
Cough secondary to drugs (angiotensin-converting enzyme inhibitors)
Vocal cord dysfunction

From ref. 7.

DIAGNOSIS

Asthma is a clinical diagnosis based on a compilation of findings from a detailed medical history, physical exam, and spirometry that establishes the presence of episodic obstructive pulmonary signs and symptoms, at least partially reversible airflow obstruction, and rules out differential diagnoses (Table 3). History should detail symptoms, their severity, frequency, and triggers, as well as explore genetic predisposition to asthma and allergies. Key indicators that increase the likelihood of diagnosis of asthma are a history of recurrent wheezing, difficulty breathing, chest tightness, and/or cough as well as a history of these symptoms occurring or worsening at night or in the presence of triggers such as exercise, viral infections, dust mites, mold, smoke, pollen, weather, strong emotions, and menses. Physical exam findings that can assist in diagnosis, though nonspecific, are wheezing during normal respiration, prolonged forced exhalation, increased nasal secretion, mucosal swelling, nasal polyps, and atopic dermatitis or eczema. Symptoms vary from patient to patient, and thus clinical judgment should be utilized to assess for the presence of asthma. Spirometry can assist in making the diagnosis of asthma. Reduced forced expiratory volume in 1 second (FEV_1), peak expiratory flow (PEF) rate, and maximal mid-expiratory flow rate suggest airway obstruction. FEV_1, forced vital capacity (FVC), and FEV_1:FVC measurements should be taken before and after the use of an inhaled short-acting bronchodilator to demonstrate reversibility. an increase of more than 12% and 200mL in FEV_1 after the use of a bronchodilator indicates reversibility of airflow obstruction. Use of spirometry is recommended for initial assessment over the use of peak-flow meters, which have a wide variability in reference values.

Table 3
Diagnosis of Asthma in Children and Adults

Episodic symptoms of airflow obstruction are present
  Difficulty breathing
  Chest tightness
  Cough (particularly worse at night)
  Symptoms occur or worsen at night, awakening the patient
  Symptoms occur or worsen in the presence of exercise, viral infections, animals, dust mites, mold, smoke, pollen, changes in weather, strong emotions, chemicals, or menses
  Wheezing

Airflow obstruction is at least partially reversible
  Diurnal variation of PEF more than 20% over 1–2 weeks
  Increase of 12% or more and 200 mL FEV_1 after bronchodilators indicates reversibility
  Reduced FEV_1 and FEV_1:FVC ratio using spirometry indicates obstruction

Alternative diagnoses are excluded
Infants and Children
  Allergic rhinosinusitis
  Cystic fibrosis
  Enlarged lymph nodes/tumor
  Foreign body
  Heart disease
  Viral bronchiolitis
  Vocal cord dysfunction
Adults
  Chronic obstructive pulmonary disease
  Congestive heart failure
  Cough secondary to angiotensin-converting enzyme inhibitors
  Mechanical obstruction of the airway
  Pulmonary embolism
  Pulmonary infiltration with eosinophilia
  Vocal cord dysfunction

PEF, peak expiratory flow; FEV_1, forced expiratory volume in 1 second; FVC, forced vital capacity.

If spirometry is normal, but the clinical suspicion for asthma is high, consider measuring diurnal variation in PEF over 1 to 2 weeks or bronchoprovocation testing. If there is a more than 20% difference in the morning PEF taken before the use of a short-acting β-agonist and the early afternoon PEF taken after the use of a β-agonist, then the diagnosis of asthma is likely. If spirometry testing continues to be unrevealing, consider bronchoprovocation testing with methacholine, histamine, cold air, or exercise challenge. Such testing should only be performed by a trained professional and done in individuals with a predicted FEV_1 more than 65%.

Other objective findings that can suggest asthma are sputum and blood eosinophilia, elevated serum IgE levels, and chest hyperinflation. Nonetheless, these findings are nonspecific and chest radiographs are more commonly normal in asthma. Chest radiographs, allergy testing, evaluation of nose for polyps and sinuses for disease, and evaluation for gastroesophageal reflux can be useful in making an accurate diagnosis. If skin allergen sensitivities are found, it is important to keep in mind that they may not necessarily correlate with allergens that trigger asthma. Finally, once the diagnosis of asthma is made and before any therapy, it is important to classify its severity to guide appropriate management (Table 4).

MONITORING

Patient should follow up as often as the clinician deems appropriate to meet the goals of therapy (Table 5). Routine assessment should evaluate for symptom control over a short period of 2 to 4 weeks, pulmonary function, quality of life/ functional status, history of exacerbations, pharmacotherapy, and patient satisfaction. Spirometry is recommended at the initial assessment, after treatment initiation, and then every 1 to 2 years to monitor pulmonary function. Home peak-flow monitoring is recommended for moderate to severe persistent asthmatics at least every morning, more frequently if PEF is less than 80% of personal best (i.e., the highest PEF over a 2 to 3 week period when asthma is well-controlled), and during acute exacerbations to determine severity and guide treatment. Peak-flow monitoring can detect airway narrowing before the onset of symptoms and appropriate management can prevent full-blown exacerbations. Although the significance of written action plans remains inconclusive, the NAEPP expert panel continues to recommend its use for asthma management, especially for patients with moderate to severe persistent asthma and for those with a history of severe exacerbations. All asthmatics should monitor symptoms and be trained to recognize inadequate control and early signs of deterioration.

Asthma control can be difficult to assess secondary to time and resource constraints in busy medical practices and is often subject to overestimation by both patients and physicians. Development of the asthma control test (ACT) (Fig. 1) looks promising because it correlates extremely well with lung function testing and can either supplement or replace lung function testing when it is not readily available. ACT is a quick five-item patient-based tool that gauges asthma symptoms, use of rescue medications, and functional impact to assess asthma control. ACT was developed using asthma specialist-treated patients, who may be better educated about asthma, and thus, still needs to be tested in a true primary care setting *(6)*.

Table 4
Asthma Classification and Preferred Medical Treatment Using a Stepwise Approach in Adults and Children

Classify severity: clinical features before treatment or adequate control	Symptoms/day Symptoms/night	PEF or FEV$_1$ (for adults)	Medications required to maintain long-term control Preferred medical treatment
Step 1 Mild intermittent	<2 days/week ≤2 nights/month	≥80%	No daily medication needed.
Step 2 Mild persistent	<2 days/week but <1×/day >2 nights/month one per day	≥80%	Low-dose inhaled corticosteroid (with nebulizer or pressurized metered dose inhaler with holding chamber with or without face mask or dry powder inhaler for children).
Step 3 Moderate persistent	Daily >1 night/week	>60%–80%	Adults and children older than 5 years Low- to medium-dose inhaled corticosteroids and long-acting inhaled β2 agonists Children 5 years and under Low-dose inhaled corticosteroids and long-acting inhaled β2 agonists or medium-dose inhaled corticosteroids.
Step 4 Severe persistent	Continual Frequent	≤60%	High-dose inhaled corticosteroids and long-acting inhaled β2 agonists.

Adapted from ref. 3.
All asthmatics should use short-acting bronchodilators on an as needed basis as "quick relievers" to diminish symptoms. Adults and children with persistent asthma should also be on a daily controller medications, intended to prevent asthma symptoms and exacerbations.

Table 5
The Goals of Asthma Therapy

- Maintain normal activity levels
- Maintain "normal" pulmonary function
- Meet patients' and families' expectations of and satisfaction with asthma care
- Prevent chronic symptoms
- Prevent recurrent exacerbations
- Provide optimal pharmacotherapy with minimal or no adverse events

Adapted from ref. 3.

The importance of patient–physician communication cannot be overemphasized. Open communication and education should begin at the time of diagnosis and continue at each follow-up visit. Patients should be taught basic facts of asthma, roles of rescue medications versus controller therapies, how to use inhalers and spacers, environmental control measures, and self-monitoring with peak-flow meters. Written materials and formal education programs should be used to supplement, not replace, education provided by physicians. Physicians should work together with the patients to formulate individualized written daily self-management and action plans that meet jointly established treatment goals. Goals should then be reviewed at each visit to assure that they are being met. Action plans and a daily asthma diary are especially important for patients with recurrent severe exacerbations and for those with moderate to severe asthma. Physicians should maintain cultural sensitivity and enlist family involvement where appropriate.

TREATMENT

Although trigger control is important and the patient should be advised to eliminate or minimize exposure to the causative agent whenever applicable, a pharmacological regimen should be initiated based on the severity of asthma (Table 4). Currently available medications are targeted largely at either reducing airway obstruction via bronchodilation or toward reducing the inflammation that leads to airway narrowing. There are multiple classes of medications, and among them are those that provide quick relief for acute exacerbations and those that provide long-term relief for persistent symptoms.

In an attempt to address the disparity between the wide availability of treatment options and the undertreatment of asthma, the NAEPP expert panel set forth clinical guidelines to establish a standard of care *(7)*. These guidelines were recently updated in 2002 to address the safety of and preference for chronic inhaled corticosteroid therapy, management of moderate persistent asthma, asthma monitoring, and the controversial role of antibiotics *(3)*. Current recom-

1. Asthma Control Test

1. In the past **4 weeks**, how much of the time did your **asthma** keep you from getting as much done at work, school or at home?

All of the time	Most of the time	Some of the time	A little of the time	None of the time
1	2	3	4	5

2. During the past **4 weeks**, how often have you had shortness of breath?

More than once a day	Once a day	3 to 6 times a week	Once or twice a week	Not at all
1	2	3	4	5

3. During the past **4 weeks**, how often did your **asthma** symptoms (wheezing, coughing, shortness of breath, chest tightness or pain) wake you up at night or earlier than usual in the morning?

4 or more nights a week	2 or 3 nights a week	Once a week	Once or twice	Not at all
1	2	3	4	5

4. During the past **4 weeks**, how often have you used your rescue inhaler or nebulizer medication (such as albuterol)?

3 or more times per day	1 or 2 times per day	2 or 3 times per week	Once a week or less	Not at all
1	2	3	4	5

5. How would you rate your **asthma** control during the **past 4 weeks**?

Not controlled at all	Poorly controlled	Somewhat controlled	Well controlled	Completely controlled
1	2	3	4	5

AMERICAN LUNG ASSOCIATION. The American Lung Association supports the Asthma Control Test™ and wants everyone 12 years of age and older with asthma to take it.

Copyright 2002, by QualityMetric Incorporated.
Asthma Control Test is a trademark of QualityMetric Incorporated.

Fig. 1. Asthma Control Test.

mendations for long-term control hail the chronic use of inhaled corticosteroids as safe and encourage their use as first-line treatment for all asthmatics with persistent symptoms, including those with mild symptoms. Furthermore, it recommends the addition of a long-acting β2-agonist to achieve symptomatic control in moderate to severe asthmatics. For acute exacerbations, short-acting β-agonists remain the mainstay and guidelines recommend short-term use of systemic corticosteroids when bronchodilator treatment alone fails to achieve symptomatic control. There are no benefits associated with the use of antibiotics in treatment of acute exacerbations, and hence, are not recommended by the NAEPP panel.

Acute Exacerbations

SHORT-ACTING β2-ADRENERGIC AGENTS

Short-acting inhaled β2-adrenergic agents, such as albuterol, are currently the mainstay for acute exacerbations, mild-intermittent asthma, and the prevention of exercise-induced bronchospasm. They stimulate β2-receptors, which in turn activate adenylate cyclase and increase cyclic adenosine monophosphate to cause smooth muscle relaxation. With an onset of action generally within minutes, they promptly improve airflow and can sustain the effects for 4 to 6 hours. The more selective β2-agonists, such as albuterol, bitolbuterol, pirbuterol, and terbutaline, are preferred over the less selective isoproterenol, metaproterenol, isoetharine, and epinephrine to maximize the action on the respiratory tract and minimize unwanted cardiac side effects that may occur, especially at high doses of the latter medications. Inhalation is the preferred route of administration because of its faster onset, fewer adverse effects, and greater effectiveness than systemic routes. Potential adverse effects include tachycardia, skeletal muscle tremor, hypokalemia, lactic acidosis, headache, and hyperglycemia. Short-acting β2-agonists should be used on an as needed basis for exacerbations and not with a regular daily dosing schedule. Use of more than one canister per month may indicate poor control and warrants the initiation or adjustment of long-term controller therapy.

ANTICHOLINERGICS

Anticholinergics, such as ipratroprium bromide, are the treatment of choice for β-blocker-induced bronchospasm and provide a good alternative for patients who are otherwise unable to tolerate β2-agonists, such as the elderly or those with co-existent cardiac disease. They provide an additive benefit when used in conjunction with inhaled β2-agonists in severe exacerbations, but are not effective for preventing exercise-induced bronchospasm. Ipratroprium bromide inhibits the effects of acetylcholine on intrapulmonary smooth muscle via competitive inhibition of muscarinic receptors. It reduces the intrinsic vagal tone in the airways and may work to decrease mucus production and to block reflex bronchoconstriction resulting from irritants or reflux esophagitis. Ipratroprium brominde helps with cough symptoms, but has a slow onset of action at about 60 to 90 minutes and is not as effective as short-acting β2-agonists in acute bronchospasm. Adverse effects may include dry mouth and airways, increased wheezing, and blurred vision with exposure to the eyes. The use of atropine, an older anticholinergic, is rare and limited by central nervous system toxicity.

SYSTEMIC CORTICOSTEROIDS

Systemic corticosteroids, such as methylprenisolone, prednisolone, and prednisone, are effective at reducing inflammation in moderate to severe exacerbations in an otherwise mild asthmatic. They prevent the progression of exacerbation, speed recovery, and prevent early recurrence. Corticosteroids have multiple anti-inflammatory actions including blocking the late reaction to allergen, reducing airway hyperresponsiveness, as well as inhibiting cytokine production, adhesion protein activation, and cell migration and activation. They also reverse β2-receptor downregulation and prevent microvascular leakage.

Systemic corticosteroids should be used in those patients whose symptoms fail to resolve after a trial of bronchodilator therapy. Steroids have a slow onset of action and improvement may not be seen for at least 4 to 6 hours, and therefore it is important to promptly start and continue aggressive bronchodilator therapy. Steroid pulse therapy can be initiated at 40 to 60 mg per day and slowly tapered to zero over 7 to 14 days (the dose should be reduced by 50% every third to fifth day) as inhaled corticosteroids are started for long-term control. The goal of short-term systemic therapy is to achieve PEF more than 80%, personal best, or symptom resolution. If symptoms recur after pulse cessation, consider alternate-day corticosteroid therapy with morning dosing as opposed to daily therapy to minimize toxicity. Adverse effects associated with short-term use of systemic corticosteroids include alterations in glucose metabolism, increased appetite, fluid retention, weight gain, mood alteration, hypertension, peptic ulcer, and potentially aseptic necrosis of the femur. Use of systemic corticosteroids can exacerbate co-existent conditions, such as herpes virus infections, varicella, tuberculosis, hypertension, peptic ulcer, and *Strongyloides*. Adverse effects associated with long-term use include adrenal axis suppression, growth suppression, dermal thinning, hypertension, diabetes, Cushing's syndrome, cataracts, muscle weakness, and immune suppression.

Long-Term Symptomatic Control

INHALED CORTICOSTEROIDS

The NAEPP recommends inhaled corticosteroid therapy as the first-line treatment for all asthmatics with persistent symptoms whether they are mild, moderate, or severe (Table 4). Corticosteroids are safe and effective anti-inflammatory agents with minimal systemic effects when used via inhalation. Although they may not prevent disease progression, they offer good long-term symptomatic control, reduce the need for oral steroids, minimize acute exacerbations, prevent hospitalizations, and dramatically decrease deaths from asthma. The mechanism of action of inhaled corticosteroids is similar to that of systemic use.

Inhaled corticosteroids include beclomethasone diproprionate, budesonide, flunisolide, fluticasone proprionate, and triamcinolone acetonide. Dexamethasone is not recommended secondary to high systemic absorption resulting in long-term side effects. The dosing is based on clinical severity and is not absolutely interchangeable among the different inhaled corticosteroids. They can take up to a week to show improvement, therefore systemic corticosteroid use should be considered if there is an urgent need for symptomatic control. Systemic therapy works well acutely when airway obstruction is not improving or worsening despite optimal bronchodilator therapy or used chronically in rare patients when standard therapy fails to achieve good control.

There has been considerable controversy regarding the safety of chronic inhaled corticosteroid use. After reviewing multiple studies examining bone mineral density, subcapsular cataracts, glaucoma, and hypothalamic–pituitary–adrenal axis suppression, the NAEPP panel found negligible adverse events from chronic inhaled corticosteroid use. They concluded that they are safe and that the benefits clearly outweighed the small potential risks. The more common adverse effects include oral candidiasis, hoarseness, and cough. Such adverse effects can be reduced with the use of aerosol spacers and rinsing the mouth after every dose.

Long-Acting β2-Adrenergic Agents

Long-acting β2-agonists, such as salmeterol and formoterol, stimulate intrapulmonary β2-receptors to cause sustained bronchodilation that can last up to 12 hours. They are effective controller agents, especially for nocturnal symptoms and exercise-induced bronchospasm, but should not be used alone or in lieu of anti-inflammatory therapy. The NAEPP panel recommends its use in combination with inhaled corticosteroids because such combination is superior to all other combinations as well as to higher dosages of inhaled corticosteroids alone for moderate to severe asthma. Long-acting β2-agonists should not be used to treat acute exacerbations as they have a slower onset of action (15–30 minutes). Adverse effects include tachycardia, tremor, hypokalemia, and a prolonged QTc interval in overdose. Inhalation is the preferred route of administration because it produces more sustained effects with less adverse reactions than oral agents such as sustained-release albuterol.

Combination medications with long-acting β2-adrenergic agents are available and serve as powerful agents in the asthma armamentarium to improve medication adherence, reduce morbidity and mortality, and health care expenditures. Recent studies demonstrate that the refill persistence for fluticasone proprionate and salmeterol combination was significantly more than for fluticasone proprionate taken alone or in combination with other controller therapies and that medication adherence was comparable to an oral agent *(8)*.

Leukotriene Modifiers

This class of medications works either by inhibiting the enzyme 5-lipoxygenase (zileuton) to prevent the synthesis of leukotrienes or by antagonizing leukotriene receptors (montelukast, zafirlukast). Anti-leukotrienes are variably effective in patients and thus, are considered alternative medications for mild persistent asthma and should only be used in combination with inhaled corticosteroids for more severe asthma. Review of current data demonstrates that the addition of anti-leukotrienes to inhaled corticosteroid therapy shows only modest improvement in lung function and are at best second-line agents when used alone compared with inhaled corticosteroids *(9,10)*. Montelukast is a leukotriene receptor antagonist, specifically inhibiting the cysteinyl leukotriene (CysLT1) receptor. It blocks leukotriene (LTD4)-mediated effects causing airway edema, bronchospasm, and inflammation. Montelukast has milder side effects such as headache, muscle aches, abdominal pain, nasal congestion, rash, and fever compared with zileuton and zafirlukast, which can also cause elevation of hepatic enzymes and reduce the metabolism of drugs such as warfarin.

METHYLXANTHINES

Methylxanthines, such as theophylline and aminophylline, are mild to moderate bronchodilators that act via phosphodiesterase inhibition. They are at best second-line medications for use either alone in mild persistent asthma or in combination with inhaled corticosteroids for moderate to severe persistent asthma. They are infrequently used as controller medications because of their wide variability in metabolism among individuals, which makes them prone to toxicity. If administered, they require close monitoring to maintain steady-state serum levels between 5 and 15 µg/mL, above which cardiac arryhthmias and seizures become more likely and can present without any milder symptoms.

CROMOLYN SODIUM AND NEDOCROMIL

Cromolyn sodium and nedocromil are nonsteroidal anti-inflammatory medications indicated as alternative treatment for mild persistent asthma or as preventative treatment before exercise or known allergen exposure. They block chloride channels, stabilize mast cell membranes, and curb eosinophilic recruitment. They both block the early and late response to allergen, but nedocromil is more effective at blocking the acute response to exercise and cold dry air. Their safety makes their use popular among the pediatric population.

FUTURE DIRECTIONS

Despite greater understanding of asthma pathophysiology and treatment options, asthma continues to remain underdiagnosed and undertreated. Although the NAEPP has set forth guidelines to address this disparity and reduce asthma exacerbations, asthma-related ED visits have remained elevated in the past decade. Studies show that the asthmatic population are largely dependent on rescue medications, such as short-acting bronchodilators and oral corticosteroids, but even more striking is that even an acute event such as an ED visit does not result in significant change in long-term controller therapies *(11)*. Given that there are 2 million asthma-related events each year in the United States, this should be a major focus for improving care. Furthermore, this study also showed that in the 12 months before the ED event, 90% presented to a primary care physician, 50% with asthma-related complaints, but nearly 75% did not receive inhaled corticosteroid controller therapy, first-line treatment for persistent asthma *(11)*. Underclassification of severity and inadequate treatment of asthma cannot be overemphasized because it is associated with a high level of morbidity and mortality, and particularly after an ED event, because continued inadequate management sustains the risk of future acute events, ED visits, and hospitalizations. This calls for a better way of monitoring patient status. Although research data is inconclusive, the NAEPP continues to recommend written action plans, peak-flow monitoring, and routine office spirometry as means for monitoring in the hopes of preventing exacerbations.

Markers for asthma severity and inflammation are also an area of investigation. Although pulmonary function tests are objective measures of lung function, they do not correlate perfectly for disease severity and are suboptimal for monitoring disease status, such as a hemoglobin A1c for diabetes or systolic blood pressure for hypertension. Nitrous oxide (NO) is produced by inflammatory cells and exhaled NO might serve as such a marker for disease status. There is evidence that NO correlates with disease severity, but significantly more data is needed.

Finally, newer therapeutic agents will be helpful. Although the safety of inhaled corticosteroids has been established, newer and theoretically safer inhaled steroids are in development. Although the methylxanthines, once a mainstay of asthma therapy, have been relegated to third- or fourth-line options, newer more specific phosphodiesterase inhibitors may provide excellent bronchodilation without the associated side effects or narrow therapeutic window. Lastly, different delivery devices and combination products will also come to the US market soon, including the combination of fomoterol (a long-acting bronchodilator) and budesonide (inhaled corticosteroids). The faster action of fomoterol over salmaterol may allow asthma control and relief in a single inhaler, possibly leading to improved compliance and control.

REFERENCES

1. Mannino DM, Homa DM, Akinbami LJ, Moorman JE, Gwynn C, Redd SC. Surveillance for asthma—1980–1999. MMWR Surveill Summ 2002;51:1–13.
2. Becker J, Rogers J, Rossini G, Mirchandani H, D'Alonzo GE, Jr. Asthma deaths during sports: report of a 7-year experience. J Allergy Clin Immunnol 2004;113:264–267.
3. National Asthma Educatoin and Prevention Program. Expert panel report: guidelines for the diagnosis and management of asthma: update on selected topics—2002. US Department of Health and Human Services, Public Health Service, National Institutes of Health, National Heart, Lung, and Blood Institute, Bethesda, MD, 1997; NIH publication no. 02-5074.
4. Leyhnaert B, Neukirch C, Kony S, et al. on behalf of the European Community Respiratory Health Survey. Association between asthma and rhinitis according to atopic sensitization in a population-based study. J Allergy Clin Immunnol 2004;113:86–93.

5. Silva G, Sherrill D, Guerra S, et al. Asthma as a risk factor for COPD in a longitudinal study. Chest 2004;126:59–65.
6. Nathan RA, Sorkness CA, Kosinski M, et al. Development of the asthma control test: a survey for assessing asthma control. J Allergy Clin Immunology 2004;113: 59–65.
7. National Asthma Education and Prevention Program. Guidelines for the diagnosis and management of asthma: expert panel report 2. US Department of Health and Human Services, Public Health Service, National Institutes of Health, National Heart, Lung, and Blood Institute, Bethesda, MD, 1997; NIH publication no. 97-4051.
8. Stoloff S, Stemple DA, Meyer J, Stanford RH, Carranza Rosenzweig JR. Improved refill persistence with fluticasone proprionate and salmeterol in a single inhaler compared with other controller therapies. J Allergy Clin Immunol 2004;113: 245–251.
9. Ducharme F, Di Salvio, F. Anti-leukotriene agents compared to inhaled corticosteroids in the management of recurrent and/or chronic asthma and children. Cochrane Database Sys Rev 2005;4.
10. Ducharme F, Schwartz Z, Hicks G, Kakuma R. Addition of anti-leukotriene agents to inhaled corticosteroids for chronic asthma. Cochrane Database Sys Rev 2004;4:CD003133.
11. Stempel D, Roberts CS, Stanford RH. Treatment patterns in the months orior to and after asthma-related emergency department visit. Chest 2004;126:75–81.

12   Exercise-Induced Bronchospasm

Khalid Jaboori and Matthew L. Mintz

CONTENTS

> CASE PRESENTATION
> KEY CLINICAL QUESTIONS
> LEARNING OBJECTIVES
> INTRODUCTION
> EPIDEMIOLOGY
> PATHOPHYSIOLOGY
> CLINICAL PRESENTATION
> DIFFERENTIAL DIAGNOSIS
> DIAGNOSIS
> TREATMENT: ACUTE, RECOVERY, AND MAINTENANCE
> NONPHARMACOLOGICAL TREATMENT OF EIA/EIB
> PHARMACOLOGICAL TREATMENT OF EIB
> FUTURE DIRECTIONS
> REFERENCES

CASE PRESENTATION

A 16-year-old high school basketball player presents with the complaint that he is not playing as well as he used to. He complains of chest tightness, coughing with wheezes, as well as the production of lots of phlegm, and slight shortness of breath during basketball practice and sometimes right after basketball games. He has no symptoms while in class but does admit that he sometimes coughs at night, especially when he has not cleaned his room in a while. This patient has no past history of asthma but does have seasonal allergies. His surgical history is significant for a tonsillectomy at age 5 and an appendectomy at age 10. The patient lives at home with his mother, who is a smoker, and his pet dog. He denies

From: *Current Clinical Practice: Disorders of the Respiratory Tract:
Common Challenges in Primary Care*
By: M. L. Mintz © Humana Press, Totowa, NJ

smoking, does not take any illegal drugs, and does not drink alcohol. Physical exam is significant for slightly erythematous and enlarged nasal turbinates. His lungs are clear to auscultation bilaterally, and the rest of the physical was normal.

KEY CLINICAL QUESTIONS

1. Does this patient have asthma?
2. Is there a difference between exercise-induced bronchospasm (EIB) and exercised-induced asthma (EIA)?
3. What would be the next step in this patient's work-up?
4. How do you determine whether you need more than a short-acting β2 agonist inhaler to treat this condition?

LEARNING OBJECTIVES

1. Understand the pathophysiology behind EIB and EIA.
2. Recognize the clinical presentation and establish differential diagnoses for EIB and EIA.
3. Diagnose EIB and EIA and learn how to determine the difference between them.
4. Understand prophylactic, acute, and long-term treatment of EIB.

INTRODUCTION

EIB and EIA are two major classifications that must be distinguished by a clinician when dealing with exercise-related breathing difficulties. Although not yet fully understood, the major difference between the two disorders is that EIA is a chronic inflammatory condition in which a patient's underlying asthma is exacerbated by exercise, whereas EIB is a bronchospastic disorder in which reversible respiratory difficulty ensues during or several minutes after exercise (Table 1). EIB can occur in otherwise healthy people, with no history of asthma or allergic diseases. Additionally, patients with EIB alone may have normal lung exams, normal peak flow, and normal spirometry at rest. Usually, patients with EIB only suffer from their symptoms (temporary bronchoconstriction) once a strenuous level of physical activity is reached and require treatment only before exercising. Patients with EIA may have a chronic mild persistent asthma that is uncontrolled. They may wheeze at rest, have abnormal peak flow and spirometry, and usually require long-term treatment both daily and before exercising.

EPIDEMIOLOGY

The prevalence of EIB ranges from 7 to 20% of the general population. Of that population, 80 to 90% of patients with asthma, and 30 to 40% of patients with allergic rhinitis have EIB *(1–3)*.

Table 1
Differences Between EIB and EIA

EIB	EIA
• May otherwise be healthy • Bronchospastic • May have no history of asthma • Normal lung exam • Normal spirometry • Only need treatment before exercise	• May have underlying untreated asthma • May have wheezing with lung exam • Abnormal spirometry[a] • Abnormal peak flow • Normal peak flow • Needs long-term daily treatment and treatment before exercise

[a]If the diagnosis is in doubt, spirometry should be done before and after exercise. A drop of FEV_1 15% or more will point the clinician to the direction of a possible underlying asthma. EIB, exercise-induced bronchospasm; EIA, exercise-induced asthma.

Although not fully known, EIB does not seem to significantly contribute to the morbidity of asthma. Studies assessing Olympic athletes and military recruits with documented EIB were done in 1984, 1998, and 2001. All conclusions showed that despite athletes/military recruits' EIB, their performance was not hindered *(4–6)*.

PATHOPHYSIOLOGY

There have been numerous theories regarding the pathophysiology of EIB, two of which are the most plausible and widely accepted theories. The first theory suggests that as one exercises, there is more air movement than usual through the airways. As the rate of breathing increases, one is forced to breathe through their mouth, bypassing the humidification that takes place through the upper airway. This increased movement of air, specifically dry or cold air, results in drying of the airways. The cold air is eventually warmed by attracting water vapor from the upper airway's respiratory epithelium. As water is lost from the respiratory epithelium, there is a change of osmolarity, temperature, and pH in pericilary fluid. The resulting change in osmolarity (hyperosmolar state) causes a cascade of events that possibly releases mediators such as prostaglandins, leukotrienes, and histamines from epithelial or mast cells. Consequently, hyperemia and increased perfusion to the airway occurs, which eventually leads to edema of the airway and bronchospasm *(7)*. The second theory suggests that the increased moving of air in the bronchial tree results in an overall decrease in temperature of the bronchi. As the exercise is terminated, the bronchial vasculature will dilate and become edematous to rewarm the airway. This reaction results in a rebound hyperemia, and eventually spasm of the bronchi.

Although it is known that inflammatory mediators exist in both theories, it is unknown which mediators occur specifically in each theory. It is hypothesized that inflammatory mediators, such as the leukotrienes LTC4, LTD4 *(8)*, histamine, and interleukin-8 *(9)* are increased in both theories. In addition, T-cells, such as Th2 (CD25) lymphocytes, and B-cells (CD 23) are increased during an episode of EIB *(10)*. The rise in these cell types facilitates the production of immunoglobulin (Ig)E, which eventually activates eosionophils. However, activation of eosionophils has not been documented in all cases of EIB *(11)*.

The difficulty in differentiating the pathophysiology of EIB versus EIA is owing in part to the design of past studies. Most research regarding this topic was done using clinical subjects with an underlying asthma. Therefore, it is difficult to ascertain if the inflammatory mediators listed above and pathophysiological mechanisms discussed are manifestations of EIB alone or are a combination of EIB with mild intermittent/persistent asthma *(12)*.

It is important to note that other studies done based on results obtained from bronchoalveolar lavage have shown an absence of mast cell activation, rising histamine levels, and signs of inflammation in patients with a diagnosis of EIB after exercise challenge *(13)*. Thus, further research is still needed to fully understand the exact pathophysiological mechanisms differentiating EIB from EIA.

CLINICAL PRESENTATION

EIB will usually occur during or immediately after some type of sustained exercise in sports such as basketball, football, long distance running, cycling, soccer, hockey, martial arts, tennis, volleyball, wrestling, and other similar sports. The symptoms usually include chest tightness 5 to 10 minutes following exercise, shortness of breath, wheezing, cough, fatigue, and possibe gastrointestinal discomfort. Triggers or exacerbating factors can be in the environment. Factors that exacerbate asthma including cold, dry, or moldy air can also trigger EIB. Allergic and non-allergic stimulants can contribute to the exacerbation of EIB. Stimulants include allergens, such as pollen, and non-allergic irritants, such as tobacco smoke and smog.

EIA or EIB is particularly common in children and adolescent athletes but can be seen in all ages *(14)*. Recognition is especially important in children. Children with EIB/EIA may have difficulty keeping up with kids their own age, often being mislabeled as lazy or out of shape. In general, EIA will present similarly in a children and adults. It is possible for EIA to be underrecognized in children because of the fact that it may not limit performance completely and that 50% of children affected with EIA become refractory to bronchoconstriction when exercise is repeated within 1 hour after initial exercise *(15)*.

There are three phases usually described during EIB *(16)*. The first phase is the immediate response, which is the initial bronchodilation followed by a bronchoconstriction that occurs 5 to 15 minutes after strenuous exercise (80% of the maximum predicted heart rate). Initially, there is a decrease in pulmonary function during this time, but pulmonary function returns to its original function 30 to 60 minutes after exercise ceases.

The second phase is the late response, which occurs in 20 to 30% of patients with EIB. In this phase, there is a drop in lung function 6 to 8 hours after exercise onset. This is thought to occur as delayed inflammatory mediators are released.

The final phase is the refractory period. In nearly half of patients with EIB, strenuous exercise 2 to 3 hours after the initial episode will result in a much weaker bronchospasm.

The exact mechanism of this refractory phase is still unknown, however, mast cell degranulation or prostaglandin release has been postulated as possible mechanisms.

DIFFERENTIAL DIAGNOSIS

The differential diagnosis of cough, dyspnea, chest tightness, and sputum production can be thought of in the categories of children and adults (Table 2). It is important to realize that any respiratory condition involving bronchospasm will be exacerbated by physical activity and other triggers discussed. It is important to appreciate that possible diagnosis of EIA/EIB can be masqueraders of other underlying pathology. For example, a patient with gastroesophageal reflux disease may present with intermittent coughing that gets worse with exercise as their presenting symptom. Patients with cardiac conditions listed above may present with difficulty breathing with exertion/physical activity, not being able to "catch their breath" with minimal exercise, and tiring quickly when active. Patients with an underlying bacterial or viral pneumonia may present with symptoms of shortness of breath, wheezing, and chest tightness with exercise. Ultimately, physicians evaluating patients for symptoms that appear to present as EIA or EIB should take a thorough history and keep other possible etiologies in mind to be certain to not overlook other similarly appearing diagnoses.

DIAGNOSIS

EIB/EIA is usually diagnosed clinically, without the need of major laboratory tests. However, if laboratory tests are done, the most definitive test involves 6 to 10 minutes of treadmill exercise testing, which raises the heart rate to 75 to 85% of the predicted maximum heart rate. A spirometry reading is obtained before exercise and every 3 to 5 minutes during and after exercise. Through spirometry, the forced vital capacity, peak expiratory flow rate, and the forced expiratory volume in 1 second (FEV_1) can be measured. Patients with EIB only will have a pre-exercise baseline FEV_1 of 80 to 100% of predicted normal values. In a patient

Table 2
Differential Diagnosis of EIB/EIA

Adults	Children
Chronic bronchitis	Asthma
Asthma	Pneumonia
Pneumonia	Croup
Emphysema	Viral bronchitis
Anaphylactic reaction	Cardiac conditions (congenital heart disease, CAD, CHF)
Gastroesophageal reflux (GERD)	
Carcinoid tumor	Gastroesophageal reflux
Pulmonary embolism	Cystic fibrosis
Chemical irritation	Anaphylactic reaction
Upper airway obstruction	Laryngeal webs
Anxiety	Vascular ring
Cardiac conditions (congenital heart disease, CAD, CHF)	Lymphadenopathy
	Foreign body aspiration
Vocal cord dysfunction	

Adapted from ref. *16*.
EIB, exercise-induced bronchospasm; EIA, exercise-induced asthma; CAD, coronary artery disease; CHF, congestive heart failure.

with chronic asthma, the FEV_1 at baseline will be less than 80% predicted. (Actually, that is not true. By definition, patients with mild asthma have normal pulmonary function tests.)

A positive test is considered as a drop in FEV_1 by 15 to 20% (mild EIB). A FEV_1 drop of 20 to 30% is considered moderate EIB and a drop of more than 30% is considered severe *(16)*.

If exercise tests are done and are inconclusive, a methacholine challenge can be done. This test is more sensitive but less specific than an exercise challenge. The test can not distinguish between EIA and EIB, however, a positive or negative result can give the clinician an idea of weather or not the patient has an underlying asthma. A normal predicted fall in a patient's FEV_1 after administration of a predetermined dose of nebulized methacholine is around 20%. In patients EIA or EIB, a low dose of methacholine (4.0 mg/mL) will incite a drop in FEV_1 of more than 20%. Conversely, in patients without EIA/EIB a high dose of methaocholine (16.0 mg/mL) will incite a modest drop in FEV_1 by about 10% *(16)*.

TREATMENT: ACUTE, RECOVERY, AND MAINTENANCE

Treatment should first be categorized into treatment of EIB alone versus patients with asthma who experience EIB (aka EIA). The treatments can then be categorized as nonpharmacological and pharmacological. The major objectives of the physician include the following:

1. Treat and prevent EIB in patients with asthma and patients with EIA without having the patient relinquish their exercise or sport.
2. Decrease the frequency of exacerbations in an patients with asthma.
3. Decrease morbidity and mortality associated with EIA.

NONPHARMACOLOGICAL TREATMENT OF EIA/EIB

Environment

A patient with EIB/EIA should be encouraged to exercise in an environment in which the air is warm and humid, not cool and dry. For example, instead of running outside in the winter, a physician should encourage the patient to run indoors or cover their faces (nose and mouth) with a scarf to facilitate humidification of the air they breathe in *(16)*.

Breathing

As most athletes increase the intensity of their exercise, a transition from nasal to mouth breathing occurs. If one can revert back to nasal breathing, less bronchospasm will occur as a result of the humidification and warming of the air breathed in. Although difficult to do at first, patients should be encouraged to attempt alternating breathing through their nose and mouth so that the air they breathe in during challenging exercise can be humidified and prevent an exacerbation.

Also, warm-up breathing before strenuous exercise should strongly be recommended to the patient with EIB. Before doing their actual work out, a patient should be advised to take part in activity that will induce short bursts of forceful breaths, such as brief sprints to encourage a high ventilation rate. Another method of warm-up breathing includes continuous moderate exercise, such as brisk walking, or anything that will have the patient breath slightly more than usual for a continuous (30–60 minutes) amount of time. These techniques aim to induce an increased level of ventilation before actual exercising takes place to eventually create a refractory period in order to better perform during their actual exercise *(17)*.

As the exercise ceases, the physician should advise the patient not to quit the exercise hastily. In other words, if a patient completes a 30-minute run on the treadmill, they should not step off as soon as the time expires. Instead, a cooling down period in which one is slowly eased out of their exercise, such as going from running to a brisk walk to normal regularly paced walk, will result in less severe EIB. The severity is decreased as the airway is gradually rewarmed, diminishing the total amount of vascular dilation, hyperemia, and edema.

Conditioning

A patient with asthma or EIB should be encouraged to undergo exercise conditioning. As the body is conditioned from continuous, regularly scheduled exercise times, a lower ventilation rate is needed for the same amount of work completed. As the ventilation rate decreases, one is less likely to induce EIB *(18)*.

Other

Some suggest encouraging cardiovascular fitness, which will eventually reduce the body's total ventilation requirements, lowering the FEV_1 and ultimately diminishing bronchoconstriction.

PHARMACOLOGICAL TREATMENT OF EIB

Treatment Summary

Patients with EIB alone should always be treated both nonpharmacologically and pharmacologically. Patients should initially use two to four puffs of a short-acting bronchodilator (β-agonist) 15 minutes before exercise, which should essentially last about 4 hours. If patients do not respond well to short-acting β-agonists, longer-acting β-agonists can be used. Specifically, salmeterol has been shown to significantly improve FEV_1, providing relief for 12 hours *(19,20)*. A problem with long-acting β-agonists, however, is that prolonged use may shorten duration of action. Second-line therapies including mast cell stabilizers, such as cromolyn sodium, and antihistamines, such as Zyrtec®, have also showed benefit in patients with EIB *(21,22)*.

If a patient is treated with the above medications and symptoms are still refractory to treatment, underlying inflammation from chronic asthma should be considered. A trial of inhaled corticosteroid (ICS; preferred) or leukotriene inhibitors (second line) is recommended in refractory cases.

β2-Agonists

β2-agonists work via adenyl cyclase, increasing the intracellular concentrations of cyclic adenosine monophosphate. As the levels of cyclic adenosine monophosphate increase, inhibition of mast cell degranulation occurs and relaxation of the bronchial and vascular smooth muscle ensues. Specific β2 agonists (slow or long acting) can be chosen and tailored to an athlete's specific requirements.

Before exercising (5–15 minutes before physical activity), prophylactic use of inhaled β2 agonists are the drug of choice. Benefits include a rapid onset of action usually no longer than 5 minutes and an extended duration of action (5–6 hours).

As a result of the rapid action of β2 agonists, it is the drug of choice in the acute setting *(7,22)*. To maximize benefit of the β2 agonist, the physician must properly educate the patient on the use of the metered dose inhaler (MDI).

The mouthpiece of the MDI should be placed about 1.5 inches in front of the patient's mouth, the patient then exhales entirely and compresses the inhaler. On inspiration, the patient should take a slow deep breath and then hold that breath for 10 seconds. After 10 seconds, the patient can exhale slowly. In younger populations, a spacer can be introduced to improve drug delivery. Side effects of β-2 agonists can include mild tremors, tachycardia, palpitations, increased wakefulness.

If patients do not respond well to the initial short-acting β-agonist, a longer-acting β-agonist may be used *(19,20)*. These β-agonists, such as salmeterol, have a slower onset but longer duration of action than shorter-acting β-agonists. These bronchodilators should be used 4 hours before exercise and can be used for up to 12 hours at a time. These longer-acting β-agonists are better choices for athletes taking part in endurance sports, such as triathlons or marathons. In addition to athletes, longer-acting β-agonists are a particularly good choice for children, offering all-day protection at school where they may take part in physical activity.

It should be noted that at the present time, it is unclear weather or not a physician can treat a person with EIB with long-acting β-agonists alone *(23)*. According to the Salmeterol Multi-Center Asthma Reseach Trial conducted in 1996 and ending in 2002, there were a "higher though not statistically significant" number of asthma-related life-threatening experiences including deaths that occurred in patients treated with salmeterol alone. Thus, a conclusion made from the study stated patients receiving salmeterol treatment should be concurrently receiving regular doses of ICS or another asthma controller medication *(24)*. There are newer longer-acting β-agonists, such as fomoterol, with a quicker onset of action than previous β-agonists, however, it is not recommended that it be used alone without ICS *(25)*. Finally, there are combination ICS plus longer-acting β-agonists soon to be available in the United States. At this time, however, there are no indications for use of this specific combination in EIA/EIB.

Cromolyn Sodium

Cromolyn sodium is a mast cell stabilizer. After administration of cromolyn sodium, there is a decreased amount of calcium that enters cells. This decrease in calcium levels in the cell eventually inhibits the degranulation of mast cells and has some anti-inflammatory effects.

Cromolyn sodium can be given as a prophylactic agent but not in an acute setting (it has no bronchodilatory effect). It is usually given 15 to 20 minutes preceding exercise and can prevent EIB in 75 to 85% of patients. A Cochrane review of nedocromil sodium showed that FEV_1 was improved by an average of 16% in most patients *(21,25)*.

Side effects of cromolyn sodium include cough, nausea, bad taste in mouth, throat dryness, and irritation. A benefit of cromolyn sodium over β2-agonists is that side effects are less noticeable and it can be used in patients whose symptoms are not relieved by β2-agonists alone. One should note that cromolyn sodium is a second-line drug and that if β-agonists alone relieve a patient's symptoms then cromolyn sodium is not needed.

Inhaled Corticosteroids

Corticosteroids are the most effective long-term pharmacological option to use to improve airway hyperresponsiveness and decrease the amount of bronchoconstriction that occurs during EIB *(26–28)*. Corticosteroids work by decreasing airway hyperresponiveness and inflammation to triggering stimuli in patients with asthma and EIB.

The difficulty in choosing whether or not a patient should be initiated on ICS therapy lies in the fact that EIB/EIA may clinically present similarly. If the clinician treats EIB with other agents listed previously (β-agonists, mast cell stabilizers) and the patient is still refractory to treatment, clinical suspicion should be high that the patient may have an underlying mild persistent asthma. At this point, treatment should be geared towards asthmatic control with β-agonists combined with ICS. Some studies have shown that regular use of an ICS can reduce exercise-induced symptoms by nearly 50% *(27)*.

Corticosteroids alone have no benefit in the acute setting, their use is primarily beneficial in the long term. Indications for use of ICS are in cases that are refractory to traditional therapy of β2-agonists or mast cell stabilizers. Side effects of ICS include candidiasis, local oropharyngeal irritation, and dysphonia.

Leukotriene Modifiers

Leukotriene modifiers are those agents that are leukotriene receptor antagonists and 5-lipooxygenase inhibitors. Leukotrienes alone are inflammatory products of phospholipid metabolites, which induces a bronchoconstrictive response 1000 times greater than histamines.

Similar to ICS, it can be difficult to distinguish between the EIB alone and EIB combined with an underlying asthma. Thus, as recommended for ICS, leukotriene modifiers are second-line therapies and should be reserved for patients refractory to initial treatment of β-agonists and mast cell stabilizers. Again, as patients become refractory to initial treatment, suspicion of underlying mild persistent asthma should be raised.

Leukotriene modifiers have been shown to be better than long-acting β-agonist in long-term therapy treating asthmatics with EIB *(29)*. Benefits of these drugs include their long half-life, which allows dosing once a day, and availability in an oral form *(30)*. In addition, tolerance occurs more frequently in long-term β2-agonists than tolerance to leukotriene modifiers. Thus, in the pediatric setting, children may frequently use their inhaled β2-agonist, rapidly becoming tolerant to its effects. Leukotriene modifiers can be used in this population.

FUTURE DIRECTIONS

Much research is needed in the area of EIB and EIA, including further understanding of the relationship between these entities and between asthma. A variety of therapies are currently under investigation and include the following:

1. Heparin: Heparin has been shown to considerably block symptoms of EIB through its direct effect on mast cells. More studies are underway at this time *(7,26)*.
2. Diuretics: Inhaled furosemide has been shown to ease the symptoms of EIB. A possible unproven mechanism postulates that the positive effect comes at the level of the lung epithelium. No conclusive evidence exists to date *(7,26)*.
3. Vitamin C: With prophylactic extremely large doses of the vitamin, a small amount of patients were protected against the symptoms of EIB. Benefits were only seen in a minority of patients and are not seen in all populations *(26,31)*.
4. Inhaled indomethacin: Indomethacin, a cyclo-oxygenase inhibitor blocks the production of prostaglandins, which can contribute to bronchoconstriction in EIB. However, a problem with this therapy is that the blockade is nonspecific, also blocking the production of prostaglandin E2, a bronchodilator *(26,32)*.

REFERENCES

1. Sinha T, David AK. Recognition and management of exercise-induced bronchospasm. Am Fam Phys 2003;67:769–774.
2. Feinstein RA, LaRussa J, Wang-Dohlman A, et al. Screening adolescent athletes for exercise-induced asthma. Clin J Sports Med 1996;6:119–123.
3. McFadden, ER Jr, Gilbert, IA. Exercise-induced asthma. N Engl J Med 1994;330:1362–1367.
4. Voy RO. The U.S. Olympic Committee experience with exercise-induced bronchospasm, 1984. Med Sci Sports Exerc 1986;18:328–330.
5. Weiler JM, Ryan EJ III. Asthma in United States Olympic athletes who participated in the 1998 olympic winter games. J Allergy Clin Immunol 2000;106:267–271.
6. Sonna LA, Angel KC, Sharp MA, et al. The prevalence of exercise-induced bronchospasm among US Army recruits and its effects on physical performance. Chest 2001;119:1676–1684.
7. Storms WW. Exercise-induced asthma: diagnosis and treatment for the recreational or elite athlete. Med Sci Sports Exerc 1999;31:S33–S38.
8. Reiss TF, Hill JB, Harman E, et al. Increased urinary excretion of LTE4 after exercise and attenuation of exercise-induced bronchospasm by montelukast, a cysteinyl leukotriene receptor antagonist. Thorax 1997;52:1030–1035.
9. Hashimoto S, Gon Y, Matsumoto K, et al. Inhalant corticosteroids inhibit hyperosmolarity-induced, and cooling and rewarming-induced interleukin-8 and RANTES production by human bronchial epithelial cells. Am J Respir Crit Care Med 2000;162:1075–1080.
10. Hallstrand TS, Ault KA, Bates PW, et al. Peripheral blood manifestations of T(H)2 lymphocyte activation in stable atopic asthma and during exercise-induced bronchospasm. Ann Aller Asthma Immunol 1998;80:424–432.
11. Kivity S, Argaman A, Onn A, et al. Eosinophil influx into the airways in patients with exercise-induced asthma. Respir Med 2000;94:1200–1205.

12. Hermansen CL, Kirchner JT. Identifying exercise-induced bronchospasm. J Postgrad Med 2004;115:6.
13. Jarjour NN, Calhoun WJ. Exercise-induced asthma is not associated with mast cell activation or airway inflammation. J Allergy Clin Immunol 1992;89:60–68.
14. Kaplan TA. Exercise challenge for exercise-induced bronchospasm. Phys Sports Med 1995;23:47–57.
15. Anderson, S. Exercise-induced asthma inchildren: a marker of airway inflammation. Medical Journal of Australia (MJA) 2002;177:S61–S63.
16. Lacroix, V. Exercise induced asthma. The Physician and Sports Medicine 1999;27:12.
17. McKenzie DC, McLuckie SL, Stirling DR. The protective effects of continuous and interval exercise in athletes with exercise-induced asthma. Med Sci Sports Exerc 1994;26:951–956.
18. Tan RA, Spector SL. Exercise-induced asthma. Sports Medicine 1998;25:1–6.
19. Coreno A, Skowronski M, Kotaru C, et al. Comparative effects of long-acting β[sub2]-agonists, leukotriene receptor antagonists, and a 5-lipoxygenase inhibitor on exercise-induced asthma. J Allergy Clin Immunol 2000;106:500–506.
20. Nelson JA, Strauss L, Skowronski M, et al. Effect of long-term salmeterol treatment on exercise-induced asthma. N Engl J Med 1998;339:141–146.
21. Spooner CH, Saunders LD, Rowe BH. Nedocromil sodium for preventing exercise-induced bronchoconstriction (Cochrane review) The Cochrane Library. Available from: http://209.242147.2/Abs/ab001183.htm. Accessed January 19, 2004.
22. Yuan Y, Wang Z, Luo Y, et al. Cetirizine improves the resistance of airway and pulmonary function in patients with asthma. Journal of West China University Medical Science 1996;27:411–414.
23. Rupp NT. Diagnosis and management of exercise-induced asthma. Phys Sports Med 1996;24:77–87.
24. National Asthma Education and Prevention Program. Guidelines for the diagnosis and management of asthma: expert panel report 2. US Department of Health and Human Services, Public Health Service, National Institutes of Health, National Heart, Lung, and Blood Institute, Bethesda, MD, 1997; NIH publication no. 97-4051.
25. Pauwels R, Löfdahl C, Postma D, et al. Effect of inhaled formoterol and budesonide on exacerbations of asthma. N Engl J Med 1997;337:1405–1411.
26. Smith BW, LaBotz M. Pharmacologic treatment of exercise-induced asthma. Clin Sports Med 1998;17:343–363.
27. Jonasson G, Carlsen KH, Hultquist C. Low-dose budesonide improves exercise-induced bronchospasm in schoolchildren. Pediatr Allergy Immunol 2000;11:120–125.
28. Jonasson G, Carlsen KH, Blomqvist P. Clinical efficacy of low-dose inhaled budesonide once or twice daily in children with mild asthma not previously treated with steroids. Eur Respir J 1998;12:1099–1104.
29. Edelman JM, Turpin JA, Bronsky EA, et al. Oral montelukast compared with inhaled salmeterol to prevent exercise-induced bronchoconstriction. A randomized, double-blind trial. Exercise Study Group. Ann Intern Med 2000;132:97–104.
30. Hansen-Flaschen J, Schotland H. New treatments for exercise-induced asthma, editorial. N Engl J Med 1998;339:192–193.
31. Cohen H A, Neuman I, Nahum H. Blocking effect of vitamin C in exercise-induced asthma. Archive of Pediatric and Adolescent Medicine. 1997;151:367–370.
32. Shimizu T, Mochizuki H, Shigeta M, Morikawa A. Effect of inhaled indomethacin on exercise-induced bronchoconstriction in children with asthma. Am J Respir Crit Care Med 1997;155:170–173.

13 Acute Cough

Karen J. Scheer and Matthew L. Mintz

CONTENTS
> CASE PRESENTATION
> KEY CLINICAL QUESTIONS
> LEARNING OBJECTIVES
> INTRODUCTION
> PATHOPHYSIOLOGY
> DIFFERENTIAL DIAGNOSIS
> DIAGNOSIS
> TREATMENT
> FUTURE DIRECTIONS
> REFERENCES

CASE PRESENTATION

A 62-year-old man, Mr. M., comes to your office with a chief complaint of a cough. He states that it started about 1 week ago with a "runny nose and scratchy throat." The cough is dry, nonproductive, and is interfering with the patient (and his wife) being able to get a full, restful night's sleep. Mr. M. denies any other symptoms, such as headache, sinus pressure, chest pain, and shortness of breath, but thinks that he may have had a fever "off and on the last few days." He has taken Tylenol® and has been drinking fluids, but his cough won't go away. The patient is requesting an antibiotic to "get this thing kicked out of my system." Mr. M. states that he is "tired of people at work looking at me like I have the plague."

Mr. M.'s past medical history is significant for hypertension and type 2 diabetes mellitus. Both his blood pressure and blood sugars have been under good control and are treated with lisinopril/hydrochlorothiazide and metformin, respectively. He takes an occasional ibuprofen for "aches and pains that come with aging." Family history is significant for a father, brother, and uncle with hypertension and a mother with diabetes. Mr. M. works full time as a postal employee, quit smoking 10 years ago (35 packs per year history), drinks occasionally, and has never used street drugs. He exercises by walking in his job as a mail carrier and has been married for 37 years with three grown, healthy children.

KEY CLINICAL QUESTIONS

1. What are the possible etiologies of this patient's cough?
2. What other history is necessary to rule out any serious causes of acute cough?
3. What is the proper evaluation for this patient?
4. Should this patient be treated with antibiotics or other prescription medications?

LEARNING OBJECTIVES

1. Understand the pathophysiology of cough.
2. Recognize the main etiological causes and symptomology of acute cough illness.
3. Become familiar with guidelines for the diagnosis of patients with acute cough illness.
4. Understand of the main treatment modalities available for acute cough illness.

INTRODUCTION

According to the Centers for Disease Control and Prevention, cough is one of the main reasons for patients to visit their physician or the emergency department. A Centers for Disease Control and Prevention survey of outpatient departments in US hospitals reported that 10.2% of the 84.6 million visits were owing to symptoms referable to the respiratory system, cough being the principal motivator for the visit. This same survey showed that the primary diagnoses for these patients were acute upper respiratory infections (URIs) *(1)*. In 2002, cough was responsible for bringing 3 of the 110 million patients to emergency departments in the United States—11.8% of which had diagnoses of ill-defined conditions and diseases of the respiratory system *(2)*. Another study conducted to examine the epidemiology of and recent trends in outpatient visits for infectious disease, reported that approximately 200 out of every 1000 office visits were related to URIs *(3)*.

Even more striking is the economic impact cough has in the United States. One study showed the cost of non-influenza-related viral respiratory tract infection to be about $40 billion annually in direct (health care resources, cost of over-the-counter [OTC] medications, outpatient physician visits, use of prescription medications) and indirect (productivity losses, absenteeism work) costs *(4)*. A 1997 study concluded that the annual cost per capita employer expenditures for patients with respiratory infections totaled $4397. The study reported estimates of the total of financial burden to employers to be a whopping sum of $112 billion spent on medical costs and lost time from work *(5)*.

The individual "cost" of cough can be high as well. There are many "cough complications" that can become problematic to patients: perceiving something is wrong (98%), exhaustion (57%), feeling self-conscious (55%), insomnia (45%), lifestyle change (45%), musculoskeletal pain (45%), hoarseness (43%), excessive perspiration (42%), and urinary incontinence (39%) *(6)*. Cough and its causes have a detrimental impact on individuals and on our health care resources.

PATHOPHYSIOLOGY

Cough is the result of the cough reflex, which can simply be described as a sudden rapid expulsion of air whose main purpose is to clear the airways from inhaled foreign bodies and to enhance mucociliary clearance in cases of impaired ciliary function and excessive mucus production *(6)*. Cough is induced by inflammation or irritation of the larynx, trachea, or bronchi. (To review the physiology of the cough reflex, please *see* Chapter 14.)

Cough is a symptom whose physical characteristics (dry, productive, whooping, staccato, and so on) can often give valuable clues to the disease underlying this symptom *(7)*. Furthermore, an effective cough depends on the ability to achieve high gas flows and velocities through the airways. Expiratory or inspiratory muscle weakness, disordered chest wall motion, altered mucus rheology, and altered mucociliary function all may affect coughing and must be kept in mind when evaluating a patient with pre-existing conditions *(6)*.

Cough is classified into categories using time as its chief differentiator. Acute cough is defined as any acute, self-limiting episodes of cough lasting less than 3 weeks. Chronic cough is a persistent cough lasting longer than 8 weeks. Subacute cough defines the period of time between acute and chronic—a 3- to 8-week intermediate period *(6,8,9)*. Although all coughs go through an "acute" phase, this chapter focuses on the most common and life-threatening causes of acute cough. The chronic causes of cough, such as gastroesophageal reflux disease, chronic obstructive pulmonary disease (COPD), asthma, postnasal drip, and cystic fibrosis, are addressed in Chapter 14.

DIFFERENTIAL DIAGNOSIS

Cough can literally be caused by hundreds of disease processes and agents—an overwhelming task to address in one chapter. One way of tackling this problem is to separate the possible etiologies into age groups. In this section, we will look at causes of acute cough in adults and children and the special circumstances to keep in mind when developing a differential diagnosis for these different age groups.

Table 1
Agents of Respiratory Illness

Virus	Bacteria
Rhinovirus	*Streptococcus pneumonia*
Adenovirus	*Haemophilus influenza*
Coronavirus	*Staphylococcus aureus*
Influenza A	*Bordetella pertussis*
Influenza B	*Mycoplasma pneumonia*
Parainfluenza	*Chlamydia pneumonia*
Respiratory syncytial virus	*Pseudomonas pneumonia*
Cocksackie A21	*Legionella pneumonia*

Adult Acute Cough

Published studies on the spectrum and frequency of causes of acute cough do not exist, but overwhelming clinical experience indicates that postnasal drip syndrome because of URIs is the most common cause *(6)*. For adults, acute cough is most commonly seen in the common cold, acute bacterial sinusitis, acute bronchitis, pertussis, COPD exacerbations, allergic rhinitis, and environmental irritant rhinitis *(6,8–10)*. Less common causes for acute cough are asthma, congestive heart failure, pneumonia, aspiration syndromes, and pulmonary emboli *(6,8,9)*.

The most common etiology of the common cold or rhinosinusitis is viral in origin *(6,8,9)*. The top suspects are usually rhinovirus, adenovirus, and coronavirus (*see* Table 1). Patients with the common cold present with an acute respiratory illness characterized by symptoms such as rhinorrhea, sneezing, nasal obstruction, postnasal drip, with or without fever, lacrimation, irritation of their throat, and a normal chest exam *(9)*.

Bacterial rhinosinusitises are sometimes difficult to clinically differentiate from their viral cousins. URI are suggestive of a bacterial cause when they have at least two of the following signs and symptoms: a maxillary toothache, purulent nasal secretions, abnormal findings on transillumination of any sinus, poor response to nasal decongestants, and a history of discolored nasal discharge *(6,9)*. Table 1 also contains the most likely agents in bacterial URIs.

Acute bronchitis is an acute cough syndrome, predominately caused by the viruses and less commonly by the bacteria listed in Table 1. Rhinovirus infection is the most common and can lead to exacerbations in asthma, COPD, and cystic fibrosis *(8)*. The mechanism of this cough is a transient bronchial hyperresponsiveness and the primary symptoms of this process include phlegm production and wheezing *(8,10,11)*.

Cough resulting from allergic rhinitis or environmental irritant rhinitis is caused by inflammation of the respiratory passages by some agent to which the patient is sensitive. There are countless numbers of irritants that cause this condition and they may be unique from patient to patient. Some of the more common agents are dog and cat hair, pet dander, dust mites, pollens, molds, and feathers. These irritants cause excess mucus production and postnasal drip, which triggers the cough reflex. A good history can identify these mechanisms as the culprits for the cough *(6)*.

Pertussis infection is present in up to 10 to 20% of adults with cough illness of longer than 2 to 3 weeks *(10)*. It initially presents as a URI during the catarrhal stage before involving the lower respiratory tract in the paroxysmal stage of the illness. No clinical features distinguish pertussis from nonpertussis infection in adults who were immunized against pertussis as children *(6,10)*.

As stated earlier in this section, acute cough can be the presenting manifestation of life-threatening disease such as pneumonia, congestive heart failure, pulmonary emboli, or aspiration *(6)*. In-depth discussion of these diseases is beyond the scope of this chapter, but ruling out pneumonia is the primary objective in evaluating adults who have acute cough with comorbidities (nursing home resident, elderly, immunocompromised, and so on) and for whom asthma is unlikely. About 5 to 10% of adult patients with acute tracheobronchitis develop bacterial infection deep in the lungs *(8)*. In adults without comorbidities, the main agents causing pneumonia are *Streptococcus pneumonia, Haemophilus influenza,* and *Moraxella catarrhalis,* and in young adults, *Mycoplasma pneumonia.*

It is especially important to have a high index of suspicion for pneumonia in the elderly and immunocompromised patients with acute cough because the classics signs and symptoms that accompany this disease sometimes do not express themselves. The abnormalities that would reveal the possible presence of pneumonia are a heart rate of more than 100 beats per minute, respiratory rate of more than 24 breaths per minute, or oral body temperature higher than 38°C *(6,8,9)*. The most common agents in elderly patients listed in order of frequency are *S. pneumonia, H. influenza,* Gram-negative agents, *Staphylococcus aureus, Chlamydia pneumonia, M. pneumonia, Legionella pneumonia,* and respiratory viruses *(8,9,12)*. For persons who are immunocompromised, especially persons with HIV, *Pneumocystis carinii* and *Mycoplasma tuberculosis* should be considered *(6)*.

Child Acute Cough

At least 90% of children with cough have a respiratory tract infection caused by common cold, croup, bronchitis, bronchiolitis, whooping cough, or pneumonia *(13)*. The most common etiologies of acute cough appear to be the common cold and environmental irritants *(6)*.

Families of children with recurrent episodes of cough frequently bring their children to their health care provider because it can be quite a disturbing and disruptive symptom to both the family and child. Although persistent moist or productive cough requires investigation, isolated nonproductive cough in the absence of evidence of airway obstruction or other evidence of systemic disease may not be abnormal *(14)*. There is evidence to suggest that persistent cough in children is more likely related to exposure to indoor and outdoor atmospheric pollution than to atopy associated with asthma *(14)*.

As in adults, the most common cause of the common cold is virus. Rhinovirus is the top culprit, responsible for 25 to 40% of the cases *(14)* and occurring in the early fall months *(15)*. Parainfluenza peaks in the late fall, respiratory syncytial virus in the early winter, and influenza in the late winter/early spring *(15)*. Children experience 3 to 8 colds per year and 10 to 15% have at least 12 colds per year, usually associated with attendance at day care center *(14)*. As in adults, the symptoms usually include rhinorrhea, cough, sore throat, with or without fever, malaise, myalgias, and mucopurulent nasal discharge. As a result of immature immune systems, infants may present with symptoms slightly different than older children, including high fevers, irritability, decreased feeding, and sleeping patterns *(14)*.

One study showed that 5 to 13% of the viral respiratory tract infections will become complicated by acute bacterial sinusitis. In children, 80% of bacterial rhinosinusitis are preceded by a viral respiratory tract infection, whereas 20% are complications from allergic rhinitis *(16)*. The leading causes are *S. pneumonia, H. influenza,* and *M. catarrhalis.* As in adults, the presence of mucopurulent nasal drainage with unilateral or maxillary face pain, fever, headache, or maxillary or periorbital swelling, most likely have a cough because of this bacterial infection *(16)*.

Croup is a URI that typically occurs in children ages 1 to 5 years and is characterized by respiratory obstruction with a characteristic barking cough with hoarseness and inspiratory stridor *(13)*. The etiology is most commonly parainfluenza virus and tends to occur the autumn. Bronchitis or tracheobronchitis, as in adults, is a syndrome involving the lower respiratory tract in which there is transient bronchial hyperresponsiveness. The primary symptom is a cough productive of phlegm and is most often caused by viral agents.

Bronchiolitis epidemics tend to occur in winter and spring with respiratory syncytial virus being implicated in many cases. It has a very similar presentation to asthma, with coughing and wheezing being the primary symptoms. Whooping cough is characterized by distinctive paroxysms of cough with vomiting and episodes of apnea in young children *(13)*.

Community-acquired pneumonia is one of the most serious infection-producing coughs in infants and children with an annual incidence of 34 to 40 cases per

Table 2
Common Causes of CAP

Age	Common causes
Birth to 20 days	*Escherichia coli*
	Group B *Streptococcus*
	Listeria monocytogenes
3 weeks to 3 months	*Chlamydia trachomatis*
	Streptococcus pneumonia
	Adenovirus
	Influenza virus
	Parainfluenza viruses 1, 2, 3
	Respiratory syncytial virus
4 months to 5 years	*Chlamydia pneumonia*
	Mycoplasma pneumonia
	S. pneumonia
	Adenovirus
	Influenza virus
	Parainfluenza virus
	Rhinovirus
	Respiratory syncytial virus
5 years to adolescence	*C. pneumonia*
	M. pneumonia
	S. pneumonia

Modified from ref. *17*.
CAP, community-acquired pneumonia.

1000 children in Europe and North America *(17)*. The etiology is age-dependant. Table 2 shows the most common causes for the specific age group. The strongest predictors of pneumonia in children are fever, cyanosis, and more than one of the following signs of respiratory distress: tachypnea, cough, nasal flaring, retractions, rales, and decreased breath sounds. Children without fever or symptoms of respiratory distress are unlikely to have pneumonia *(17,18)*.

Another cause of acute cough in children that can be potentially life threatening is the inspiration of a foreign body *(6)*. This particular etiology should be on top of a differential list, especially with children 6 months to 3 years of age.

As with adults, there may be acute cough as an indicator of the onset of a more chronic condition in a child. Congenital malformation, reactive airway disease, asthma, cystic fibrosis, congestive heart failure and gastroesophageal reflux disease need to be kept in the differential diagnosis of a child with acute cough *(18)*. These conditions tend to produce a more chronic cough in children and are discussed in Chapter 14.

DIAGNOSIS

In children or adults, a clinical approach is recommended for the initial evaluation of acute cough *(6,8,9,13,14)*. As with all other evaluations, this approach consists of history and physical exam. In addition, keeping in mind the estimated frequency of conditions, based on the epidemiological data as well as clinical experience is key to a successful diagnosis *(6,9)*. Most patients who present to their physician with a cough of less than 3 weeks' duration, rhinorrhea, sneezing, nasal obstruction, postnasal drip, with or without fever, lacrimation, irritation of their throat, and a normal chest exam will most likely have a viral respiratory infection *(6,8,9)*.

In the diagnosis of a patient with acute cough, the important questions become the following:

1. Is this acute cough is a symptom of something that may be life threatening to the patient?
2. Is this a high-risk patient for which I have to look at less common causes for acute cough?
3. Does this patient have any symptoms besides acute cough that raise a red flag?

The evaluation of the seriousness of a patient's condition begins as the soon as the practitioner enters the room with observations such as the patient's disposition, breathing pattern, and speech patterns (Table 3). High-risk patients, such as the very young, elderly, nursing home patients, and the immunocompromised, receive an automatic high index of suspicion for a more in-depth look.

Normal history questions should include: past medical history (conditions, medications, hospitalizations, and so on); recent immunizations (pneumovax, influenza); and social history (tobacco, alcohol, drugs, recent travel, occupation, environmental exposures). Red flags in the history of present illness and physical exam such as fever, shortness of breath, orthopnea, tachypnea, tachycardia, pleuritic chest pain, rales, rhonchi, mucopurulent nasal discharge, sinus pain and pressure, and mental status changes should trigger further exploration beyond the simple clinical evaluation. Complete blood count, Chem 7, and chest X-rays would be warranted in many cases to determine if a more malevolent process than the common cold is at work. It cannot be overstressed that ruling out pneumonia is a primary objective in evaluating high-risk adults.

In the case of infants and children important information to find out in the history would include prenatal and birth history, growth and development, hospitalizations, immunizations, day care attendance, exposure to infectious agents, family history, antibiotic treatment within the previous month, recent travel, recent choking episodes and changes in feeding, and sleeping and diapering patterns *(6,17,18)*. Red flags on the physical exam that warrant further investigation would be fever, cyanosis, pallor, dehydration, tachycardia, grunting, nasal

Table 3
Signs and Symptoms of a Life-Threatening Cough

Adults/children	Infants/young children
Position—lying down/sitting?	Irritable/crying?
Coloring?	Inconsolable?
Affect/mood?	Listlessness? Moving?
Level of distress?	Able to produce a smile?
Breathing rapidly?	Working to breathe?
Sweating/shivering?	Coloring?
Able to talk without effort?	Sweating/shivering?

flaring, mucopurulent nasal discharge, rales, retractions, tachypnea, use of accessory muscles for breathing, and wheezing *(6,13,17,18)*.

As in adults, when history and physical exam indicate it, complete blood count, Chem 7, and chest X-rays would be helpful in determining the more serious causes of cough, especially pneumonia.

TREATMENT

As a first line in therapy, most practitioners will recommend OTC medications as a way of initially addressing acute cough. These OTCs include antitussives, expectorants, mucolytics, antihistamines, antihistamine–decongestion combinations (Table 4). Practitioners will typically recommend a trial of these OTCs and if the patient does not improve or worsens, he or she will then look to other causes for the illness.

No good evidence for or against the effectiveness of OTC medications for acute cough exists. Even when randomized, control trials treating adults and children with acute cough had significant results, the effect size was small, there was doubt of clinical relevance, or there were conflicting results between trials in each medication group *(8,19,20)*. Most preparations, however, appear to be safe based on those studies reporting side effects *(8,19,20)*.

Despite the predominately viral cause of acute cough, antibiotics are frequently prescribed to children and adults *(4,10,11)*. At times, patients expect and demand a medicine that will alleviate or end their symptoms and many times practitioners give into this pressure. Antibiotic prescriptions for acute bronchitis, which are primarily viral and cause an acute cough illness, range from 50 to 80% *(11)*. Because of the lack of efficacy and low complication rates, antibiotic treatment of children with URIs is not supported by current evidence from randomized trials *(21)*. Specifically, randomized, placebo-controlled trials conducted in the past 25 years have failed to support the role of antibiotics in the treatment of

Table 4
Examples of Commonly Used OTC Medications

Category	OTC medication
Antitussives	Dextromethorphan
	Codeine
Expectorants	Guaifensin
Mucolytics	Bromohexine hydrochloride
Antihistamines	Loratidine
	Chlorpheniramine
	Bromopheniramine
Decongestants	Pseudoephedrine

OTC, over the counter.

acute bronchitis, either in the reduction of severity of symptoms (acute cough) or the duration of this condition *(10,11)*. Meta-analysis of these trials report no impact of antibiotics on illness duration, activity limitation, or work loss, but have shown that the inhaled bronchodilator albuterol decreases the duration of the cough *(8,10,11)*.

Figure 1 shows one proposed algorithm for the evaluation and management of adults with acute cough illness *(10)*. Although the end point on the right side of this flow chart is "acute bronchitis," common cold or URI with its appropriate treatment can easily be substituted.

The treatment of other common causes of acute cough are summarized below:

1. In allergic rhinitis/environmental irritant, the simple treatment is avoiding the offending allergens or agents and using an antihistamine, such as loratidine, to alleviate symptoms *(9)*.
2. In acute bacterial sinusitis, treatment includes dexbrompheniramine plus pseudoephedrine, oxymetazoline and an antibiotic directed against *S. pneumonia* and *H. influenza (8,9)*.
3. In the case of COPD exacerbation, the recommendations are an antibiotic directed against *S. pneumonia* and *H. influenza*, systemic corticosteroids tapered over 2 weeks, continuous O_2 if PaO_2 is 55 mmHg or less or SaO_2 is 88% or less, and ipratropium plus albuterol treatments *(9)*.
4. In acute bronchitis, it is recommended to treat acute cough with dextromethorphan or codeine, a bronchodilator, nonsteroidal anti-inflammatory drugs or acetaminophen for pain relief. Because one of the most common causes of acute cough is the influenza virus, a flu vaccine will help prevent the condition in the first place. If influenza is suspected as the cause, the antiviral amantidine or rimantidine can be used but must be initiated within 48 hours of diagnosis *(10,11)*.
5. For *Bordetella pertussis* infections, a 14-day course of erythromycin or bactrim is the recommended treatment for acute cough *(9)*.

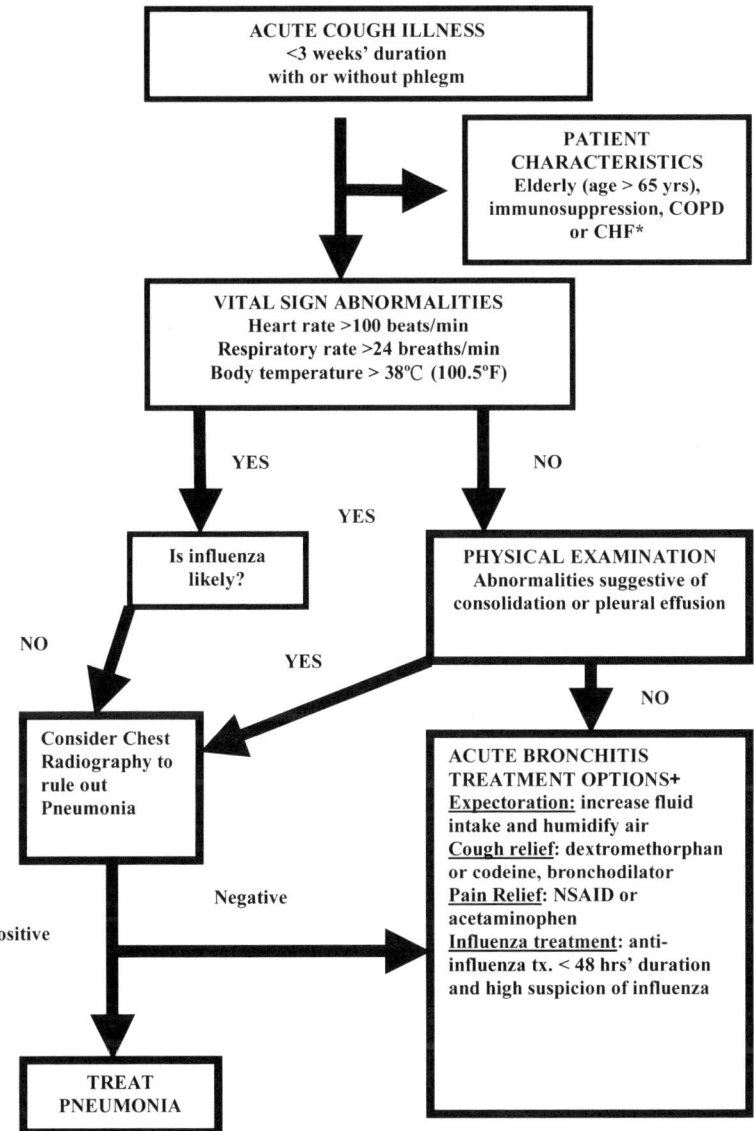

Fig. 1. Evaluation and treatment of acute cough.

Finally, prevention and prophylaxis is an important component in the care of our patients, especially our elderly and at-risk patients. Annual immunization against influenza is standard practice for these two groups. Vaccination against *S. pneumonia* with the Pneumovax® is also recommended for at-risk groups and will help to prevent many of the acute cough illnesses described earlier *(8)*.

FUTURE DIRECTIONS

There is much work to be done to address the symptom of acute cough and provide effective means to alleviate patient suffering from this malady. First and foremost, there needs to be further study to fully define the scope and causes of the problem. Much of the information in this chapter is based on clinical experience only. Although this experience is valuable, published studies on the frequency and spectrum of causes of acute cough in both adults and children are needed.

Although there is an array of OTC medications that may help to improve the effectiveness of cough or shorten its duration, large, randomized, controlled clinical studies documenting improvement in patient morbidity and mortality are lacking *(6,8–10,19–21)*. Lost work days, absenteeism from school, money spent on ineffective OTC treatments, and time and resources wasted in emergency departments and primary care offices would be significantly curtailed if we could identify effective self-care treatments with rigorously designed studies. Future studies using outcome measures that can be easily assessed in a primary care setting and that produce clinically meaningful results, such as patient satisfaction, relief of nighttime disturbance, side effects, or time to return to normal daily activities, are needed *(6,9,19,20)*.

According to clinical experience, viruses are the chief agent causing the URIs that lead to the acute cough illness. Although the OTC options for treatment try and reduce the severity of certain symptoms, they do nothing to address the underlying cause of the URI—the virus. There are five treatments under development that target the most common viruses implicated in non-influenza-related URI, including three virus capsid-binding agents: pleconaril, pirodavir, and tremacamra *(4)*. It is an exciting prospect for practitioners to possibly have a therapeutic option someday that actually addresses the etiology of the acute cough by reducing the viral load.

REFERENCES

1. Ly N, McCraig L, Burt C. National hospital ambulatory medical care survey: 1999 outpatient department summary. Centers for Disease Control and Prevention, Bethesda, MD, 2001; 321.
2. McCraig L, Burt C. National hospital ambulatory medical care survey: 2002 emergency department summary. Centers for Disease Control and Prevention, Bethesda, MD, 2004; 340.
3. Armstrong GL, Pinner RW. Outpatient visits for infectious diseases in the united states, 1980 through 1996. Arch Intern Med 1999;159:2531–2536.
4. Fendrick AM, Monto AS, Nightengale B, Sarmes M. The econonmic burden on non-influenza-related vial respiratory tract infections in the United States. Arch Intern Med 2003;163:487–494.
5. Birnbaum HG, Morley M, Geenburg P, et al. Economic burden of respiratory infections in an employed population. Chest 2002;122:603–611.

6. Irwin RS, Boulet L-P, Cloutier MM, et al. Managing cough as a defense mechanism and as a symptom. A consensus panel report of the American College of Chest Physicians. Chest 1998;114:133S–181S.
7. Pirila P, Sovijarvi ARA. Objective assessment of cough. Eur Respir J 1995;8:1949–1956.
8. Widdicombe J, Kamath S. Acute cough in the elderly: aetiology, diagnosis and therapy. Drugs Aging 2004;21:243–258.
9. Irwin R, Madison J. Primary care: the diagnosis and treatment of cough. N Eng J Med 2000;343:1715–1721.
10. Gonzales R, Sande MA. Uncomplicated acute bronchitis. Ann Intern Med 2000;133:981–991.
11. Gonzales R, Winker MA. A 65-year-old woman with acute cough illness and an important engagement. JAMA 2003;289:2701–2708.
12. Furman CD, Rayner AV, Tobin EP. Pneumonia in older residents of long-term care facilities. Am Fam Physician 2004;70:1495–1500.
13. Hay AD, Schroeder K, Fahey T. Acute cough in children. BMJ 2004;328:1062.
14. West JV. Acute upper respiratory infections: childhood respiratory infections. Br Med Bull 2002;61:215–230.
15. Monto AS. Occurrence of respiratory virus: time, place and person. Pediatr Infect Dis J 2004;23:S58–S64.
16. Conrad DA, Jenson HB. Management of acute bacterial rhinosinusitis. Curr Opin Pediatr 2002;14:86–90.
17. Ostapchuk M, Roberts DM, Haddy, R. Community-acquired pneumonia in infants and children. Am Fam Physician 2004;70:899–907.
18. Margolis P, Gadomski A. Does this infant have pneumonia? JAMA 1998;279:308–313.
19. Schroeder K, Fahey T. Systematic review of randomized controlled trials of over the counter cough medicines for acute cough in adults. BMJ 2002;324:329–334.
20. Schroeder K, Fahey T. Over-the-counter medications for acute cough in children and adults in ambulatory settings. Cochrane Database Syst Rev 2004;4:CD0018310.
21. Fahey T, Stocks N, Thomas T. Systematic review of the treatment of upper respiratory tract infection. Arch Dis Child 1998;79:225–230.

14 Chronic Cough

Clara Peck and Matthew L. Mintz

CONTENTS

    CASE PRESENTATION
    KEY CLINICAL QUESTIONS
    LEARNING OBJECTIVES
    BACKGROUND
    ANATOMY AND PHYSIOLOGY OF COUGH
    DIFFERENTIAL DIAGNOSIS OF COUGH
    COMMON CAUSES OF CHRONIC COUGH IN ADULTS
    COMMON CAUSES OF CHRONIC COUGH IN CHILDREN
    DIAGNOSTIC APPROACH TO THE PATIENT WITH CHRONIC COUGH
    TREATMENT OPTIONS
    FUTURE DIRECTIONS
    REFERENCES

CASE PRESENTATION

Mrs. J. is a 47-year-old female who presents with 2 months of persistent nagging cough that is nonproductive and unresponsive to over-the-counter antitussives. She has been unable to get restful sleep as a result of her cough, and her declining focus at work has prompted her visit. The patient's past medical history is significant for hypertension, mild intermittent asthma, seasonal allergies that are associated with rhinitis and chronic sinusitis, and smoking less than two cigarettes per day for the past 20 years. With the exception of cigarette smoke, there is no known exposure to environmental irritants. She does not report any wheezing or chest tightness over the past 2 months and has no history of heartburn or regurgitation after eating. Her current medications include lisinopril, hydrochlorothiazide, and inhaled albuterol as needed.

From: *Current Clinical Practice: Disorders of the Respiratory Tract:
Common Challenges in Primary Care*
By: M. L. Mintz © Humana Press, Totowa, NJ

KEY CLINICAL QUESTIONS

1. What are the most likely causes of prolonged cough in this patient?
2. What further history would be helpful in formulating a differential diagnosis?
3. How often can the etiology of chronic cough be correctly identified in adults?
4. What is the next step in the evaluation of this patient?
5. Are any diagnostic investigations appropriate at this time?

LEARNING OBJECTIVES

1. Review the physiology of the cough reflex.
2. Define acute, subacute, and chronic cough.
3. Become familiar with the common causes of chronic cough in adults and children.
4. Adopt a systematic approach to the patient with chronic cough.
5. Recognize the role of diagnostic tests in the routine evaluation of chronic cough.

BACKGROUND

Cough is the single most common presenting symptom for which patients seek outpatient medical services in the United States *(1)*. As such, cough has a considerable financial impact on our health care system. In the United States the cost of treating cough associated with the common cold alone accounts for more than $1 billion annually *(2)*. The clinical significance of this complaint in primary care medicine underscores the need to have an effective diagnostic strategy for patients who present with cough of unknown etiology. This chapter reviews the current recommendations for the evaluation and treatment of chronic cough persisting for more than 8 weeks. It is estimated that chronic cough affects 14 to 23% of nonsmoking adults and more than 50% of heavy smokers (more than two packs per day) *(3)*. A systematic approach to the patient with prolonged cough is essential for accurately identifying the underlying disease process and targeting therapy.

ANATOMY AND PHYSIOLOGY OF COUGH

Cough is a symptom that encompasses a broad spectrum of diseases that all share a common physiological mechanism, the activation of the central cough reflex. A basic awareness of this reflex and the mechanics of effective coughing is vital to understanding how various disease processes induce chronic cough. In healthy individuals, mucociliary action removes mucus and foreign material from the tracheobronchial tree. When large amounts of material accumulate in the airways, or when the mucociliary system is impaired, cough is the primary mechanism of clearance. For example, cough becomes essential for airway clearance in patients with chronic bronchitis (CB) because smoking causes both abnormal mucus secretion and impaired ciliary function *(4)*.

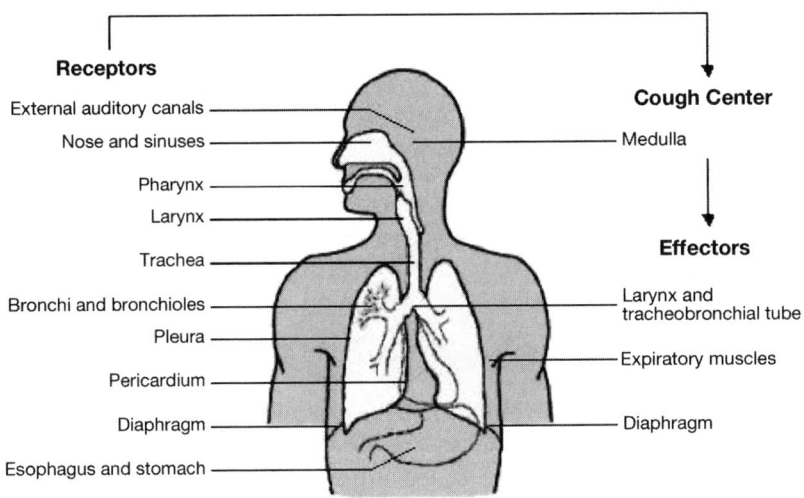

Fig. 1. The cough reflex arc. (From ref. *1*.)

The cough reflex arc (Fig. 1) consists of peripheral receptors, vagal afferent fibers, a medullary cough center, and efferent fibers that transmit signals to the airways and respiratory muscles to achieve a concerted cough response. Irritant receptors are located throughout the lower airways from the larynx to respiratory bronchioles *(5)*. These chemical and mechanical receptors respond to a variety of stimuli such as noxious gases, edema fluid, foreign bodies, and bronchospasm *(6)*. Cough receptors are also found outside of the lower respiratory system. In the setting of an upper respiratory tract infection, cough is the result of pharyngeal receptor stimulation by postnasal drip and throat clearing *(7)*. Extrapulmonary receptors that can elicit the cough reflex have also been reported in the paranasal sinuses, external auditory canals, diaphragm, pleura, pericardium, esophagus, and stomach *(6)*.

Once a reflex response has been initiated, the complex interaction between gas flow and mucus within the airways must be coordinated to produce an effective cough. The sequence of events during a typical cough begins with deep and rapid inspiration, followed by the achievement of high intrathoracic pressures, and explosive expiration. The ability to generate high expulsive velocities is critical for successful airway clearance. This in turn requires high intrathoracic pressures, which are achieved with a large inspiratory volume, glottal closure, and adequate muscle contraction. The central conducting airways transiently constrict during the expiratory phase of cough, further augmenting flow. Expiratory velocities of more than 500 miles per hour can be generated during vigorous coughing *(6)*.

In addition to high gas velocities, the surface properties of airway secretions are key determinants of cough effectiveness. Mucus must be mobilized into droplets in the passing stream of expiratory gas to clear the airways. The level of ease with which mucus can be separated from the epithelial lining depends on its depth, as well as its adhesiveness and cohesiveness. It is well recognized that the abnormally thick and viscous respiratory secretions in patients with cystic fibrosis (CF) cause poor airway clearance. Similarly, altered mucus properties in asymptomatic smokers result in less effective coughing compared with nonsmokers *(8)*.

DIFFERENTIAL DIAGNOSIS OF COUGH

The first step in the evaluation of cough is to differentiate patients based on symptom duration into one of three categories: acute, subacute, or chronic cough (Table 1) *(9)*.

Acute cough is defined as lasting less than 3 weeks and is often infectious in nature. The bulk of acute cough is comprised of upper respiratory tract infections, such as the common cold, acute bacterial sinusitis, chronic obstructive pulmonary disease exacerbations, allergic and non-allergic rhinitis, as well as pertussis *(9)*. The common cold, as a result of self-limited viral infections of the upper respiratory tract, is by far the most likely diagnosis in an adult with acute cough. Less common but potentially lethal causes of acute cough include pneumonia, pulmonary embolism, congestive heart failure, asthma exacerbation, and aspiration *(6,9)*. In children with acute cough, aspiration of a foreign body should always be considered *(10)*.

Subacute cough, 3 to 8 weeks in duration, often shares etiologies with acute cough. When subacute cough develops after an upper respiratory tract infection, postinfectious cough, bacterial sinusitis, asthma, and pertussis are among the most common diagnoses to consider *(9)*. A pertussis-like syndrome with prolonged spasmodic cough can be seen in children with some viral and atypical bacterial infections such as adenovirus, chlamydia, and mycoplasma *(10)*. Subacute cough that is not clearly associated with an infection should be treated in the same manner as chronic cough.

Adults with chronic cough, lasting more than 8 weeks, are less likely to have a respiratory infection. Ninety-five percent of cases are caused by postnasal drip syndrome (PNDS), asthma, CB, gastroesophageal reflux disease (GERD), sinus and nasal disease, angiotensin-converting enzyme (ACE) inhibitor use, eosinophilic bronchitis, and bronchiectasis *(9)*. Unlike acute cough, subacute and chronic cough can result from more than one etiology in 18 to 62% of cases *(6)*. Rare causes of chronic cough that should be considered in patients who are refractory to treatment include malignancy, congestive heart failure, aspiration, sarcoidosis, and tuberculosis (TB) *(2)*. The differential diagnosis of prolonged cough in an immunocompromised patient is beyond the scope of this chapter.

Table 1
Common Causes of Cough in Adults and Children

	Acute (less than 3 weeks)	Subacute (3–8 weeks)	Chronic (more than 8 weeks)
Adults	Upper respiratory tract infection Acute bacterial sinusitis Exacerbation of chronic obstructive pulmonary disease Asthma exacerbation Allergic rhinitis Non-allergic rhinitis Pertussis	Postinfectious cough Bacterial sinusitis Asthma Pertussis	Postnasal drip syndrome Asthma Chronic bronchitis GERD Angiotensin-converting enzyme inhibitor use Sinus and nasal disease Eosinophilic bronchitis Bronchiectasis
Children	Upper/lower respiratory tract infection Asthma exacerbation GERD Foreign body aspiration	Postinfectious cough Pertussis-like syndrome Asthma	Recurrent viral bronchitis Asthma Sinusitis/postnasal drip syndrome GERD Environmental exposures Congenital anomalies

Adapted from refs. *1*, *2*, and *10*.
GERD, gastroesophageal reflux disease.

The triad of PNDS, asthma, and GERD accounts for essentially all cases of chronic cough in adults who do not smoke or take an ACE inhibitor, and who have a normal or near-normal chest X-ray *(1)*.

In the pediatric population, respiratory infections, asthma, PNDS, and GERD are the most common causes of both acute and chronic cough *(6)*. Recurrent viral bronchitis is an important etiology of cough that parents often perceive to be chronic, although symptoms should actually subside between infections *(10)*. Asthma is probably the most common cause of truly persistent cough in children. Sinusitis with subsequent PNDS is the next most frequent etiology, followed by GERD, which accounts for 15% of chronic cough in children *(11)*. Less common causes include environmental exposures, congenital anomalies, aspiration (including foreign bodies), congenital heart disease, psychogenic cough, and serious underlying lung disease *(6,10)*.

COMMON CAUSES OF CHRONIC COUGH IN ADULTS

Postnasal Drip Syndrome

PNDS is the single most common cause of chronic cough in nonsmoking adults with a normal chest X-ray. Underlying conditions that predispose patients to PNDS include chronic sinusitis, allergic and non-allergic rhinitis, vasomotor rhinitis, and postinfectious rhinitis. Unfortunately, upper respiratory signs and symptoms have proven to be unreliable evidence of PNDS *(6)*. Classic findings such as pharyngeal drainage, frequent throat clearing, and a cobblestone appearance to the pharynx are nonspecific, and PNDS often presents simply as a syndrome of cough and phlegm *(12)*. Therefore, this diagnosis should not be based exclusively on a suggestive history or physical examination. Currently, the most conclusive demonstration of PNDS as a cough etiology is response to a first-generation H_1-antagonist combined with a decongestant *(9)*. The newer generation antihistamines are less effective.

Asthma

Asthma is second only to PNDS as a cause of chronic cough in adult nonsmokers with a normal chest X-ray. It is also the second most common cause in children after recurrent viral bronchitis. Cough is a symptom that occurs in all asthmatics *(6)*, but it can be the sole manifestation of disease in up to 57% of cases *(13)*. This cough-variant asthma has the same prognosis as typical asthma and responds to therapy in the same way. Asthma management involves the identification and avoidance of triggers, as well as the use of medications such as bronchodilators and corticosteroids. Other inflammatory conditions may respond to corticosteroids, but the resolution of cough with inhaled bronchodilators is diagnostic of asthma *(6)*. Although targeted therapy can be used to diagnose cough-variant asthma, pulmonary function testing with a methacholine challenge is the most effective means of ruling it out. This test measures flow rates after inhalation of methacholine, an agent that provokes bronchospasm. Subsequent measurements after treatment with an inhaled bronchodilator document the degree of reversible airway obstruction. The negative predictive value of a methacholine challenge is 100% and many experts encourage its routine use in primary care *(9)*.

Gastroesophageal Reflux Disease

The third most common cause of chronic cough in nonsmoking adults with a normal chest X-ray is GERD. Gastroesophageal reflux can be "silent"in up to 75% of cases, lacking the typical symptoms of heartburn and regurgitation *(14)*. Persistent cough may be the only indication of disease in these patients. In the setting of GERD, the cough reflex is primarily initiated by extrapulmonary irritant receptors in the distal esophagus. Repeated micro-aspiration of gastric contents can irritate the airways directly and induce both chronic cough and wheeze, but this mechanism is probably less common *(6)*. GERD is also an important cause of chronic cough in children, but it is rare for cough to be the sole manifestation of disease in this population. Most children with GERD have typical reflux symptoms as well as irritability, chest pain, and wheezing *(6,10)*. Ambulatory esophageal pH monitoring over a 24-hour period is the most sensitive and specific method for diagnosing GERD-induced cough *(6)*. However, the inconvenience and limited availability of this test prevents its routine use. Establishing GERD as a cause of chronic cough with empirical trials of therapy can be difficult as well, because lifestyle changes and medical management may not be effective initially. Symptomatic improvement can take 2 to 3 months and cough resolution usually requires at least 6 months of therapy. If given adequate time, the cough does resolve in 70 to 100% of patients treated medically *(6)*.

Chronic Bronchitis

CB is a form of chronic obstructive pulmonary disease characterized by progressive airflow obstruction that is not completely reversible with treatment. CB is one of the most frequent causes of chronic cough in the United States, but most people with this disease do not seek medical attention for their cough. In fact, CB is only diagnosed in 5% of patients who present for evaluation of persistent cough *(12)*. When CB is suspected, the key to diagnosis is a focused history. The defining feature of this condition is recurrent productive cough that is particularly severe in the morning. The cough should be present on most days during at least 3 months of the year for at least 2 consecutive years. Typically, the age of onset is 50 to 60 years of age. CB occurs almost exclusively in patients with a history of significant exposure to tobacco smoke or other irritants. Smoking induces impaired mucociliary clearance, airway inflammation, and mucus hypersecretion. This combination of derailments ultimately results in chronic activation of the cough reflex *(6)*. There is a dose-related relationship between cigarette smoking and the prevalence of productive cough *(15)*. Symptomatic improvement following smoking cessation or irritant avoidance demonstrates that CB is either partly or completely responsible for the patient's cough. This cough will resolve or significantly improve after abstaining from smoking in 94% of cases, often within 4 weeks *(16)*.

ACE Inhibitors

ACE inhibitors are typically well tolerated in the management of hypertension, chronic renal disease, and congestive heart failure. However, a persistent dry cough can develop in 5 to 20% of patients on an ACE inhibitor *(17)*. Although the mechanism of this side effect is not known, one hypothesis links cough to the accumulation of kinins in the lungs, which results from ACE blockade. Kinins, such as bradykinin, can directly activate pulmonary irritant receptors and sensory afferents involved in the cough reflex. Moreover, increased bradykinin levels promote a general inflammatory state in the respiratory system of susceptible individuals, resulting in bronchospasm and local edema *(17)*. These changes further augment the cough reflex by stimulating mechanical receptors in the airways. ACE inhibitor-induced cough is more common in females and usually develops within a few weeks of therapy, although it can be delayed by up to 6 months *(17)*. Discontinuation of the drug should eliminate or substantially improve symptoms within 4 weeks *(9)*. Because the cough is likely to return with rechallenge, an alternate drug class is preferred in these patients. Angiotensin II receptor blockers do not cause cough *(17)*.

Other Etiologies

Eosinophilic bronchitis may be responsible for up to 13% of chronic cough in adults *(18)*. This is a condition of chronic airway inflammation in which eosinophils make up at least 3% of non-squamous cells on sputum smear *(18)*. It is not associated with bronchospasm, which distinguishes it from asthma. Thus, eosinophilic bronchitis responds to inhaled and systemic corticosteroids but not to bronchodilators. Eosinophilic bronchitis has not been reported in children *(6)*.

In bronchiectasis, severe airway inflammation results in progressive bronchial dilation, impaired mucociliary clearance, and subsequent chronic bacterial colonization. These persistent bacteria perpetuate a cycle of further inflammation and damage. Conditions that can lead to bronchiectasis include severe or poorly treated infections, aspiration, and impaired host defenses. CF is the most common cause of childhood bronchiectasis in the United States *(6)*. Patients with bronchiectasis typically present with chronic productive cough, often with copious amounts of thick sputum. Hemoptysis and wheeze are also common. The diagnosis should be confirmed with a high-resolution computed tomography (CT) scan of the chest, which is both sensitive and specific *(6)*.

Fewer than 20% of smokers develop bronchogenic carcinoma, but it remains the leading cause of cancer death in the United States *(19)*. Lung cancer is an uncommon cause of cough, but smokers who develop a persistent or changing cough warrant careful evaluation because early detection improves survival *(19)*. Additional findings that raise concern for malignancy in a smoker include hemoptysis, hoarseness, dysphagia, localized wheeze, stridor, and evidence of metastatic disease or paraneoplastic syndromes. Chest radiography is one of the first steps in the evaluation of a smoker with chronic cough. If the cough persists despite smoking cessation and the chest X-ray is normal, bronchoscopy is indicated *(6)*.

TB remains one of the most common causes of chronic cough worldwide. In the United States, an estimated 15 million people are infected with *Mycobacterium tuberculosis*, comprising a significant reservoir for the development of new cases of active disease *(20)*. Most TB in non-HIV-infected patients is confined to the lungs, and the most common symptom of pulmonary TB is cough *(20)*. This cough tends to become productive of sputum, but hemoptysis is rare at presentation. The tuberculin skin test is a screening tool for identifying individuals with latent infection, but because of limited sensitivity and specificity it should not be used as evidence of active disease. When there is high clinical suspicion, the diagnosis of active TB must be confirmed by culture and detection of acid-fast bacilli in the sputum. Essentially all cases of pulmonary TB cause an abnormal chest X-ray or CT scan, but these modalities are not always diagnostic of active disease and should not replace sputum studies *(20)*.

Sarcoidosis is a multi-organ granulomatous disease that primarily affects the lung and lymphatic systems. It is an important cause of chronic cough with an estimated 1 to 40 cases per 100,000 in the United States *(21)*. Sarcoidosis shows a strong predilection for adults less than 40 years old, with a slightly higher incidence among women and African Americans *(21)*. Although the etiology of sarcoidosis is unknown, it is thought that the inciting event may be certain environmental exposures or infections in genetically susceptible individuals. Pulmonary sarcoidosis tends to present with nonproductive cough, dyspnea, and chest pain associated with bilateral hilar lymphadenopathy. Parenchymal infiltrates or evidence of advanced fibrosis with honeycombing may also be seen *(21)*. Constitutional symptoms such as fever and weight loss are probably more common in African Americans. The diagnosis of sarcoidosis is confirmed when the characteristic clinical presentation and radiological findings are supported by histological evidence of noncaseating granulomas *(21)*.

COMMON CAUSES OF CHRONIC COUGH IN CHILDREN

As in adults, the triad of asthma, PNDS, and GERD accounts for most cases of chronic cough in children *(6)*. Recurrent bouts of viral bronchitis should also be among the first diagnoses to consider in a child with chronic cough. Although it is probably not truly chronic in nature, lower respiratory tract infections are thought to be the single most common cause of persistent cough in children *(10)*. Younger children are more prone to developing viral bronchitis, which is frequently caused by respiratory syncytial virus. The onset of bronchitis is usually associated with signs and symptoms of an upper respiratory tract infection, and in cases of prolonged cough these upper respiratory symptoms may be intermittent. A careful history might reveal transient cough-free periods, worsening in the winter months or with exposure to tobacco smoke at home *(10)*.

Environmental exposures, particularly parental smoking, play an important role in pediatric cough. Of children younger than 11 years of age with two smoking parents, 55% have chronic cough *(22)*. This is partially because of the increased frequency of viral upper respiratory tract infections in children who are exposed to cigarette smoke *(10)*. As in adults, smoke-induced cough should resolve with irritant avoidance. Other environmental risk factors include dampness in the home and air pollution. Isolated persistent cough in children strongly correlates with a lower socioeconomic status *(10)*.

Chronic cough in infants may be the first presentation of congenital anatomical abnormalities that affect the respiratory system. An anomalous aorta or pulmonary artery that compresses the central airways can cause cough with wheeze or stridor. Tracheobronchomalacia similarly results in collapse of the large airways and subsequent cough *(6)*. Cough caused by chronic aspiration is common in the setting of a tracheoesophageal fistula or laryngeal cleft *(10)*. Even with normal anatomy, a wide spectrum of disorders, including GERD and swallowing abnormalities, can lead to chronic pulmonary aspiration and cough.

Foreign body aspiration is a noteworthy cause of persistent cough in toddlers and young children. Food and other objects lodged in an airway usually presents acutely, but 20% of cases go unrecognized until 1 week or more after the event *(6)*. This can result in a syndrome of chronic cough and may lead to secondary infection. Children under 4 years of age, especially boys, are most at risk for aspirating foreign bodies *(10)*.

Congenital heart disease that results in pulmonary edema or bronchial compression can cause chronic cough associated with wheeze or respiratory distress in young children. Examples of such lesions include a patent ductus arteriosus, ventricular septal defect, and tetralogy of Fallot *(1)*.

Psychogenic or "habit" cough is relatively common in children and is thought to be a manifestation of underlying stress or conflict *(1)*. However, it is not well-studied and remains a diagnosis of exclusion. Psychogenic cough is typically described as abating during sleep or with distraction and worsening with attention. Children with this habitual cough tend to be females who are older than 5 years of age *(10)*. Suggestion therapy or other psychiatric intervention is the principal mode of treatment, but a short course of nonspecific antitussives may be indicated *(6)*.

Serious underlying lung disease as in CF is an important cause of pediatric cough, although cough is rarely an isolated finding in these patients. CF may present with failure to thrive in the setting of chronic purulent cough of early onset *(10)*. A sweat test is strongly recommended for the evaluation of children with chronic cough whenever CF is even remotely considered *(6)*.

DIAGNOSTIC APPROACH TO THE PATIENT WITH CHRONIC COUGH

The cause of persistent cough can be correctly identified in 88 to 100% of adults *(6)*. Arriving at a diagnosis in the patient with chronic cough should be a systematic process using a directed history, targeted diagnostic testing, and trials of empirical therapies for common etiologies (Fig. 2).

The timing, quality, and character of chronic cough are rarely useful in establishing a diagnosis *(9)*. Rather than focusing on cough as a symptom (e.g., whether or not it is productive), the clinician should seek out key elements in the history that would suggest an underlying cause. In particular, the initial evaluation of an adult with chronic cough becomes straightforward when there is a history of smoking, exposure to environmental irritants, or ACE inhibitor use. If the history is suggestive of CB, smoking cessation or irritant avoidance should be strongly recommended. A potential temporal relationship between the initiation of an ACE inhibitor and cough onset warrants discontinuation of the drug. If the cough persists for 4 weeks or more after these interventions, further evaluation is necessary.

There is a larger role for diagnostic studies in patients with chronic cough than for those with acute and subacute cough. In the absence of any suggestive findings in the history, the initial work-up of an adult with prolonged cough should be guided by chest radiography. A normal or near-normal chest X-ray (with a stable and clearly unrelated abnormality) would effectively rule out bronchogenic carcinoma, sarcoidosis, TB, and bronchiectasis as a cause of cough *(6,19)*. Any concerning lung pathology noted on chest X-ray necessitates prompt evaluation and specialist referral.

For the subset of adults who do not smoke or take an ACE inhibitor, and who have an essentially normal chest X-ray, trials of empirical therapy provide critical diagnostic information. In these patients, a definitive cause of cough can only be established when there is a documented response to specific treatment. A series of systematic therapeutic trials should be started in order of the most to

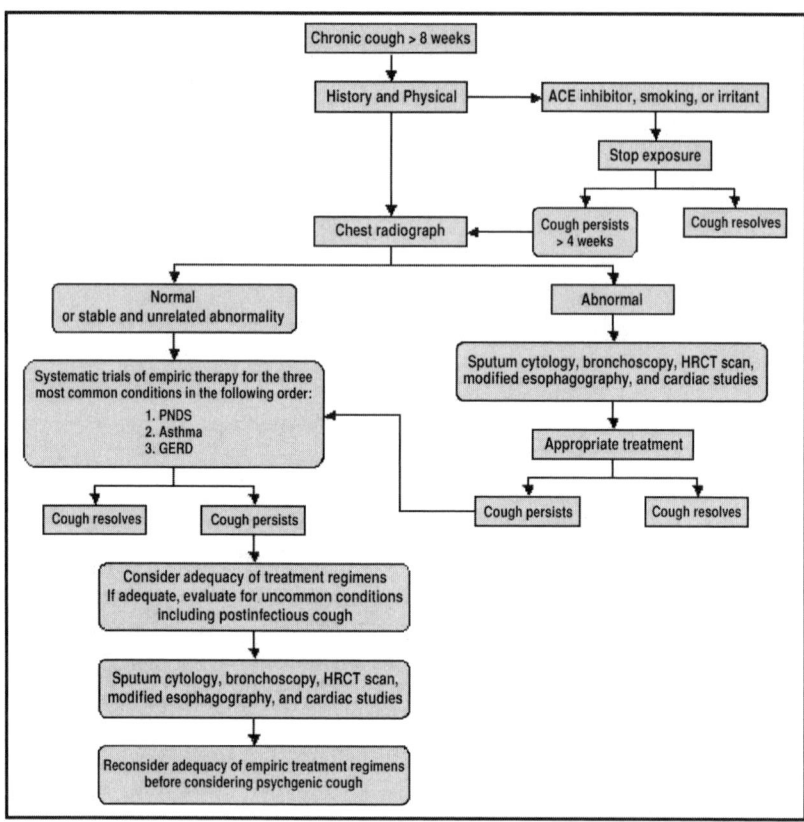

Fig. 2. Diagnostic approach to the patient with chronic cough.

least common etiologies (Table 1) until some degree of symptomatic relief is achieved. Nearly all adults with chronic cough will be diagnosed with PNDS, asthma, GERD, or some combination of these conditions *(6)*. Therefore, the clinician must focus on this triad of disorders during the initial evaluation. PNDS-induced cough should be suspected first and an antihistamine/decongestant combination should be started. If there is suspicion that a patient has PNDS as a result of chronic sinusitis, there may be a role for antibiotics in addition to antihistamine/decongestant therapy. Although definitive studies are lacking, sinus CT scanning beofre initiating therapy is probably appropriate for the evaluation of sinusitis as a cause of chronic cough *(6)*. Incomplete cough resolution after an adequate trial of PNDS therapy should not be discounted because chronic cough often results from multiple conditions simultaneously *(6,9)*. Rather, a second empirical trial can be added to the partially effective one. The most likely comorbid diagnosis in this scenario is cough-variant asthma. If there is any doubt as to the response to bronchodilator therapy, a methacholine challenge test can be employed to exclude asthma. The next diagnosis to consider is GERD. The pressures generated by chronic coughing from any etiology may precipitate GERD, resulting in a self-perpetuating cycle of cough and reflux *(6)*. Thus, GERD should always be considered as a contributory factor in chronic cough. In addition to lifestyle changes, acid suppression with a proton pump inhibitor or H_2-blocker should be implemented for at least 2 months, but ideally 6 months or more, before assessing response *(6)*.

This systematic diagnostic approach applies to the pediatric population as well. To some extent, chronic cough is "normal" in childhood and most cases tend to resolve spontaneously *(10)*. However, if a child's cough is unusually severe or persistent the possibility of an underlying disorder must be addressed (Table 2). As with adults, the goal of the history is to elicit key findings that might suggest a cough etiology. Chronic cough that is associated with feeding suggests GERD or chronic pulmonary aspiration. A strong family history of asthma or atopy may be helpful supporting evidence of cough-variant asthma. Acute onset of persistent cough in a previously asymptomatic child may indicate foreign body aspiration, especially if the cough began after a choking episode. Neonatal onset of cough should raise concern for either infection aquired *in utero*, congenital anomaly, or underlying lung disease. Chronic purulent cough and failure to thrive are always worrisome for a serious pulmonary disease, such as CF. A child's home environment, including parental smoking behavior, should always be sought in the history *(10)*. Past immunizations and any potential exposure to TB are important factors as well.

The physical examination of a child with chronic cough may reveal signs of infection, atopy, failure to thrive, or abnormal lung auscultation consistent with underlying disease. Failure to thrive is an especially important finding to document. The patient's ears should always be examined, as foreign bodies in the external auditory canal or fluid in the middle ear can elicit the cough reflex *(6)*.

In the initial work-up of childhood chronic cough, a chest radiograph should be obtained to rule out lower respiratory tract, cardiac, and vascular abnormalities *(6)*. Sputum can be sent for Gram stain and culture or rapid viral assay if an infectious etiology is suspected. Pulmonary function testing is appropriate in children older than 5 years of age, but empirical bronchodilator therapy should be used to diagnose asthma in younger children *(6)*. As in adults, 24-hour esophageal pH monitoring is the gold standard for diagnosing GERD as a cough etiology. If a foreign body is suspected, rigid bronchoscopy is both diagnostic and therapeutic *(10)*. A chloride sweat test for CF is indicated in cases of childhood chronic cough when the diagnosis is unclear.

Table 2
History Suggestive of Chronic Cough Etiology

Adults	Children
Smoking	Family history of asthma or atopy
Exposure to environmental irritants	Cough associated with feeding
Angiotensin-converting enzyme inhibitor use	Cough after a choking episode
	Neonatal onset
	Chronic purulent cough with failure to thrive
	Parental smoking

Adapted from refs. *1* and *10*.

TREATMENT OPTIONS

The series of empirical therapeutic trials outlined in the previous section represent the most effective treatment strategy for chronic cough. When an efficacious regimen is found, both the underlying diagnosis and appropriate management are established. This pathophysiology-based protocol is successful in 84 to 98% of cases *(6)*, limiting the utility of nonspecific treatments. The goal of nonspecific therapy is to control rather than eliminate cough, but in fact many of the available nonspecific antitussive agents offer minimal symptomatic relief. Opiates, such as morphine, are very effective at inhibiting the cough reflex both centrally and peripherally, but their use is limited by dependence, respiratory depression, and gastrointestinal side effects at therapeutic doses. There is no strong evidence to support that low doses of weaker opiates, such as codeine, are effective at suppressing cough *(23)*. The nonsedating opiate dextromethorphan is at least as effective as codeine and is the most commonly used antitussive in the United States *(23)*. Another commonly used agent, guaifenesin, is thought to act as an "expectorant" that enhances cough effectiveness by increasing sputum volume and decreasing its viscosity. Guaifenesin has also been shown to have antitussive properties in the setting of an upper respiratory tract infection, but it did not alleviate cough in healthy volunteers *(24)*. Inhaled local anesthetics such as lignocaine delivered directly to the airways provide transient relief from cough *(25)*, but the resulting oropharyngeal anesthesia increases aspiration risk. Menthol has a mild antitussive effect *(26)* but to a lesser extent than local anesthetics. In the specific setting of postinfectious cough following a viral upper respiratory tract infection, inhaled ipratropium bromide has shown some benefit *(27)*. Based on the comprehensive diagnostic approach detailed in this chapter, the treatment of chronic cough in adults and children should always be directed at the underlying cause. For those rare circumstances in which an etiology cannot be identified, it is appropriate to start a course of nonspecific therapy with dextromethorphan, guaifenesin, and/or ipratropium.

FUTURE DIRECTIONS

In contrast to the adult literature, limited data is available regarding chronic cough in children. Further research is needed to better elucidate the prevalence pediatric asthma, PNDS, GERD, and other conditions that cause cough. This information would be very useful for the diagnostic work-up of a child with persistent cough, particularly for directing empirical trials of therapy.

The diagnosis and treatment of GERD-induced cough in both adults and children can be challenging. Although the clinical suspicion for GERD may be high, patients often have a delayed response to an empirical trial with a proton pump inhibitor. The gold standard for diagnosis is to monitor 24-hour esophageal pH, but this test is not widely used. Future research may provide a better diagnostic tool for GERD that would markedly improve current strategies for the evaluation of chronic cough.

Most nonspecific antitussives are generally regarded to be ineffective. Promising new drugs that are being developed include opiates that specifically target sensory fibers in the airways, as well as bradykinin and neurokinin receptor antagonists *(23)*. Although there is a limited role for nonspecific therapy in chronic cough, these future drugs may provide better relief for cough of unknown or untreatable etiologies.

Despite how common chronic cough occurs, work-up continues to remain somewhat challenging for the primary care provider. Newer, office-based techniques to diagnose the individual etiologies of chronic cough are in the process of development. For example, nitrous oxide is a marker of airway inflammation and may one day be able to assist with the diagnosis of asthma. Ambulatory pH monitoring can be helpful in diagnosing GERD, but is inconvenient for the patient. New techniques to diagnose GERD would also be of value. Finally, new therapeutic agents that suppress chronic cough are greatly needed. As mentioned, research into drugs that work like opiates without the addictive properties and side effects are currently underway.

REFERENCES

1. Schappert S. National ambulatory medical care survey: 1991 summary. Vital Health Stat 1994;13:1–110
2. Couch R. The common cold: control? J Infect Diseases 1984;150:167–173.
3. Philp E. Chronic cough. Am Fam Physician 1997;56:1395–1404.
4. Puchelle E, Zahm J, Girard F, et al. Mucociliary transport in vivo and in vitro. Relations to sputum properties in chronic bronchitis. Eur Respir J 1980;61:254–264.

5. Tatar M, Sant'Ambrogio G, Sant'Ambrogio F. Laryngeal and tracheobronchial cough in anesthetized dogs. J Appl Physiol 1994;76:2672–2679.
6. Irwin R, Boulet L, Cloutier M, et al. Managing cough as a defense mechanism and as a symptom. A consensus panel report of the American College of Chest Physicians. Chest 1998;114:133S–181S.
7. Curley F, Irwin R, Pratter M, et al. Cough and the common cold. Am Rev Respir Dis 1988;138:305–311.
8. Bennett W, Chapman W, Gerrity T. Ineffectiveness of cough for enhancing mucus clearance in asymptomatic smokers. Chest 1992;102:412–416.
9. Irwin R, Madison J. Primary care: the diagnosis and treatment of cough. N Engl J Med 2000;343:1715–1721.
10. de Jongste J, Shields M. Cough 2: chronic cough in children. Thorax 2003;58:998–1003.
11. Holinger L, Sanders A. Chronic cough in infants and children: an update. Laryngoscope 1991;101:596–605.
12. Irwin R, Curley F, French C. Chronic cough. The spectrum and frequency of causes, key components of the diagnostic evaluation, and outcome of specific therapy. Am Rev Respir Dis 1990;141:640–647.
13. Irwin R, Corrao W, Pratter M. Chronic persistent cough in the adult: the spectrum and frequency of causes and successful outcome of specific therapy. Am Rev Respir Dis 1981;123:413–417.
14. Irwin R, French C, Curley F, Zawacki J, Bennett F. Chronic cough due to gastroesophageal reflux. Clinical, diagnostic, and pathogenetic aspects. Chest 1993;104:1511–1517.
15. Morice A, Kastelik J. Cough 1: chronic cough in adults. Thorax 2003;58:901–907.
16. Wynder E, Kaufman P, Lesser R. A short-term follow-up study on ex-cigarette smokers: with special emphasis on persistent cough and weight gain. Am Rev Respir Dis 1967;96:645–655.
17. Israili Z, Hall W. Cough and angioneurotic edema associated with angiotensin-converting enzyme inhibitor therapy. A review of the literature and pathophysiology. Ann Intern Med 1992;117:234–242.
18. Brightling C, Ward R, Goh K, Wardlaw A, Pavord I. Eosinophilic bronchitis is an important cause of chronic cough. Am J Respir Crit Care Med 1999;160:406–410.
19. Brashers V, Haden K. Differential diagnosis of cough: focus on lung malignancy. Lippincott's Primary Care Practice. 2000;4:374–389.
20. American Thoracic Society. Diagnostic standards and classification of tuberculosis in adults and children. Am J Respir Crit Care Med 2000;161:1376–1395.
21. American Thoracic Society. Statement on sarcoidosis. Am J Respir Crit Care Med 1999;160:736–755.
22. Charlton A. Children's coughs related to parental smoking. BMJ 1984;288:1647–1649.
23. Belvisi M, Geppetti P. Cough 7: current and future drugs for the treatment of chronic cough. Thorax 2004;59:438–440.
24. Dicpinigaitis P, Gayle Y. Effect of guaifenesin on cough reflex sensitivity. Chest 2003;124:2178–2181.
25. Choudry N, Fuller R, Anderson N, Karlsson J. Separation of cough and reflex bronchoconstriction by inhaled local anaesthetics. Eur Respir J 1990;3:579–583.
26. Morice A, Marshall A, Higgins K, Grattan T. Effect of inhaled menthol on citric acid induced cough in normal subjects. Thorax 1994;49:1024–1026.
27. Holmes P, Barter C, Pierce R. Chronic persistent cough: use of ipratropium bromide in undiagnosed cases following upper respiratory tract infection. Respir Med 1992;86:425–429.

15 Chronic Obstructive Pulmonary Disease

Anna Person and Matthew L. Mintz

CONTENTS
> CASE PRESENTATION
> KEY CLINICAL QUESTIONS
> LEARNING OBJECTIVES
> BACKGROUND
> PATHOPHYSIOLOGY
> DIFFERENTIAL DIAGNOSIS
> DIAGNOSIS
> STAGING
> TREATMENT
> FUTURE DIRECTIONS
> REFERENCES

CASE PRESENTATION

A 56-year-old Caucasian male presents to his primary care physician (PCP) complaining of a 6-month history of shortness of breath when walking a few blocks or up stairs. Accompanying these symptoms are feelings of tightness in the chest and wheezing throughout the day. He also complains of a productive cough for the past several months and a recent upper respiratory infection requiring treatment with antibiotics. He denies chest pain, nausea, vomiting, diarrhea, fever, chills, recent weight loss, or syncope. He has a past medical history significant for hypertension and hyperlipidemia for which he takes hydrochlorothiazide, an angiotensin-converting enzyme inhibitor, and a statin. He has no known drug allergies, no history of asthma, and states he has mild "hay fever" each spring, for which he takes over-the-counter antihistamines. He says he generally gets two to three respiratory illnesses each winter, but states that "they're nothing

From: *Current Clinical Practice: Disorders of the Respiratory Tract:
Common Challenges in Primary Care*
By: M. L. Mintz © Humana Press, Totowa, NJ

out of the ordinary." The patient has worked for the past 35 years as a dock worker in Baltimore, MD. He lives with his wife and has four adult children. He has a 60 pack per year tobacco history, drinks two to three beers per night, and six beers on weekends. He has no history of illicit drug use. Review of systems is negative. The patient says he has recently had to miss more and more work because of his shortness of breath and limitations on his activity, and notes that he is beginning to "feel a bit depressed" about the effects his symptoms have taken on his life.

On physical exam, the patient's vital signs are normal except for a respiratory rate of 21. He is an obese white male, breathing is shallow through pursed lips on expiration, some use of sternocleidomastoid muscles with respiration. He has a broad anterior–posterior diameter of chest. There is prolonged expiration with expiratory wheezes bilaterally and decreased breath sounds throughout. Labs are unremarkable.

KEY CLINICAL QUESTIONS

1. What further testing would be required to make a diagnosis in this patient?
2. How would the PCP classify the severity of this patient?
3. What are the medications of choice for this patient?
4. Besides medications, what else can a PCP do for this patient?
5. What is the burden of disease for chronic obstructive pulmonary disease (COPD) (cost to society, patient, and so on)?

LEARNING OBJECTIVES

1. Know the classification schema for COPD as proposed by current guidelines.
2. Understand the various therapies for COPD, including the role of inhaled corticosteroids (ICS) and bronchodilators.
3. Know the pathogenesis of COPD, and understand its relationship to asthma.
4. Recognize the burden to society that chronic respiratory disorders, such as COPD, contribute.

BACKGROUND

According to the Global Initiative for Chronic Obstructive Lung Disease (GOLD) in 2001, the definition of COPD is "A disease state characterized by airflow limitation that is not fully reversible. Airflow limitation is usually both progressive and associated with an abnormal inflammatory response of the lungs to noxious particles or gases. Symptoms, functional abnormalities, and complications of COPD can all be explained on the basis of this underlying inflammation and the resulting pathology."

It is thought that data for prevalence of COPD greatly underestimates the actual effect of the disease on society. Underdiagnosis is common, because patients do not generally present to their PCPs until the course of the disease is quite advanced. Another complicating factor in diagnosing COPD is that the definition has fluctuated greatly over the last several years, and clinicians are not always aware of the latest classification or staging criteria of the disease.

According to the National Center for Health Statistics, there was an estimated 15.7 million cases of COPD in the United States in 1994 *(1)*. In 1997, COPD was named as the fourth leading cause of death in the United States, and the sixth worldwide *(2)*. In 2000, reported figures estimated that 1.5 million emergency room visits were made because of COPD. That same year, there were 726,000 hospitalizations and 119,000 deaths attributed to COPD. Eight million patients visited their PCPs with COPD-related complaints *(3)*.

These numbers, however, do not allow for an assessment of the true burden of COPD on society. The 1996 World Bank/World Health Organization Global Burden of Disease Study tried to investigate this further using a unit called the disability-adjusted life year (DALY). The DALY unit was intended to estimate years lost as a result of premature disability and the severity of such disability. The study showed that in 1990, COPD was the 12th leading cause of lost DALYs worldwide (2.1% of total lost years owing to illness). Projections were then made that indicated COPD in 2020 would jump to the fifth leading cause of lost DALYs in the world. The study concluded that the dramatic increase of COPD's effect on lives was largely owing to the increasing use of tobacco across the globe *(2)*. However, few studies quantifying COPD incidence and prevalence are available owing to the confusion in defining COPD.

Disability caused by COPD has a dramatic impact on our society economically and physically. The Department of Health and Human Services reports that in 1993 the annual monetary burden of COPD to the United States was $23.9 billion. They state that $14.7 billion of the total was a result of direct expenditures for health care services. Indirect costs were estimated at $9.2 billion, calculated from lost productivity at work, caregiver costs, and disability payments. It was calculated that each patient with COPD per year costs society $1522 *(4)*. The economic burden is just one of the ways COPD weighs heavily on our society, but it is clearly a significant load to carry.

PATHOPHYSIOLOGY

Much has been learned about the pathophysiology of COPD, including its relationship to other airway diseases. As a result of these discoveries, it is thought that perhaps some of these diseases may no longer represent discrete entities, but instead may fall on a continuum. Where each disease process may fall on the continuum depends on the pathological changes inherent in the disease. The pathological changes, in turn, lead to physiological changes. It is the physiological changes of COPD, such as mucus production and airflow limitation (not fully reversible), that cause the symptomatology that often brings patients to their PCP.

COPD, as it is newly defined, is a disease characterized by inflammatory changes throughout the airways and lung parenchyma in response to noxious particles or gases (usually tobacco smoke). The inflammation is stimulated by a number of cells present at increased levels in patients with COPD. Acute exacerbations generally correspond with high levels of neutrophils, which secrete proteinases that possibly contribute to the chronic secretion of mucus and destruction of lung parenchyma. It is thought that macrophages augment the inflammatory process by releasing tumor necrosis factor-α, interleukin-8, and leukotrienes *(5)*. Patients may also have eosinophils present in small and large airways, but generally only during acute exacerbations *(6)*.

In addition to the effects of inflammation in COPD, the pathological changes found are also thought to be owing to an imbalance of proteinases and antiproteinases. This is shown in the hereditary α-1-antitrypsin defeciency. Without the inhibition of proteinases that α-1-antitrypsin provides, there is destruction of aleveolar walls and other evidence of lung parenchymal changes that are characteristic of emphysema. Oxidative stress is thought to add to this imbalance and promote inflammation *(7)*.

The hallmarks of COPD include hypersecretion of mucus and airflow limitation. The production of mucus and sputum is thought to be a result of hypertrophy of the mucus-secreting glands as mediated by leukotrienes and proteinases. Mucociliary clearance of debris is also limited because of changes induced in the epithelial cells. Airflow limitation is partly reversible, but it does have an irreversible component. It is thought that the irreversible changes are a result of remodeling of the smaller airways (<2 mm in diameter) *(8)*. The inflammation and remodeling of these airways lead to a significant increase in peripheral airway resistance. Additionally, the destruction of alveoli and other parts of lung parenchyma cause decreased elastic recoil of the lung, contributing further to the dysfunction of the lung and airways.

All of these changes contribute to another component of COPD—decreased proficiency of gas exchange because of a mismatch of ventilation and perfusion. In the areas of airway remodeling or lung parenchymal destruction, shunting occurs and hypoxemia is induced as a result of fewer functioning gas-exchange units. The vasoconstriction increases pulmonary artery pressures that, in advanced disease, can lead to pulmonary hypertension or cor pulmonale *(9)*.

Although they share many of the same inflammatory mediators, COPD differs from asthma in several ways. There are some very clear differences in pathology at the microscopic level. The inflammatory cells in COPD are mostly macrophages, neutrophils, and $CD8^+$ T-lymphocytes, whereas asthma is characterized by eosinophils and $CD4^+$ lymphocytes. The clinical picture and patient profile of those with asthma and COPD differ, as do responses to treatment. However, a theory proposed originally in 1961 called the Dutch hypothesis, argues for the consideration of asthma and COPD as two diseases on the same continuum. It is usually considered true that the airway obstruction in COPD is irreversible, whereas asthma's obstruction may be reversed. As we learn more about the two diseases, however, there is evidence that many people with asthma may have at least some irreversible component to their disease, and that the reversibility of airflow obstruction following bronchodilator use in COPD demonstrates that the disease shares some similarities with asthma. The Dutch hypothesis focuses on the similarities instead of the differences of asthma and COPD, and has three components *(10)*:

1. Various forms of obstructive lung disease have overlapping clinical features.
2. One form of obstructive lung disease may evolve into another.
3. The development of obstructive lung disease is based on allergy (i.e., inflammation), bronchiohyperesponsiveness, and endogenous factors determined by heredity, but is modulated by exogenous factors (e.g., allergens, infections, smoking, pollution, and age).

Despite disagreement in the scientific community about these tenets, the idea that asthma and COPD share similarities is again being revisited. The overlap between these two diseases is yet another reason why early and appropriate diagnosis and treatment of COPD is such a challenge to PCPs.

DIFFERENTIAL DIAGNOSIS

The differential diagnosis for COPD is broad and includes asthma, chronic bronchitis, emphysema, community acquired pneumonia, cystic fibrosis, congestive heart failure, bronchiectasis, tuberculosis, asbestosis, and many others. Many of the diseases included in the differential for COPD fall into the category of obstructive lung disorders. Obstructive lung disorders are defined by a reduced ratio of forced expiratory volume in 1 second to forced vital capacity (FEV_1:FVC); the degree of reduction estimates the severity of the disease. This is opposed to restrictive airway disorders, which are known for FEV_1:FVC ratios that are normal or increased, because of lung stiffness or chest wall stiffness. Restrictive ventilatory defects can be noted by a reduction in vital capacity and total lung capacity.

Chronic bronchitis and emphysema are classic obstructive disorders. Chronic bronchitis is defined by sputum production for at least 3 months a year for at least 2 consecutive years. It is characterized by inflammation of the bronchi and hypersecretion of mucus. Emphysema, on the other hand, consists of alveolar destruction and disrupted air exchange. Although these two diseases may have very different radiographic presentations, they often co-exist.

Other etiologies for a patient's symptoms must also be explored. Sputum cultures and Gram stains as well as chest X-rays can identify pneumonia. Tuberculosis must be explored in patients who are homeless, imprisoned, immigrants, or in people who may have contact with these populations. Associated symptoms and an echocardiogram may reveal congestive heart failure. Work and home conditions must be explored for possible exposures to asbestos or other chemicals. History will often provide the appropriate clues for a diagnosis of COPD or another etiology for a patient's presentation.

DIAGNOSIS

In the past, identifying COPD has centered around the diagnosis of either emphysema or chronic bronchitis. The global initiative for COPD has made the diagnostic criteria more broad.

The GOLD guidelines suggest that "a diagnosis of COPD should be considered in any patient who has cough, sputum production, or dyspnea, and/or a history of exposure to the risk factors of the disease," the most common being tobacco smoke. The use of spirometry is necessary, and is considered the gold standard. Values of $FEV_1:FVC$ less than 70% of predicted and FEV_1 less than 80% of predicted indicate that there is significant airflow limitation that is obstructive in nature *(11)*. COPD is consistent with an increased total lung capacity and residual capacity because of the increased air trapping in the lungs. However, there is a decrease in vital capacity, and the effectiveness of alveoli gas exchange, measured with carbon dioxide, is decreased. This information, combined with the clinical picture of a patient who is older, most likely has a history of smoking (usually at least a 20 pack-year history), who complains of shortness of breath and sputum production, should lead to a tentative diagnosis of COPD. Hemoptysis may occur, and the clinician should perform a work-up for carcinoma if there is high clinical suspicion. During an acute exacerbation a patient may present to his or her physician with fever, chills, and purulent sputum production. Patients may have been told at some point that they have asthma. If so, it is important to ascertain if the patient's findings on spirometry fail to normalize after bronchodialator use, a finding that would point away from asthma as a diagnosis. All of this is information that should be obtained during the history, with a special focus on how symptoms have affected the patient's life.

On physical exam, a patient may show visible work of breathing, with the use of accessory muscles of respiration. They may be breathing at a rapid rate. The anterior–posterior diameter of the chest may be increased; the patient may have a so-called "barrel chest." In advanced disease, pursed lip breathing may be evident, in an attempt to create the positive pressure needed to keep alveoli open as long as possible. On auscultation, the physician may hear expiratory wheezes or rhonchi *(12)*. As COPD progresses, the most evident finding on auscultation

Table 1
Pulmonary Function Values and Staging

Stage 0	At risk; normal lung function.
Stage I	Mild COPD; FEV_1:FVC less than 70% predicted. FEV_1 more than 80% predicted.
Stage II	Moderate COPD; FEV_1 30–80% predicted.
Stage III	Severe COPD; FEV_1 less than 30% predicted.

COPD, chronic obstructive pulmonary disease; FEV_1, forced expiratory volume in 1 second; FVC, forced vital capacity.

of chest is the striking lack of air movement. Heart sounds may be displaced medially. End-stage findings include evidence of cyanosis, right heart failure, hepatomegaly, jugular vein distension, and even asterixis because of severe carbon dioxide retention. However, the physician cannot base a diagnosis of COPD on physical exam findings alone *(13)*.

The physical exam and spirometry findings must be correlated with radiographic findings. Chest X-rays may show hyperlucent, hyperexpanded lungs, with flattened diaphragms. Computed tomography functions only in identifying panacinar from centrilobar emphysema, and is generally not used. Sleep studies, α-1-antitrypsin deficiency screening, and routine arterial blood gas measurements should be done at the discretion of the physician.

STAGING

Once a diagnosis is established, it is crucial to determine the stage of the patient's COPD. The global initiative for COPD has created criteria by which to stage a patient's disease and use as a way to measure the patient's progression and decide what treatment is necessary (Table 1).

The stages created are stages 0 to III *(14)*. Stage 0 indicates that a patient still has normal lung function, but is at risk for COPD. The most likely risk factor is a history of tobacco use, but could include genetic predisposition owing to α-1-antitrypsin deficiency or other factors. The patient at this stage may start to develop a chronic cough or may begin producing sputum. He or she may attribute this to tobacco use, and think it is "normal." The patient may not realize that he or she is in fact in the beginning stage of a very progressive and debilitating disease.

Stage I indicates that the patient suffers from mild COPD. This criterion carries with it a specific value on lung function tests, emphasizing the importance of spirometry when treating a patient with COPD. The airflow limitation is mild at this time, and again, most patients will not express concern to their physician.

Table 2
Strategies to Help the Patient Willing to Quit Smoking

ASK	Systematically identify all tobacco users at every visit.
ADVISE	Strongly urge all tobacco users to quit.
ASSESS	Determine willingness to make a quit attempt.
ASSIST	Aid the patient in quitting.
ARRANGE	Schedule follow-up contact.

It is often very difficult for clinicians to diagnose COPD at this stage, in part because few patients present to the office until symptoms are much worse.

Stage II is moderate COPD. Moderate disease denotes more advanced airflow limitation, and patients will thus begin to experience the symptoms such as dyspnea on exertion that will likely bring them to a physician. Exacerbations are characterized by FEV_1 less than 50% predicted.

Stage III is severe, or end-stage, COPD. A patient's activities of daily living will be markedly impaired, and he or she may have signs of cor pulmonale or frank respiratory failure. Mortality from acute exacerbations at this stage is high—approximately 10% if admitted to the hospital. Once a patient reaches stage III disease the 1-year mortality ranges from 40 to 59% *(15)*.

TREATMENT

Smoking Cessation

The first step in management of a patient with COPD should be to advise smoking cessation. Many physicians may skip this step altogether, figuring that the patient "would never quit anyway." In fact, one large study has shown that if education on smoking cessation is provided to the patient on a consistent basis, a full 25% may be able to quit and continue to abstain on a long-term basis *(16)*. It is of paramount importance to have a conversation with each patient regarding a plan for smoking cessation, because it is the single most beneficial thing they can do to limit airflow obstruction and progression of disease *(17)*. The physician can follow the "ask, advise, assess, assist, arrange" method (Table 2). In routine office visits for patients who smoke without COPD it is also important to emphasize the risk of developing COPD or some degree of airflow impairment. Nonsmokers will have a rate of decline in FEV_1 of 30 mL per year, whereas smokers average an annual decline in FEV_1 of 60 mL per year *(18)*. As the GOLD guidelines state, "The common statement that only 15 to 20% of smokers develop clinically significant COPD is misleading. A much higher proportion develop abnormal lung function at some point if they continue to smoke" *(19)*.

Medications

There are several pharmacological treatment agents at the physician's disposal. The very important point about all these medications is that they only act to control a patient's symptoms—there is no evidence that these agents modify the course of the disease *(16,20)*. Additionally, given that lung function is primarily irreversible in COPD, changes in FEV_1 and other parameters are limited, even in agents that are effective. Thus, other markers in addition to lung function, such as quality of life and decreases in exacerbations must be used to determine benefit. There are a number of options to treat the symptoms of COPD, and according to the GOLD guidelines, each agent should be added in a stepwise increase in treatment as needed (Table 3).

Bronchodilators (β2-agonists, anticholinergics, and theophylline) are the mainstay of treatment. They are given on a regular basis, with special attention paid to teaching the patient how to use the metered dose inhaler, if necessary. Short- or long-acting β2-agonists may be used with equal effectiveness; one must consider compliance and cost when choosing an agent. Both salmeterol (at 50 µg bid) and an inhaled anticholinergic (such as ipratropium qid) have been shown to improve a patient's quality of life dramatically *(21)*. Theophylline and other methylxanthines do not have the data behind it as do the β2-agonists and anticholinergics. The risk of sometimes fatal cardiac arrythmias has limited their use. Seizures are also an uncommon, but reported, side effect. Theophylline is sometimes used in combination with a β-agonist and an anticholinergic, although better studied and more effective is the combination of a β2-agonist and an anticholinergic (ipratropium) alone. This regimen has been shown to produce greater improvements on lung function tests than either drug used on its own *(22)*.

A new long-acting anticholingeric medication, tiotropium, is a recently developed agent that can be used with once-a-day dosing. Side effects are similar to ipatropium and salmeterol, with dry mouth being the most common complaint. In a randomized, double-blind, multicenter study testing tiotropium versus salmeterol in the treatment of stable COPD, tiotropium appeared superior. Patients noted better quality of life, better lung function on spirometry, and improved dyspnea *(23)*. Another large study was done comparing tiotropium with ipratropium, showing tiotropium again to have better outcomes in FEV_1 and peak expiratory flow measurements *(24)*. Both studies recommended tiotropium as first-line therapies for COPD.

The role of corticosteroids depends on the patient's stage of severity as well as whether or not the patient is stable or having an acute exacerbation. Stable COPD and corticosteroid treatment is an area of rigorous research in recent years. The results of such studies have been mixed. The majority of studies conclude that oral steroids are not recommended for long-term use owing to side effects of myopathy. It was once thought that a short course of oral corticoster-

Table 3
Therapy at Each Stage of COPD

Stage	Characteristics	Recommended treatment
All		Avoidance of risk factors Influenza vaccine
0: At risk	Cough, sputum Normal spirometry Exposure to risk factors	
I: Mild COPD	FEV_1:FVC less than 70% FEV_1 more than 80% predicted With or without symptoms	Short-acting bronchodilator when needed
II: Moderate COPD	IIA: FEV_1:FVC less than 70% 50% less than FEV_1 less than 80% With or without symptoms	Regular treatment with one or more bronchodilators Rehabilitation Inhaled corticosteroids if significant symptoms and lung function response
	IIB: FEV_1:FVC less than 70% 30% less than FEV_1 less than 50% With or without symptoms	Regular treatment with one or more bronchodilators Rehabilitation Inhaled corticosteroids if significant symptoms and lung function response
III: Severe COPD	FEV_1:FVC less than 70% FEV_1 less than 30% or presence or respiratory failure or right heart failure	Regular treatment with one or more bronchodilators Rehabilitation Inhaled corticosteroids if significant symptoms and lung function response Treatment of complications Long-term oxygen therapy

COPD, chronic obstructive pulmonary disease; FEV_1, forced expiratory volume in 1 second; FVC, forced vital capacity.
Adapted from GOLD guidelines.

oids would be a good predictor for a patient's response to ICS. The data on this, however, is inconclusive and it is not currently recommended that a patient be placed on a short course of oral steroids before initiation of inhaled steroid treatment *(25)*.

Many studies have investigated the role of ICS treatment with varying results. Information that has been consistent in these trials is that there are two indications for their use: only use ICS in patients who are symptomatic and who show an improvement on lung function tests by spirometry after use and use in patients who have an FEV_1 less than 50% of predicted and repeated exacerbations *(26)*. These criteria remain under investigation, and it remains to be seen if they will continue to be the most appropriate conditions under which ICS should be used. The use of ICS in stable COPD has been shown to slow the decline in FEV_1. However, the average decline obtained by ICS is still less than that which can be achieved by smoking cessation, which can slow the rate of deterioration by 50% *(18)*.

ICS may be best used to improve quality of life. Many physicians will add ICS to a patient's regimen to maximize the patient's ability to live a regular life and perform his or her activities of daily living. However, it has been shown in many studies that ICS do not decrease airway inflammation in COPD, and in four recent clinical trials ICS have shown no benefit in this capacity against placebo. Yet, some of those same studies demonstrated that treatment with ICS alleviated patient's symptoms, reduced the frequency of exacerbations, and improved health status. Therefore, adherence to the GOLD guideline critieria may not be necessary if there is suspicion that a patient's life may be improved with the addition of these drugs.

Given all these pharmacological options, the order in which to use them may be overwhelming. According to one treatment algorithm, the most common strategy is to begin with either a long-acting anticholinergic or β-agonist. Tiotropium bromide, an anticholinergic, has a duration of action of more than 24 hours; the β-agonists formoterol fumarate and salmeterol xinafoate both act for 8 to 12 hours *(27)*. A short-acting bronchodilator must be prescribed for relief of acute symptoms. Then, if a single long-acting bronchodilator does not result in sufficient symptomatic relief, combination therapy of a long-acting β-agonist and an anticholingeric, such as albuterol and ipratroprium, are used. Theophylline may be considered if further relief is needed, although vigilance for possible adverse drug reactions is necessary. Following failure of these regimens, most clinicians will initiate therapy with a long-acting β-agonist and ICS at that time.

Managing exacerbations requires different tactics. The most common cause of such exacerbations are pollution-related or an infection of the airways. Onethird of the time a source will not be identified. Patients will present with complaints of shortness of breath, purulent sputum, and increase in cough. The significance of the exacerbation depends on the patient's stage of disease before the exacerbation. To assess severity it is crucial to take a thorough history of present illness, perform lung function tests, arterial blood gases, and chest X-rays. An FEV_1 less than 1 L is indicative of a severe exacerbation unless the patient has had long-term severe disease *(28)*. On arterial blood gas measurement, a PaO_2 less than 50 mmHg, a $PaCO_2$ more than 70 mmHg, and a pH less than 7.3 can indicate a life-threatening state *(29)*.

Table 4
Criteria for Admission to Hospital

Indications for hospital assessment or admission for acute exacerbations of COPD

Marked increase in intensity of symptoms, such as development of resting dyspnea
Severe background COPD
Onset of new physical signs (cyanosis, peripheral edema)
Failure of exacerbation to respond to initial medical management
Significant comorbidities
Newly occurring arrhythmias
Diagnostic uncertainty
Older age
Insufficient home support

COPD, chronic obstructive pulmonary disease.
Adapted from GOLD guidelines.

Pharmacological treatment of exacerbations depends on the regimen a patient is already on. The patient should continue bronchodilator use, and add an anticholinergic or other agent until improvement. Nebulizer treatments can be supplemented, if necessary. There is widespread agreement that corticosteroids are beneficial in treating exacerbations. They show the most efficacy when administered systemically, and the GOLD guidelines suggest prednisone at 40 mg per day for 10 days. Admit to the hospital for closer monitoring if indicated (*see* Table 4). For those with severe COPD and dangerous exacerbations, noninvasive intermittent positive pressure ventilationis known to be very successful at increasing pH, reducing $PaCO_2$, decreasing intubation rates, and length of hospital stay *(30)*.

Antibiotics play an important role in the treatment of acute exacerbations. One large clinical trial showed that when antibiotics were used for an exacerbation, symptoms resolved within 21 days in 68% of the patients *(31)*. For those who received placebo, symptoms resolved in that same time period in only 55%. The most common pathogens are *Streptococcus pneumonia*, *Moraxella catarrhalis*, and *Haemophilus influenzae*. There is a tendency to initiate treatment with broad-spectrum antibiotics, however, no studies have shown these to be more beneficial than more narrow-spectrum drugs such as trimethoprim-sulfamethoxazole, doxycycline, or amoxicillin. Additionally, the preservation of the broader spectrum antibiotics prevents resistance and affords physicians other drug options down the line, should they prove necessary. Both Gram stain and sputum culture are usually not done unless a patient does not respond to initial empirical therapy. Most clinicians choose to treat for 5 to 10 days.

Oxygen therapy is a mainstay in the treatment of acute exacerbations of COPD. It is thought that oxygen saturation levels should be maintained from 90 to 92% to ensure optimal hemoglobin saturation. Higher levels of saturation are not necessary, and in fact may be detrimental to those who are "CO_2 retainers," or those for whom some degree of hypercapnia drives respiration. Long-term oxygen therapy (>15 hours per day), although costly, has been shown in at least two large trials to reduce mortality and improve quality of life in patients with severe COPD. It has not been demonstrated that long-term use of oxygen is beneficial in patients with partial pressure of arterial oxygen values of less than 55 mmHg *(32)*. Because of its costliness, it is important to determine who would benefit from continuous oxygen therapy based on severity of hypoxemia.

Another nonpharmacological intervention that may be helpful is pulmonary rehabilitation. Generally consisting of lower and upper extremity exercise conditioning, breathing retraining, education, and psychosocial support, pulmonary rehabilitation has been shown by the GOLD guidelines to have several benefits in COPD. These include improving exercise capacity, reducing breathlessness, and reducing the number of hospitalizations *(30)*. It has also been shown to prolong survival and assist with the depression and anxiety that often accompanies living with a chronic and debilitating illness.

FUTURE DIRECTIONS

As the knowledge about the pathophysiology of COPD grows, new pharmacological agents are being developed in accordance with findings about how the disease progresses. One area of new research continues to be about the definition of COPD itself. Its relationship to asthma and other airway diseases is incompletely understood, as is its natural progression. The clearer the picture of COPD as a disease, the better researchers and clinicians are able to combat it. The definition, staging criteria, and treatments put forth by the GOLD guidelines will need to be amended as new discoveries engender yet another concept of COPD.

Pharmacologically, there is clearly an urgent need for agents that actually slow or halt the destruction of lung airways and parenchyma, instead of simply managing symptoms. Possible areas of research include the use of antioxidants, because oxidative stress is found to be one of the components of the disease. The imbalance of proteinases and antiproteinases has been studied in detail, and many of the enzymes responsible for alveolar damage have been identified. Proteinase inhibitors may one day be used as prevention or treatment of this type of lung destruction. The hypersecretion of mucus is another topic of interest, and there have been some mucoregulatory drugs in development, such as tackykinin antatgonists and mucin gene suppressors. There is even investigation into repair of destroyed alveoli through retinoic acids that have reversed elastase-induced damage in mice. Hepatocyte growth factor is used to stimulate alveoli growth in the fetus, and there is question as to how this might translate into an effective therapy in patients with COPD *(33)*. Phosphodiesterase 4 inhibitors, which act to inhibit neutrophil-mediated inflammation, have been under investigation for some time. Many of these trials have shown improvement in symptoms and quality of life for patients with COPD, although side effects, such as nausea, may slow the introduction of this class of drugs. The combination of budesonide and formoterol has been shown to reduce severe exacerbations in asthma by 40% in one study *(34)*; its use in COPD is also being investigated.

However, much of the investigation that needs to be done regarding COPD is not pharmacological in nature. What is needed is an assessment of the natural progression of the disease over time and across the globe. Accurate information on the true cost (economic and societal) of COPD needs to be ascertained. Data on the methods and effectiveness of screening and primary prevention of COPD must be available for PCPs so they can incorporate this into daily practice. A protocol on how to educate patients about COPD is needed. How can education best help with compliance, coping with the illness, and reducing the number and frequency of acute exacerbations? Finally, although tobacco smoke is known to be the most important risk factor for COPD, others must be identified. As COPD is poised to affect more people than ever on a national and global scale, we must understand the role that our changing world might play in reducing the scope of this disease.

REFERENCES

1. Singh GK, Matthews TJ, Clarke SC. Annual summary of births, marriages, divorces, and deaths: United States, 1994. Monthly Vital Statistics Report 43(13). National Center for Health Statistics, Hyattsville, MD: 1994.
2. Murray CJL, Lopez AD. The global burden of disease: a comprehensive assessment of mortality and disability from diseases, injuries and risk factors in 1990 and projected to 2020. Harvard University Press, Cambridge, MA: 1996.
3. Mannino DM. Chronic obstructive pulmonary disease surveillance—United States, 1971–2000. MMWR Surveill Summ 2002;51:1.
4. National Heart, Lung, and Blood Institute. Morbidity mortality: chartbook on cardiovascular, lung, and blood diseases. US Department of Health and Human Services, Public Health Service, National Institutes of Health, Bethesda, MD, 1998.
5. Finkelstein R, Fraser RS, Ghezzo H, Cosio MG. Alveolar inflammation and its relation to emphysema in smokers. Am J Respir Crit Care Med 1995;152:1666.
6. Saetta M, Di Stefano A, Maestrelli P, et al. Airway eosinophilia in chronic bronchitis during exacerbations. Am J Respir Crit Care Med 1994;150:1646–1652.
7. Carp H, Miller F, Holdal JR, Janoff A. Potential mechanism of emphysema: alpha 1-proteinase inhibitor recovered from lungs of cigarette smokers contains oxidized methionine and has decreased elastase inhibitory capacity. Pro Nat Acad Sci USA 1982;126:2041–2045.
8. Hogg JC, Macklem PT, Thurlbeck WM. Site and nature of airway obstruction in chronic obstructive lung disease. N Engl J Med 1968;278:1355–1360.

9. MacNee W. Pathophysiology of cor pulmonale in chronic obstructive pulmonary disease. Part two. Am J Respir Crit Care Med 1994;150:1158.
10. Bleecker E. Similarities and differences in asthma and COPD: the Dutch hypothesis. Chest 2004;126:93S–95S.
11. Global strategy for the diagnosis, management, and prevention of chronic obstructive pulmonary disease, Executive Summary. Global Initiative for Chronic Obstructive Lung Disease (GOLD) National Heart, Lung, and Blood Institute (US), Federal Government Agency (US) World Health Organization, International Agency. 2001 (revised 2005), section 3, pp. 6–8.
12. Kanner RE, Connett JE, et al. Effects of randomized assignment to a smoking cessation intervention and changes in smoking habits on respiratory symptoms in smokers with early chronic pulmonary disease: the Lung Health Study. Am J Med 1999;106:410–416.
13. Badgett RG, et al. Can moderate chronic obstructive pulmonary disease be diagnosed by historical and physical findings alone? Am J Med 1993;94:188–196.
14. Pauwels RA, Buist AS, Ma P, Jenkins CR, Hurd Ss, GOLD Scientific Committee. Global strategy for the diagnosis, management, and prevention of chronic obstructive pulmonary disease: National Heart, Lung, and Blood Institute and World Health Organization Global Initiative for Chronic Obstructive Lung Disease (GOLD): executive summary. Respir Care 2001;46:798–825.
15. Seneff MG, Wagner DP, Wagner RP, Zimmerman JE, Kraus WA. Hospital and 1 year survival of patients admitted to intensive care units with acute exacerbation of chronic obstructive pulmonary disease. JAMA 1995;274:1852–1857.
16. Anthonisen NR, Connett JE, Kiley JP, et al. Effects of smoking intervention and the use of an inhaled anticholinergic bronchodilator on the rate of decline of FEV1. The Lung Health Study. JAMA 1994;272:1497–1505.
17. Stewart MA. Effective physician-patient communication and health outcomes: a review. CMAJ 1995;152:1423.
18. Sutherland ER. Inhaled corticosteroids reduce the progression of airflow limitation in chronic obstructive pulmonary disease: a meta-analysis. Thorax 2003;58:937.
19. Global strategy for the diagnosis, management,a nd prevention of chronic obstructive pulmonary disease, Executive Summary. Global Initiative for Chronic Obstructive Lung Diesease (GOLD) National Heart, Lung, and Blood Institute (US), Federal Government Agency (US) World Health Organization, International Agency. 2001 (revised 2005), section 1, pp. 2–4.
20. Vestbo J, et al. Long-term effect of inhaled budesonide in mild and moderate chronic obstructive pulmonary disease: a randomized controlled trial. Lancet 1999;353:1819–1823.
21. Jones PW, et al. Quality of life changes in COPD patients treated with salmeterol. Am J Respir Crit Care Med 1997;155:1283–1289.
22. In chronic obstructive pulmonary disease, a combination of ipratropium and albuterol is more effective than either agent alone. An 85-day multicenter trial. COMBIVENT Inhalational Aerosol Study Group. Chest 1994;105:1411.
23. Donohue JF, van Noord JA, Batemen ED, et al. A 6-month, placebo-controlled study comparing lung function and health status changes in COPD patients treated with tiotropium or salmeterol. Chest 2002;122:47–55.
24. Van Noord JA, Bantje TA, Eland ME, Korducki L, Cornelissen PJ. A randomized controlled comparison of tiotropium and ipratropium in the treatment of chronic obstructive pulmonary disease. Thorax 2000;55:289–294.
25. Senderovitz T, Vestbo J, Frandsen J, et al. Steroid reversibility test followed by inhaled budesonide or placebo in outpatients with stable chronic obstructive pulmonary disease. The Danish Society of Respiratory Medicine. Respir Med 1999;93:715–718.

26. Global strategy for the diagnosis, management, and prevention of chronic obstructive pulmonary disease, Executive Summary. Global Initiative for Chronic Obstructive Lung Disease (GOLD) National Heart, Lung, and Blood Institute (US), Federal Government Agency (US) Health Organization, International Agency. 2001 (revised 2005), section 3, pp. 11–16.
27. Sutherland ER. Inhaled corticosteroids reduce the progression of airflow limitation in chronic obstructive pulmonary disease: a meta-analysis. Thorax 2003;58:937.
28. Emerman CL. Use of peak expiratory flow rate in emergency department evaluation of acute exacerbation of chronic obstructive pulmonary disease. Ann Emer Med 1996;27:159.
29. Emerman CL. Relationship between arterial blood gases and spirometry in acute exacerbations of chronic obstructive pulmonary disease. Ann Emer Med 1989;18:523.
30. Clinical indications for noninvasive positive pressure ventilation in chronic respiratory failure due to restrictive lung disease, COPD, and nocturnal hypoventilation—a consensus conference report. Chest 1999;116:521.
31. Stoller JK. Acute exacerbations of chronic obstructive pulmonary Disease. N Engl J Med 2002;346;13.
32. Barnes PJ. Chronic Obstructive Pulmonary Disease. N Engl J Med 2000;343:4.
33. Global strategy for the diagnosis, management, and prevention of chronic obstructive pulmonary disease, Executive Summary. Global Initiative for Chronic Obstructive Lung Disease (GOLD) National Heart, Lung, and Blood Institute (US), Federal Government Agency (US) World Health Organization, International Agency. 2001 (revised 2005), section 4, p. 21.
34. Pauwels RA. Effects of inhaled formoterol and budesonide on exacerbations of asthma. N Engl J Med 1997:337:1405.

16 Lung Cancer

Mohammad A. Raza and Matthew L. Mintz

CONTENTS

　　CASE PRESENTATION
　　KEY CLINICAL QUESTIONS
　　LEARNING OBJECTIVES
　　EPIDEMIOLOGY
　　PATHOGENESIS
　　DIFFERENTIAL DIAGNOSIS
　　MANAGEMENT
　　PREVENTION
　　FUTURE DIRECTIONS
　　REFERENCES

CASE PRESENTATION

Mrs. J., a 58-year-old woman, views herself as health conscious. After smoking for 30 years, she quit smoking "cold turkey" almost 4 years ago. She sees her primary care physician (PCP) annually for a complete physical. During her most recent physical, Mrs. J. mentioned to her PCP that she has had a mild but persistent cough for the past 6 months and has lost 10 lb. over the last month. After further questioning, Mrs. J. reports that she occasionally sees red streaks in her sputum but this never lasts more than 2 to 3 days at a time. She attributes the coughing to dry air in her home. Her PCP orders a chest X-ray, which is remarkable for a suspicious spot on the right lung. Mrs. J. then undergoes chest computed tomography (CT) imaging, which shows a probable tumor with accompanying lympadenopathy. Mrs. J. undergoes a needle biopsy, which confirms a diagnosis of small-cell lung cancer (SCLC).

From: *Current Clinical Practice: Disorders of the Respiratory Tract:
Common Challenges in Primary Care*
By: M. L. Mintz © Humana Press, Totowa, NJ

KEY CLINICAL QUESTIONS

1. What is the next step in the work-up for this patient?
2. What is the likelihood that this patient will have complications, such as hypercalcemia, caused by tumor-secreted parathyroid hormone analog?
3. What is the 5-year survival rate among patients with SCLC?
4. How should PCPs screen current or former smokers for lung cancer?

LEARNING OBJECTIVES

1. Become familiar with the incidence of lung cancer in the United States and worldwide.
2. Understand the relationship between lung cancer and smoking.
3. Adopt appropriate screening recommendations for lung cancer.
4. Recognize the clinical presentation of a patient with lung cancer.
5. Become familiar with the evaluation of lung nodule discovered on chest X-ray.

EPIDEMIOLOGY

Lung cancer is a significant public health problem and is of particular interest to primary care physicians because smoking, major attributable cause, is a modifiable risk factor. Despite the fact that the death rate from lung cancer has decreased modestly in recent years, the annual incidence of lung cancer, both in the United States and worldwide, continues to rise. As a result, lung cancer is now the leading cause of cancer death in both men and women. According to estimates by the American Cancer Society, there were approximately 160,000 deaths owing to lung cancer in the United States in 2004 *(1)*. This is more than the combined mortality from colorectal, breast, and prostate cancer, which in 2004 was estimated to be approximately 125,000 deaths. Bronchogenic carcinoma, the focus of this chapter, is by far the most common form of lung cancer and is responsible for approximately 1 million deaths worldwide each year. This includes one-third of all cancer-related deaths in men and approximately 5 to 10% of all cancer deaths in women. As population size increases and ages, it is likely that the number of new lung cancer cases per year will continue to rise. Of all lung cancers, 35 to 40% are adenocarcinoma, 20 to 30% are squamous cell carcinoma, 10% are large carcinoma, and 15 to 20% are SCLC. Bronchogenic carcinoma occurs more often in men than women, but studies have shown that women are at a higher risk for developing lung cancer than men when data is adjusted for amount of tobacco exposure. Furthermore, women develop adenocarcinoma disproportionately to men *(2)*.

PATHOGENESIS

Types

Bronchogenic carcinoma is divided into two groups: non-small cell lung cancer (NSCLC) and SCLC. NSCLC is further categorized as adenocarcinoma, squamous cell carcinoma, and large cell carcinoma. SCLC is further categorized as oat cell, mixed cell, intermediate, and undifferentiated carcinoma. Approximately 75% of all lung cancers represent NSCLC. Classification of primary malignant tumors of the lung, specifically bronchogenic carcinomas, is extremely useful because the various neoplastic diseases in a subgroup share a similar natural history, prognosis, and expected response to therapy. For example, the cancers grouped as NSCLC have different clinical presentations and histopathologies, but share similar prognoses and treatment approaches. SCLC, on the other hand, has a markedly different prognosis and treatment approach than NSCLC.

Neoplastic diseases of the lung, specifically malignant neoplasms, most commonly arise in response to carcinogenic insult or irritation. The mucosal lining of the lung parenchyma is vulnerable to chemical injury. Cigarette smoke alone has been found to contain more than 1000 chemical entities, many of which can initiate and/or promote carcinogensis. A complex process initiated by exposure to carcinogens results in a transformation of normal mucosal cells into malignant cells. There are many different theories that explain how this transformation occurs, most revolving around genetic alteration caused by carcinogens, such as activation and amplication of oncogenes and inactivation of tumor suppressor genes, and several investigations have found that most pulmonary neoplastic lesions contain many of these genetic alterations. Enzopyrene from tobacco smoke has been shown to cause inactivation of *p53*, one of the most commonly inactivated tumor suppressor genes in bronchogenic carcinoma *(3)*. The molecular pathogenesis of NSCLC is believed to be mutations in the *ras* oncogenes and, to a lesser extent, aberrant anti-apoptotic pathways and mutations causing abnormal activation of epithelial growth factor receptor *(4,5)*.

Adenocarcinomas are the most common lung cancers among nonsmokers and include bronchial-derived adenocarcinoma and bronchioalveolar carcinoma. The difference between these two subtypes of adenocarcinomas, as their names imply, is the specific epithelial location from which the lesions arise. These are usually slower growing as compared with other forms of NSCLC and tend to be peripherally located in the lung. Histologically, adenocarcinomas range from well-differentiated glandular structures to poorly differentiated papillary lesions and masses.

Squamous cell carcinoma, also known as epidermoid carcinoma because its keratin-containing structure resembles skin, follows adenocarcinoma as the second most common bronchogenic carcinoma. Whereas adenocarcinoma is the type of NSCLC found in nonsmokers and women, squamous cell carcinoma is often found in men with a long history of smoking. Recent evidence suggests that human papillomavirus may have an etiological role in squamous cell lung cancer, however, further investigation is necessary *(6)*. Squamous cell carcinoma arises in a central area (perihilar), such as the larger bronchi, and grows rapidly. Squamous cell carcinomas are encountered in different stages of differentiation, ranging from keratin- and intercellular bridge-containing structures to poorly differentiated masses.

Large cell carcinoma is so named because relative tumor cell size is larger than those encountered with other types of NSCLC. These tumors contain anaplastic cells and are poorly differentiated. Grossly, the tumors can be found peripherally or centrally in the lung. Large cell carcinomas include clear cell carcinoma and giant cell carcinoma, with the latter being notable for extremely poor survival resulting from the rapid rate of disease progression.

Small cell carcinoma is a high malignant neoplasm that arises from specialized neuroendocrine bronchial epithelial cells called Kulchitsky's (argentaffin) cells. It is extremely rare for SCLC to occur in nonsmokers. The subtypes of SCLC are oat cell, intermediate cell, mixed, and undifferentiated. SCLC characteristically arises in central regions of the lung and is staged differently than NSCLC because of its highly metastatic nature. Histologically, SCLC cells are small with scant cytoplasm. The cells often contain neurosecretory granules.

Risk Factors

Tobacco smoke has long been recognized as the primary risk factor for developing lung cancer. Although early evidence for the link between tobacco smoke and lung cancer was largely anecdotal in nature, an article published by Doll and Hill in 1950 showed an epidemiological association between the development of lung cancer and history of exposure to tobacco smoke *(7)*. Since the publication of Doll and Hill's seminal study, a significant amount of research has proven the association between tobacco smoke and bronchogenic carcinoma. In 2004, the US Department of Health and Human Services released a comprehensive update of the Surgeon General's report regarding the health consequences of smoking. This report conclusively states that there is a causal relationship between cigarette smoke and the development of many kinds of neoplastic diseases including lung cancer *(8)*. Although not all individuals who smoke will develop lung cancer, the relative risk of developing bronchogenic carcinoma in an individual with history of chronic cigarette smoking compared with nonsmokers ranges between 10- and 40-fold *(9–11)*.

Not only is cigarette smoking a strong risk factor for developing lung cancer, the risk of lung cancer is also influenced by the age at which one begins smoking, as well as the tar and nicotine content of cigarettes. One study estimated that for a 35-year-old man who is a chronic smoker, the likelihood of dying from lung cancer before the age of 85 doubles from 9 to 18% if he smokes more than 25 cigarettes per day *(9)*. One study found that among current smokers, the risk of lung cancer risk doubles for every 10 cigarettes per day up to 30 to 40 cigarettes *(12)*. Although there is a myriad of evidence to prove that the relationship between cigarette smoking and lung cancer is not merely a coincidental one, many smokers underestimate their own risk of developing lung cancer and even believe that their risk of developing lung cancer is less than that of some non-smokers *(13)*.

Although cigarette smoking is that single biggest risk factor for developing lung cancer, other types of smoking, including second-hand smoke, are also risk factors. Studies have shown that cigar smoking increases the risk of lung cancer and has a dose–response relationship, however, cigar smoking appears to be a weaker risk factor for developing lung cancer *(14,15)*. Various hypotheses exist as to why this is so, with one generally accepted explanation being that cigar smoking sends smaller amounts of particulate carcinogens deep into the lungs. Environmental tobacco smoke (ETS) exposure, or second-hand tobacco smoke, has also been shown to increase the risk of developing lung cancer. Studies investigating the relationship between ETS and lung cancer have shown that there is a 30 to 75% higher risk of developing lung cancer among individuals exposed to ETS for long periods of time *(16)*. One study showed that 25 or more years of ETS exposure in the home doubled the risk of lung cancer, whereas less exposure had no effect *(17)*.

Many chemicals encountered in the occupational setting are known to be carcinogens, which can increase the risk of developing bronchogenic carcinoma. These carcinogens include asbestos, radon, chromium, formaldehyde, radiation, nickel, polycyclic aromatic hydrocarbons, hard metals, and various plastic polymers, such as vinyl chloride *(18)*. Among the most alarming of these substances has been asbestos because of its ubiquitous use in older factories, schools, apartment buildings, and houses. A causal relationship exists between asbestos and lung cancer. Prolonged asbestos exposure is known to be a risk factor for cancer, especially mesothelioma. The risk is further magnified if asbestos exposure is accompanied with smoking. Most of these occupational carcinogens have been shown to have a dose-dependent relationship with regard to cancer incidence among those exposed. Recent case reports of lung cancer incidence in clusters in which household radon exposure is high have spurred further investigation into this area, but insufficient data is currently available to conclusively establish a causal association and quantify risk.

Clinical Presentation

Bronchogenic carcinoma is an insidious process in which disease progression is rapid and patients are usually symptomatic at time of presentation, except when lung masses are found incidentally. Typically, patients are 50 to 60 years old and have endured symptoms for 6 to 9 months. Symptoms are caused by endobronchial obstruction, recurrent pneumonias secondary to endobronchial obstruction, mass effects from a peripheral nodule or central lesion, and tumors of the lung apex (Pancoast's tumor). Symptoms can also results from lesions other than the primary lung lesion, such as distant metastases and paraneoplastic syndromes. In some cases, metastases may be the cause of symptoms and the patient may have no complaints resulting from the primary lung lesion.

In order of frequency, the most common presenting symptoms of lung cancer are cough, weight loss, chest pain, and dyspnea. Fifty to seventy-five percent of patients present with cough *(19)*. Other presenting symptoms include hoarseness, hemoptysis, wheezing, and fever. The presence of multiple symptoms may indicate a worse prognosis. The presence or absence of sputum production with cough is usually nonspecific. Pulmonary and pericardial effusions result from pleural invasion by tumor cells. Weight loss occurs in 40 to 50% of patients, and unintended weight loss can result from paraneoplastic phenomonenon.

As many as 50% of all patients with bronchogenic carcinoma complain of chest pain on initial presentation. Pain is usually dull and is indicative of intrathoracic spread. Sharp pain from bronchogenic carcinomas is an ominous sign reflecting advanced disease or invasion of the pleura. Approximately 30% of patients present with dyspnea. Endobronchial obstruction, atalectasis, and pleural effusion are all potential causes of dyspnea in bronchogenic carcinoma patients. Hemoptysis, when present, usually consists of small volumes of blood-tinged sputum and is caused by underlying chronic pneumonia or bronchitis rather than blood extravasation from large vessels. Hoarseness results from impingement of the recurrent laryngeal nerve.

Apical lung tumors can cause a mass effect syndrome. Pancoast tumors occur in the superior sulcus and invade surrounding sympathetic ganglia and intercostals nerves as well the brachial plexus. This results in shoulder pain, weakness or numbness of the ipsilateral upper extremity, and Horner syndrome (ptosis, miosis, anhidrosis). Compression of the superior vena cava (SVC) can lead to SVC syndrome manifested by upper extremity edema, facial plethora, and dyspnea *(20)*. Paraneoplastic syndromes (Table 1), caused by secretion of hormones or hormone-like chemicals by the tumor or in response to the tumor, occur in approximately 10 to 15% of patients.

Metastases to distant bones, especially vertebrae, may result in significant bone pain. Cancer metastasis to the liver is an extremely negative prognostic factor and can result in signs of hepatic insufficiency, such as metabolic abnormalities,

Table 1
Paraneoplastic Syndromes

Cancer subtype	Syndrome	Clinical manifestation
Small-cell carcinoma	Cushing syndrome	Central weight gain, facial/nuchal adiposity, hypertension, abdominal striae, glucose intolerance, electrolyte abnormalities
	Syndrome of inappropriate antidiuretic hormone secretion	Hyponatremia
Squamous-cell carcinoma	Parathormone, parathyroid hormone-related peptide excess	Hypercalcemia
Large-cell carcinoma	Human chorionic gonadotropin, human chorionic gonadotropin-like peptide syndrome	Gynecomastia

because of decreased processing of biochemical wastes and coagulopathies resulting from decreased clotting factor production. Bronchogenic carcinoma, especially NSCLC, may metastasize to the brain before a patient presents for initial clinical evaluation *(21)*. Symptoms of brain metastasis include headaches, nausea, vomiting, neurological deficits, and seizures.

Rare systemic manifestations of disease include hypertrophic pulmonary osteoarthropathy, peripheral neurophathy, and a myasthenic syndrome caused by anti-calcium ion channel auto-antibodies (Lambert-Eaton syndrome).

DIFFERENTIAL DIAGNOSIS

The differential diagnosis of signs and symptoms associated with bronchogenic carcinoma is vast. Causes of dyspnea alone range from chronic obstructive pulmonary disease in the smoker to heart failure. Similarly, hemoptysis is seen in conditions ranging from bronchiectasis to Goodpasture's Syndrome. However, it is often the discrete lung lesion that is most challenging for the primary care physicians. The term *solitary pulmonary nodule* describes a lung lesion less than 4 cm in size; larger lesions are referred to as lung masses. Although lung masses seen on plain chest radiograph and CT scans usually represent malignant neoplastic disease, the same is not true of lung nodules.

Approximately 40% of all solitary pulmonary nodules in clinical practice are found to be malignant *(22)*. Lung adenocarcinoma often presents as a solitary peripheral lung nodule. Cancer metastatic to the lung and carcinoid tumors may also present as solitary lung nodules. Benign lung neoplasms, such as hematomas, often appear as solitary pulmonary nodules. It is also important to keep in mind the non-neoplastic etiologies of solitary pulmonary nodules. Mycobacterium infection and fungal infections such as histoplasmosis, cryptococcosis, and *Pneumocystis carinii* can present as solitary nodules on chest radiograph or CT imaging *(23)*. Parasitic infections of the lung also cause appearance of a solitary pulmonary nodule. *Echinococcus granulosus* and *Dirofilaria immitis* (dog "heartworm") in humans can present as solitary pulmonary nodules, with the latter sometimes being confused for malignant disease on initial imaging *(24)*. The vast majority of multiple pulmonary nodule cases represent metastatic cancer to the lung. However, fungal and parasitic infections may also manifest as multiple pulmonary nodules. Similarly, septic emboli and pulmonary abcesses may have the appearance of multiple nodules on plain chest radiograph. Autoimmune diseases, such as Wegener's granulomatosis, and reactive diseases, such as pneumoconiosis, also appear as multiple lung nodules.

MANAGEMENT
Diagnostic Evaluation

Solitary pulmonary nodules vary slightly in terms of nodular shape and size. Benign lesions often have well-defined borders. In contrast, malignant lesions have irregular edges and varying densities. However, accurate characterization of pulmonary nodules is a diagnostic dilemma and remains controversial. Because the chances for successful lung cancer treatment are best when malignancy is discovered early, all efforts should be made towards achieving proper diagnosis. When interpreted by a skilled radiologist, helical CT imaging is an excellent follow-up to the discovery of pulmonary nodules. Helical CT has the advantage of reducing artifacts and more precisely depicting the size and shape of a lesion. Computer software also exists to aid in the radiographic characterization of the lesions. One study demonstrated 90% sensitivity for detecting solid lung nodules early in the disease course through use of computer algorithms with CT imaging *(25)*. After CT imaging, some type of cell or tissue sample must be obtained if the history and physical and radiographic assessment do not yield enough data to indicate a diagnosis. Tissue sample is obtained by fiberoptic bronchoscopy, fluoroscopic/CT-guided transthoracic needle biopsy, video-assisted thoracic surgery, or thoracotomy. The advantage of the former two techniques is that they are less invasive, whereas the latter two allow for wider sampling and excision. Thoracotomy for lesion characterization has become increasingly rare as video-assisted thoracic surgery has been shown to be a safe diagnostic method with good patient acceptance and tolerance *(26,27)*. The method of tissue sampling is chosen by pulmonologists and thoracic surgeons based on lesion size and location.

Table 2
Defining Tumor (T), Node (N), and Metastasis (M) Characteristics

Tumor description	T
Presence of malignant cells in sputum or bronchial washings but tumor not seen on direct or indirect imaging	TX
Primary tumor not evident	T0
Carcinoma *in situ* (no invasion of adjacent tissue)	Tis
Tumor or 3 cm or less, no evidence of invasion beyond lobar bronchus	T1
Tumor more than 3 cm, invasion of main bronchus or visceral pleura, limited bronchial obstruction	T2
Invasion of chest wall, diaphragm, pleura, parietal pericardium, but not carina	T3
Tumor invasion of mediastinal/chest structures not already listed above	T4

Node description	N
Nodes not assessed	NX
No lymph node involvement	N0
Metastasis to ipsilateral peribronchial, hilar, or intrapulmonary nodes	N1
Metastasis to ipsilateral mediastinal or subcarinal nodes	N2
Involvement of contralateral hilar or mediastinal nodes or any scalene or supraclavicular nodes	N3

Assessment of metastasis	M
No distant metastasis	M0
Distant metastasis	M1

Adapted from ref. 28.

Staging and Prognosis

Treatment approaches for bronchogenic carcinoma depend on cancer subtype and stage. Staging of bronchogenic carcinoma is different for NSCLC and SCLC. Staging of the cancer is useful because it provides information about prognosis and helps define the best course of treatment.

NSCLC is staged using the tumor (T), node (N), metastases (M) system (Tables 2 and 3). SCLC is not staged using the TNM system. Rather, the designations *limited disease* and *extensive disease* are used to describe SCLC. In general, if SCLC involves only the ipsilateral hemithorax with no invasion or metastasis beyond that point, it is referred to as limited stage SCLC. If the cancer extends to beyond the ipsilateral hemithorax, it is referred to as extensive stage SCLC.

Without treatment, the prognosis for lung cancer is extremely poor. Most patients live less than 1 year if no treatment is given. Patients with NSCLC tend

Table 3
Staging of NSCLC

TNM	Stage
Tis	0
T1	IA
T2	IB
T1N1	IIA
T2N1	IIB
T3	IIB
T3N1	IIIA
T1N2	IIIA
T2N2	IIIA
T3N2	IIIA
T4	IIIB
T4N1	IIIB
T4N2	IIIB
T1N3	IIIB
T2N3	IIIB
T3N3	IIIB
T4N3	IIIB
M1 (any T, any N)	IV

Adapted from ref. 28.
NSCLC, non-small cell lung cancer; TNM, tumor, node, metastasis.

to have better overall long-term survival than those with SCLC because two-thirds of patients with SCLC have extensive stage cancer when diagnosed. The 5-year survival for untreated bronchogenic carcinoma is less than 1% (29). Fortunately, treatment improves long-term survival. The 5-year survival for treated limited stage SCLC and extensive stage SCLC is 5 to 8% and 0.8%, respectively. The 5-year survival for treated NSCLC is better as shown in Table 4. Five-year survival for NSCLC is better with histopathology staging as compared with clinical staging.

Treatment

NON-SMALL CELL LUNG CANCER

Treatment for NSCLC depends on disease staging. Currently, patients with stage I disease are treated by surgical resection of the primary tumor. Those with stage II disease also undergo surgical resection, but they may or not receive chemotherapy or radiation. Patients with stage III disease require chemotherapy

Table 4
Clinically Staged NSCLC 5-Year Survival (Posttreatment)

Stage	Five-year survival % (after treatment)
IA	67
IB	41
IIA	34
IIB	26
IIIA	14
IIIB	6
IV	2

NSCLC, non-small cell lung cancer.
Adapted from ref. 28.

or radiotherapy followed by surgical resection. One consensus development conference recommended against adjuvant chemotherapy and/or radiotherapy in completely resected stage I-II-IIIA for N1 based on current clinical evidence (30). The management of metastatic NSCLC (i.e., stage IV) is more challenging. It ranges from palliative measures to chemotherapy. Surgical resection of the primary lesion or metastatic lesion is generally not done because it does not significantly improve survival. However, some oncologists propose that if only a single metastatic lesion exists, surgical resection may be appropriate.

Patients with advanced NSCLC (e.g., stage IIIB or IV) are often managed with palliative care alone. The guidelines for palliative care are less standardized. Palliative care usually means chemotherapy but may also include other appropriate measure such as radiation therapy to ameliorate spinal cord compression caused by metastasis to the vertebra and partial resection of lesions causing mass effect symptoms. The reasoning behind chemotherapy is to use chemical agents that are capable of destroying cancer cells either without harming normal cell, or more frequently, giving normal cells a better chance to recover from the chemotherapeutic insult. Typical chemotherapy for NSCLC involves a platinum-based regimen (31). Cisplatinum or carboplatin is given in a regimen with other agents, such as etoposide, irinotecan, paclitaxel, or gemcitabine. Numerous clinical trials have been published discussing the properties and survival benefits associated with different combination chemotherapy regimens. Although much controversy exists, platinum-based combination regimens seem to be the most effective and are recommended by the American Society of Clinical Oncology.

SMALL-CELL LUNG CANCER

Management of SCLC is different from that of NSCLC in that resection is rarely done, and treatment involves chemotherapy and radiation therapy. Surgical resection is not a good option unless the primary lesion is discovered early in the course of disease. Chemotherapy usually involves two or more regimens administered in accordance with a predetermined cycle. The goal, once again, is to destroy cancer cells while giving normal cells an opportunity to recover. Cancer cells have a higher rate of cell division and growth and thus are more susceptible to cytotoxic effects of chemotherapeutic agents. The initial response to chemotherapy for SCLC has been shown to be consistently good in clinical studies. However, remission is usually short lived. Chemotherapy agents used in the treatment of SCLC include doxorubicin, cyclophosphamide, etoposide, cisplatin, gemcitabine, topotecan, vinorelbine, amrubicin, and irinotecan. Taxanes are not effective in SCLC *(32)*.

PREVENTION

Smoking Cessation

In order to convince smokers to consider quitting, physicians should apprise their patients about the health consequences of smoking as well as the positive effects of smoking cessation on overall health and reduction in lung cancer risk. Many studies that examine the long-term effect of smoking cessation show that among ex-smokers, the odds ratio of developing lung cancer decreases with increasing time since quitting, with maximum benefit occurring among heavy smokers. A report issued by the US Surgeon General after examining studies regarding the health benefits of smoking cessation concluded that risk reduction for lung cancer varies from 20 to 90%, and the risk of developing lung cancer decreases as years of smoking abstinence increase. Additionally, former smokers who had quit smoking 15 or more years ago had 80 to 90% less risk of developing lung cancer as compared with their peers who continued smoking *(33)*. The potential risk reduction achieved with smoking cessation is encouraging, but people who successfully quit smoking still have a higher risk of developing lung cancer compared with those who never smoke.

Screening for Lung Cancer

Screening refers to the identification of an asymptomatic disease by means of patient history/interview, physical exam, lab test, or routine procedure. Keeping in mind that symptomatic lung cancer is associated with significant mortality, it would seem that screening for lung cancer would decrease the lung cancer mortality. Unfortunately, studies thus far have not shown this to be the case. Plain chest radiography has been suggested by some as a means to screen for lung cancer. The Mayo Lung Project and the Czechoslovakia lung cancer screening trial examined the screening value of plain chest X-ray. The experimental group in each study received chest radiographs every 4 months and every 6 months, respectively. Although both studies demonstrated that the screened groups had a greater number of cancers detected in early stage and had higher 5-year survival rates, neither trial showed an improvement in lung cancer mortality *(34,35)*. The Memorial Sloan-Kettering Lung Project had patients in the experimental group receive chest radiographs every 6 months and sputum cytology every 4 months, whereas the comparison group received only a single annual chest radiograph. This study showed no difference in cancer deaths between the screened group and the comparison group, in essence proving that sputum cytology also has little value as a screening test *(36)*.

CT scanning of the chest has also been suggested by some as a possible screening device for lung cancer. A landmark Mayo Clinic/National Cancer Institute study is currently underway to determine the benefit, if any, of using CT scanning as a lung cancer screening method. As would be expected, initial results indicate that a greater number of lung lesions are detected with CT scanning than with plain chest radiograph. However, not all detected lesions represent neoplastic disease. It may turn out that CT scanning is an effective tool for lung cancer screening, however, the study has many years to go before reaching its end point. Therefore, no conclusions can be drawn as of yet *(37)*. Other trials are planned to evaluate the use of positron emission tomography scans for lung cancer screening.

The US Preventive Services Task Force (USPSTF) has published a recommendation statements regarding lung cancer screening. In 1996, the USPSTF recommended against screening for lung cancer, stating that the USPSTF found at least fair evidence that screening for lung cancer through conventional techniques is ineffective or that harms outweigh benefits. In 2004, the USPSTF slightly revised its recommendation regarding lung cancer screening, giving it an "I" recommendation (evidence is insufficient to recommend for or against routinely providing the service). As stated in the 2004 guidelines:

> *The USPSTF found fair evidence that screening with Low Dose CT, chest radiograph, or sputum cytology can detect lung cancer at an earlier stage than lung cancer would be detected in an unscreened population; however, the USPSTF found poor evidence that any screening strategy for lung cancer decreases mortality. (38)*

The USPSTF guidelines emphasize that although low-dose CT has greater sensitivity in detecting lung lesions as compared to plain chest radiograph, it is also associated with more false-positive results, which may result in unnecessary invasive procedures. Additionally, the USPSTF considers patient anxiety with false-positive results and false sense of security with negative results as potential harms of screening. Routine screening for lung cancer is not currently recommended by any major health organizations including the American Cancer Society and the American Academy of Family Physicians.

FUTURE DIRECTIONS

The best way to manage lung cancer is to prevent it. Unlike many other cancers, the major risk factor for lung cancer, smoking, is a modifiable one. New methods are continually being introduced to prevent people from becoming smokers and to aid existing smokers in smoking prevention. As professionals who promote avoidance of tobacco and encouraging smoking cessation, PCPs can play a larger role in lung cancer management than medical or surgical oncologists. Although lung cancer screening is not currently standard of care, development of new assays detecting serum markers of lung cancer may change expert opinion on screening. New developments in lung cancer focus on more effective treatments for bronchogenic carcinoma. Regarding NSCLC, significant research is underway to develop chemical entities that target reception tyrosine kinases and epithelial growth factor receptors found in cancer cells. Gefitinib (Iressa) and cetuximab are two agents that target epithelial growth factor receptors *(39)*. The *Her2/neu* protooncogene is also being targeted to treat NSCLC. In the realm of SCLC, monoclonal antibodies targeting CD56 seem promising for treatment of SCLC. Thalidomide, although not a new drug, is being re-examined for a role in treating lung neoplastic disease because of the drug's anti-angiogenesis properties. The future will bring to the forefront antibodies and chemical agents that more specifically target lung cancer cells resulting in improved outcomes and fewer side effects of treatment.

REFERENCES

1. Jemal A, Tiwari R, Murray T, et al. Cancer statistics, 2004. CA Cancer J Clin 2004;54:8–29.
2. United States Preventive Services Task Force. Lung cancer screening: Recommendation statement. Ann Intern Med 2004;140:738.
3. Sundaresan V, Rabbits P. Genetics of lung tumors. In: Hasleton, ed. Spencer's Pathology of the Lung, 5th Ed. McGraw-Hill, New York, 1996; pp. 975–1008.
4. Denlinger CE, Rundall BK, Jones DR. Modulation of antiapoptotic cell signaling pathways in non-small cell lung cancer: the role of NF-kappaB. Semin Thorac Cardiovasc Surg 2004;16:28–39.
5. Massague J. G1 cell-cycle control and cancer. Nature 2004;432:7015.
6. Syrjanen KJ. HPV infections and lung cancer. J Clin Path 2002;55:885–891.
7. Doll R, Hill AB. Smoking and carcinoma of the lung; preliminary report. BMJ 1950;2:739.
8. United States Department of Health and Human Services. The health consequences of smoking: a report of the Surgeon General. Washington, DC: USDHHS, Center for Disease Control. CDC Publication number 7829. Available from: http://www.cdc.gov/tobacco/sgr/sgr_2004/chapters.htm. Accessed: December 27, 2005.
9. Mattson ME, et al. What are the odds that smoking will kill you? Am J Public Health 1987;77:425.
10. Crispo A, Brennan P, Jockel KH, et al. The cumulative risk of lung cancer among current, ex- and never-smokers in European men. Br J Cancer 2004;91:1280–1286.
11. Villeneuve PJ, Mao Y. Lifetime probability of developing lung cancer, by smoking status, Canada. Can J Public Health 1994;85:385–388.

12. Rachet B, Siemiatycki J, Abrahamowicz M, Leffondre K. A flexible modeling approach to estimating the component effects of smoking behavior on lung cancer. J Clin Epidemiol 2004;57:1076–1085.
13. Weinstein ND, Marcus SE, Moser RP. Smokers' unrealistic optimism about their risk. Tob Control 2005;14:55–59.
14. Baker F, Ainsworth SR, Dye JT, et al. Health risks associated with cigar smoking. JAMA 2000;284:735–740.
15. Shapiro JA, Jacobs EJ, Thun MJ. Cigar smoking in men and risk of death from tobacco-related cancers. J Natl Cancer Inst. 2000;92:333–337.
16. Fontham ET, Correa P, Reynolds P, et al. Environmental tobacco smoke and lung cancer in nonsmoking women. A multicenter study. JAMA 1994;271:1752–1759.
17. Janerich DT, Thompson WD, Varela LR, et al. Lung cancer and exposure to tobacco smoke in the household. N Engl J Med 1990;323:632–636.
18. Grimsrud TK, Berge SR, Haldorsen T, Andersen A. Can lung cancer risk among nickel refinery workers be explained by occupational exposures other than nickel? Epidemiology 2005;16:146–154.
19. Schrump D, Altorki N, et al. Cancer of the lung. In: DeVita V, Helman S, Rosenberg S, eds. Cancer: Principles and Practice of Oncology, 7th Ed. Lippincott, Williams, and Wilkins, New York, 2005, pp. 753–800.
20. Arcasoy SM, Jett JR. Superior pulmonary sulcus tumors and Pancoast's syndrome. N Engl J Med 1997;337:1370–1377.
21. Bajard A, Westeel V, Dubiez A, et al. Multivariate analysis of factors predictive of brain metastases in localised non-small cell lung carcinoma. Lung Cancer 2004;45:317–323.
22. Lillington GA, Caskey CI. Evaluation and management of solitary and multiple pulmonary nodules. Clin Chest Med 1993;14:111–119.
23. Rolston KV, Rodriguez S, Dholakia N, Whimbey E, Raad I. Pulmonary infections mimicking cancer: a retrospective, three-year review. Support Care Cancer 1997;5:90–93.
24. Rena O, Leutner M, Casadio C. Human pulmonary dirofilariasis: uncommon cause of pulmonary coin-lesion. Eur J Cardiothorac Surg 2002;22:157–159.
25. Paik DS, Beaulieu CF, Rubin GD, et al. Surface normal overlap: a computer-aided detection algorithm with application to colonic polyps and lung nodules in helical CT. Trans Med Imaging 2004;23:661–675.
26. Ludwig C, Zeitoun M, Stoelben E. Video-assisted thoracoscopic resection of pulmonary lesions. Eur J Surg Oncol 2004;30:1118–1122.
27. Midthun DE. Solitary pulmonary nodule: time to think small. Curr Opin Pulm Med 2000;6:364–370.
28. Mountain CF. Revisions in the international system for staging lung cancer. Chest 1997;111:1710–1717.
29. Scagliotti G. Consensus development conference on the medical treatment of non-small cell lung cancer: treatment of the early stages. Lung Cancer 2002;38:S23–S29.
30. Scagliotti GV, De Marinis F, Rinaldi, M, et al. Phase III randomized trial comparing three platinum-based doublets in advanced non-small-cell lung cancer. J Clin Oncol 2002;20:4285–4291.
31. Popat S, O'brien M. Chemotherapy strategies in the treatment of small cell lung cancer. Anticancer Drugs 2005;16:361–363.
32. United States Department of Health and Human Services (USDHHS). The health benefits of smoking cessation: a report of the Surgeon General. USDHHS, Washington, DC,.
33. Fontana R, Sanderson DR, et al. Screening for lung cancer: the Mayo program. J Occup Med 1986;28:746.

34. Kubik A, Polak J. Lung cancer detection: results of a randomized prospective study in Czechoslovakia. Cancer 1986;57:2427.
35. Melamed MR, Flehinger BJ, Zaman MB, Heelan RT, Perchick WA, Martini N. Screening for early cancer: results of the Memorial Sloan-Kettering study in New York. Chest 1984;86:44–53.
36. Swensen SJ, Jett JR, et al. Lung cancer screening with CT: Mayo Clinic experience. Radiology 2003:226:756–761.
37. United States Preventive Services Task Force. Lung cancer screening: recommendation statement. Ann Intern Med 2004;140:738.
38. Pao W, Miller VA. Epidermal growth factor receptor mutations, small-molecule kinase inhibitors, and non-small-cell lung cancer: current knowledge and future directions. J Clin Oncol 2005;23:2556–2568.

17 Sarcoidosis

Danielle Davidson and Matthew L. Mintz

CONTENTS

    CASE PRESENTATION
    KEY CLINICAL QUESTIONS
    LEARNING OBJECTIVES
    EPIDEMIOLOGY
    PATHOPHYSIOLOGY
    CLINICAL PRESENTATION
    CLINICAL COURSE
    DIFFERENTIAL DIAGNOSIS
    DIAGNOSIS
    TREATMENT
    FUTURE DIRECTIONS
    REFERENCES

CASE PRESENTATION

A 41-year-old African-American woman with a history of asthma presents to her primary care physician's office complaining of a rash on her arm. The rash has been there for approximately 1 month and is pruritic. She denies the use of new detergents, new clothing, or recent insect bites. The patient feels well, other than generalized fatigue. She states that her asthma, which was diagnosed 5 years ago, is slightly worse. She continues to feel short of breath with exertion, and her inhalers help minimally. She had a recent cardiac work-up that was negative.

On exam, the rash is well-circumscribed and limited to the forearm. It is violaceous and plaque-like in appearance. There is suspicion of tinea corporis and therefore a topical antifungal medication is prescribed.

From: *Current Clinical Practice: Disorders of the Respiratory Tract: Common Challenges in Primary Care*
By: M. L. Mintz © Humana Press, Totowa, NJ

The patient returns 2 weeks later, and her rash has not improved. She also complains that her dyspnea and dry cough seem to be worsening. You refer her to dermatology where a biopsy is performed. Noncaseating granulomas are noted on biopsy. A chest radiograph is also done, which reveals evidence of bilateral interstitial process.

KEY CLINICAL QUESTIONS

1. When should the diagnosis of sarcoidosis be suspected in a patient?
2. How does sarcoid normally present, and what are atypical but not uncommon presentations?
3. What is the appropriate treatment of this patient?
4. What is the appropriate follow-up and management of this patient?

LEARNING OBJECTIVES

1. Review the epidemiology of sarcoidosis.
2. Understand the pathophysiology of the disease.
3. Recognize diverse clinical presentations of sarcoidosis.
4. Describe the clinical predictors for disease progression and outcomes.
5. Provide a differential diagnosis and delineate a diagnostic pathway for sarcoid.
6. Understand the risk and benefits of current treatment options for sarcoidosis.

EPIDEMIOLOGY

Sarcoidosis is a multi-organ inflammatory disease characterized by noncaseating granulomas. The disease affects people of all ages, races, and genders. Despite more than a century of observation and research, sarcoidosis continues to perplex researchers and clinicians. The clinical appearance and presenting symptoms are diverse, and the clinical course is equally varied. For some patients, the disease will spontaneously remit, whereas in others the symptoms and organ involvement progresses to cause significant morbidity and mortality.

The age-adjusted annual incidence rate of sarcoidosis in the United States is approximately 10.9 per 100,000 in whites and 35.5 per 100,000 in blacks *(1)*. Sarcoid can affect persons of all ages, races, and sexes. It most commonly presents in young adults under the age of 40, although it may emerge at any age. A second peak incidence after the age of 50 has been described most commonly in the Japanese and Scandinavian populations *(2)*. Sarcoidosis tends to have a slightly greater proclivity for women than for men and presents predominately in the winter and early spring months. Sarcoidosis is more prevalent among certain racial groups as well. US blacks, Swedes, and Danes are more commonly affected by sarcoidosis, whereas US whites, Japanese, Indians, Spaniards, Portuguese, and South Americans are less likely to become afflicted with the disease.

The true incidence among all populations remains in question because it is likely that this complex disease, with its variability in organ involvement and specific symptoms, goes misdiagnosed frequently *(2)*.

PATHOPHYSIOLOGY

The exact cause for the noncaseating granulomas of sarcoidosis is not currently known. Initiating events such as infectious contacts, environmental exposure, and genetic predisposition have all been proposed, and all three theories have some degree of evidence that support their claims. Diseases such as mycobacterium and fungi produce a similar clinical and histological picture to sarcoid. The infectious theory is further supported by observation that sarcoidosis and certain infections have a predilection for the early spring and winter months *(1)*. Microbes including human herpesvirus, retrovirus, Epstein-Barr virus, coxsackie B, cytomegalovirus, mycobacterium, *Borrelia burgdorfi*, propionibacterium, *Chlamydia pneumonia*, and *Rickettsia helvetic* have all been proposed as inciting agents of sarcoid's granuloma formation *(3)*. However, culture of microbes among patients afflicted with sarcoid has not been revealing. Exposure to certain environmental toxins can also result in disease clinically indistinguishable from sarcoid, and it has been suggested that toxins, such as berrylium, aluminum, zirconium, pine tree pollen, and talc, place patients at risk for the development of sarcoidosis. Several case reports describe increased incidence of sarcoidosis among people living in close-quartered environments where there is significant exposure to one of these toxins. A higher incidence of sarcoidosis has been reported among firefighters, aircraft personnel, and hospital employees, all of whom had been exposed to environmental culprits *(4)*. Although environmental exposure, infection, or toxin may contribute to the development of sarcoid, current investigation points strongly towards genetic predisposition as the major etiology behind sarcoidosis. There is a fivefold increase in the relative risk of developing sarcoid among first-degree relatives *(5)*. Moreover, certain ethnic and racial groups such as African Americans are at greater risk of developing sarcoid (four times greater than whites) and tend to have a more protracted course *(3)*. Thus far, researchers have discovered that human leukocyte antigen and major histocompatibility complex on the short arm of chromosome 6 play a role in both the risk of developing sarcoid and predicting its clinical course *(3)*. Interleukin (IL)-1 and tumor necrosis factor (TNF)-α genes have also been linked to the pathogenesis of granuloma formation *(3)*.

The sarcoid granuloma is a discrete noncaseating granuloma consisting of giant cells (mononuclear phagocytes and lymphocytes). The place of granulomatous deposition (i.e., lungs versus lymph nodes versus nervous system) affects the clinical course and prognosis. The exact mechanism of granuloma formation is not known, but it is clear that the T-helper-1 cell and various cytokines play a major role in the immunopathogenesis. From the start, the host is exposed to one or several inciting antigens. The antigen(s) are recognized by an antigen-presenting cell. The antigen–antigen-presenting cell interaction promotes a nonspecific, over-exuberant inflammatory response involving T-helper-1 cells, macrophages, various cytokines, chemokines, and growth factors including interferon-λ, IL-2, TNF-α, IL-6, and IL-1. Eventually, T-cells and mononuclear inflammatory cells, which differentiate into epitheloid and multinucleated giant cells, accumulate in the target organ. In later stages, a band of fibroblasts, mast cells, collagen fibers, and proteoglycans form a perimeter around the inflammatory cells, culminating in granuloma formation. Some of theses inflammatory cells not only promote the inflammatory cascade, but also promote fibrosis. For many afflicted with sarcoidosis, this results in irreversible organ damage and dysfunction *(1)*.

CLINICAL PRESENTATION

The clinical presentation and picture of sarcoidosis is heterogenous. Approximately 30% of patients are asymptomatic; they are discovered to have sarcoidosis when a characteristic chest radiograph is performed for other reasons. The majority of patients afflicted with sarcoidosis, however, do complain of nonspecific constitutional symptoms including fever, weight loss, anorexia, and malaise. Sarcoid can affect numerous organs in the body (Table 1).

The lungs are involved in more than 90% of patients with sarcoidosis, even if subclinical *(1)*. Dyspnea, cough, and chest pain are the most common respiratory symptoms noted by patients. The symptom of dyspnea varies; some patients complain of shortness of breath with great exertion, whereas others are breathless at rest. The cough is usually dry. Sputum production and hemoptysis is rare and may point to additional diagnoses. The cause of the cough is not currently known. Sarcoidosis is most often an interstitial lung disorder and dry rales are appreciated on physical exam in advanced stages. Airway hyperactivity and expiratory wheezing can also be noted in up to 20% of patients, making sarcoidosis a diagnostic challenge *(2)*. Chest pain is most often retrosternal in position. The reason for this symptom is also not clear. Experts have speculated that mediastinal lymphadenopathy causes this nonspecific pain. This theory was disputed by a study performed by Highland et al. who compared the incidence of adenopathy seen on chest computed tomography (CT) with subjective pain. The study showed no correlation between the presence of adenopathy and complaint of chest pain *(6)*.

As previously mentioned, systemic or constitutional symptoms are not uncommon in sarcoidosis. These symptoms occur in approximately 33% of patients *(2)*. Fever is usually low grade. Night sweats, fatigue, malaise, and minimal weight loss are also noted with a fair degree of frequency *(1)*.

Table 1
Organs Affected by Sarcoid

Organ	Affected (%)	Clinical signs/symptoms
Lungs	>90	Cough, dyspnea, chest pain
Constitutional	20–35	Fevers, weight loss, malaise, night sweats
Cardiac	5–20	Conduction abnormality, cardiomyopathy, congestive heart failure, sudden death
Skin	25	Maculopapular eruption, plaques, nodules, erythema nodosum, lupus pernio
Ocular	20–80	Anterior/post-uveitis, conjunctival invasion, lacrimal gland enlarged
Msk	20–35	Polyarthritis, muscle granulomas, proximal myopathy
Spleen	50–80	Asymptomatic, splenomegaly, thrombocytopenia
Liver	20	Asymptomatic, granulomas in portal triad, elevated alk phos and bili
Kidney/Endo	10–20	Renal granuloma, hypercalcemia, hypercalciuria, nephrolithiasis, renal insufficiency
Neurological	2–7	Cranial neuropathy, CN VII most common, granulomatous basal meningitis, parenchymal masses ± hydrocephalus, peripheral neuropathy, aseptic meningitis

Cn, cranial nerve; MSK, musculoskeletal; Endo, endocrine.

Lymphadenopathy is a hallmark of sarcoidosis with hilar lymph node involvement occurring in 90% of patients with sarcoid *(1)*. Peripheral lymph nodes, such as cervical, axillary, epitrochlear, and inguinal nodes, are also commonly affected *(2)*. Peripheral nodes are usually non-tender and mobile. The lymphadenopathy causes little clinical impairment unless it obstructs other organs. Splenic involvement can cause abdominal pressure, anemia, and thrombocytopenia, although these complications are rare *(2)*.

Although an uncommon presentation of sarcoidosis, myocardial involvement can result in significant morbidity and mortality if not recognized early. Clinical evidence of cardiac involvement occurs in approximately 5% of patients *(2)*. Clinical manifestations include congestive heart failure owing to infiltrative disease, pericarditis, papillary muscle dysfunction, heart block, and ventricular tachycardia. Approximately 50% of myocardial sarcoidosis have abnormal electrocardiogram. These anomalies include nonsinus rhythms, conduction disturbance, and repolarization disturbances *(1)*.

Table 2
Clinical Features Associated With Poor Prognosis

Lupus pernio	Progeressive pulmonary disease
Chronic uveitis	Nasa mucosal involvement
Over age 40	Cystic bone lesion
Chronic hypercalcemia	Neurosarcoid
Nephrocalcinosis	Myocardial involvement
Black race	Stage III and IV on chest X-ray

Some form of skin pathology is found in 25% of sarcoid patients *(2)*. Dermatological manifestations are diverse. Maculopapular eruptions, plaques, subcutaneous nodules, alopecia, hypo- and hyperpigmentation represent the range of skin findings. Skin lesions generally do not cause pain or pruritis and do not ulcerate *(2)*. Two dermatological conditions that should prompt clinicians to suspect an underlying presence of sarcoidosis are erythema nodosum and lupus pernio. Erythema nodosum is a condition characterized by the presence of raised, red, tender nodules on the anterior aspect of legs. Adjacent joints are often edematous, erythematous, and painful. Lupus pernio are violaceous lesions that appear most frequently on or near the face. Cheeks, nose, lips, ears, and nasal mucosa are commonly involved *(2)*. Erythema nodosum and lupus pernio portend important prognostic indicators (Table 2).

Sarcoidosis can also affect the ophthalmological system causing significant morbidity for some patients. Anterior uveitis, resulting in blurred vision, photophobia, and increased lacrimation, are the most common complaints. All parts of the eye have the potential to be affected. Conjuctival follicles (small, pale, yellow nodules), lacrimal gland enlargement (aka Mikulicz syndrome), keratoconjunctiva sicca, and retinal vasculitis are all possible presentations of sarcoid in the eye.

The musculoskeletal system is commonly affected by sarcoid as exemplified by the presence of granulomas in 50% of patients diagnosed with sarcoidosis. Fortunately, not nearly as many are symptomatic. Joint pains can occur, although deforming arthritis is rare. Knees, ankles, elbows, wrists, and small joints of the hands and feet are the most common areas involved. Proximal muscle weakness is also present, but this symptom must be distinguished from steroid-induced myopathy *(1)*.

Like the musculoskeletal system, clinically apparent liver disease is very rare, despite the frequency of granulomas noted on liver biopsy. Portal hypertension and liver failure is exceedingly rare, whereas mild liver function abnormalities are common *(2)*. Approximately one-third of patients have an elevated alkaline phosphatase and/or hyperbilirubinemia *(1)*. The remainder of the gastrointestinal tract is involved in less than 1% of patients with sarcoidosis.

Various lines of the hematological system may be affected by sarcoidosis. Between 4 and 20% of patients are noted to be anemic. Leukopenia, although mild, can occur in up to 40% of patients with sarcoidosis. Leukonpenia is thought to be secondary to the sequestration of T-cells at the site of disease, thus reducing the total white blood cell count in the serum. Finally, thrombocytopenia can occur in the setting of significant splenomegaly *(1)*.

The endocrine system, glands, and electrolytes can all be altered as a result of sarcoidosis. The parotid gland, for example can be enlarged in sarcoidosis. A syndrome known as Heerfordt's syndrome or uveo-parotid fever consists of fever, parotid gland enlargement, facial palsy, and anterior uveitis *(1)*. Hypercalcemia and hypercalciuria have been associated with sarcoidosis and granulomatous diseases in general. Macrophages present within the granuloma can cause a dysregulation and overproduction of 1,25 (OH)2-D3 (calcitiol) resulting in elevated calcium levels. Nephrolithiasis and nephrocalcinosis can further result from this electrolyte disturbance. Hypo- and hyperthyroidism, adrenal suppression, and pituitary dysregulation can all occur in the presence of noncaseating granulomas.

Like many of the systems described, the nervous system is unfortunately vulnerable to sarcoid infestation. Between 5 and 16% of patients with sarcoid have neurological complaints. If neurological symptoms emerge, they tend to appear within the first 2 years of diagnosis *(7)*. Cranial nerve VII neuropathy, or Bell's palsy, is the most common form of neurosarcoidosis. Encephalopathy, dementia, seizures and headaches, aseptic meningitis, peripheral neuropathy, and hypothalamic and pituitary involvement can all occur in neurosarcoidosis *(2,7)*. The neurological system is rarely the sole system involved. Most people have other organ systems concomitantly affected by sarcoidosis *(7)*. Acute onset of neurosarcoidosis is usually a cranial neuropathy or aseptic meningitis. Conversely, chronic presentation of neurosarcoidosis usually implies parenchymal involvement, hydrocephalus, or peripheral neuropathies *(7)*.

Lastly, a condition known as Löfgren's syndrome is associated with sarcoidosis. The syndrome presents with bilateral hilar lymphadenopathy, ankle arthritis, erythema nodosum, and fever, malaise, and weight loss. Fortunately, this conglomeration of physical findings signify an excellent prognosis *(8)*.

CLINICAL COURSE

Sarcoidosis not only has a large spectrum of initial presentation, but its clinical course and prognosis is also diverse and varied. Spontaneous remission or stabilization of the disease occurs in approximately two-thirds of cases *(3)*. On the other side of the continuum, 10 to 30% suffer from a chronic and progressive course, and at least 20% have permanent clinical sequele *(2)*. Mortality rates have been reported as high as 1 to 5%, the majority occurring at referral centers

(2,3). Respiratory failure followed by sudden cardiac death and severe neurosarcoidosis are the most common causes of mortality *(3)*. Why some people have favorable outcomes and others progress to severe ailment remains a subject for further research and discussion.

Pattern of extrapulmonary involvement and overall prognosis seems to vary depending on race, age, and ethnic background. Additionally, certain initial clinical manifestations of sarcoid, including chest radiograph, portend a better prognosis than others. African Americans have been reported to present with more acute and severe forms of sarcoidosis, whereas whites are more likely to be asymptomatic. The diagnosis in whites is more often made on chest radiographs performed for other reasons *(1)*. Extrathoracic presentations are also more common in non-white ethnic groups. Blacks tend to present with more musculoskeletal and constitutional symptoms. They also have a higher incidence of cystic bony lesions, extrathoracic lymphadenopathy, skin involvement with lupus pernio, and chronic uveitis. Relapse rate among African Americans is also higher. Puerto Ricans are more likely to present with lupus pernio, which, again, portends a worse prognosis. Cardiac and ocular involvement appears commonly in those of Japanese descent *(2,4)*. Erythema nodosum and Lögren's syndrome are most commonly seen in whites and these clinical presentations are good prognostic markers *(2)*. Although mortality rates among the different ethnic groups have not been reported, morbidity is clearly higher among those individuals of certain ethnicities whose multiple organs are affected by this disease process. Table 2 lists clinical features that predict prognosis.

DIFFERENTIAL DIAGNOSIS

The often subclinical nature of sarcoidosis, as well as its seemingly unrelated multi-organ involvement, makes sarcoidosis a diagnostic dilemma for clinicians. One case–control study of sarcoid patients showed that nearly 50% of patients were diagnosed with sarcoidosis after 3 months of symptoms and more than 25% after 6 months of symptoms *(4)*. Although there is no definitive test specific for sarcoid, using the following criteria can aide in making the diagnosis: the presence of a clinical constellation of symptoms as described above, a chest radiographic typical of sarcoid, the presence of noncaseating granulomas on histology, and the exclusion of other granulomatous diseases. Because sarcoidosis can present in numerous organs, the differential diagnosis is quite extensive. Tuberculosis, atypical mycobacterium, and fungal diseases, such as histoplasmosis, coccidiomycosis, and blastomycosis can produce granulomas in the lung, lymph nodes, skin, and bone marrow. Other systemic diseases, such as lymphoma, Crohn's disease, rheumatoid arthritis, lupus, Wegener's granulomatosis, and a reaction to foreign bodies and drugs can all present like sarcoidosis *(8)*. A

Table 3
Sarcoid Staging

Stage	X-ray appearance	Chance of remission (%)
Stage 0	Normal	—
Stage I	Adenopathy (bilateral hilar)	50–90
Stage II	Adenopathy + infiltrates (bilateral)	40–70
Stage III	Infiltrates (bilateral) alone	10–20
Stage IV	Fibrosis (honey-combing, hilar retraction, bullae cysts, and emphysema)	0

thorough family, environmental, and occupational history as well as a complete review of systems is essential in the diagnostic pathway.

DIAGNOSIS

More than 40 years ago, Wurm and Scadding developed a staging system by chest radiograph that is still used today (Table 3). If the clinician suspects sarcoidosis and the chest radiograph is not clear, a CT scan can often more clearly depict the extent of disease. Features such as bilateral hilar and right paratracheal lymphadenopathy, pulmonary nodules along bronchovascular bundles, and fibrosis in later stages can all be seen on chest CT scan (4).

After acquiring a clinical history suggestive of sarcoid and imaging compatible with this disease, the next step in the diagnostic pathway is to obtain tissue confirmation of noncaseating granulomas. The most appropriate site of biopsy for histological confirmation is that which is least invasive. Skin lesions (except erythema nodosum) and peripheral lymph nodes are easily accessible for biopsy, safe, and can rule out lymphoma. If such sites are not available, endobronchial and transbronchial lung biopsy via bronchoscopy is the next recommended procedure in most scenarios. This is generally safe, however, a limited sample can miss granulomas or be insufficient for culture of fungus or mycobacterium (6). Mediastinoscopy can also be performed with biopsy of the right paratrachael lymph nodes when seen on chest CT, and is very helpful in distinguishing sarcoid from lymphoma. Open lung biopsy via video-assisted thoracoscopy is usually performed in an effort to distinguish between other causes of interstitial pulmonary fibrosis, but this procedure is associated with significantly greater risk than brochoscopy (6).

If biopsy and histology confirmation is not reasonable (e.g., if the patient refuses or lung disease is too severe to tolerate a procedure), other clinical markers can be used. Nonspecific labs such as anemia, leukopenia, thrombocytopenia, hypercalcemia, hypercalciuria, an elevated alkaline phosphatase, and hyperbilirubinemia are often seen in sarcoidosis. Broncho-alveolar lavage may show a predominance of lymphocytes with an increase CD4 to CD8 ratio higher than 3.5 *(2)*. This ratio is associated with alveolitis as seen in sarcoidosis. Cultures can also be sent from the broncho-alveolar lavage washings. A gallium-67 scan can further provide diagnostic information. Bilateral hilar and right paratrachael lymph node uptake is known as the "lambda pattern." Lung parenchyma, lacrimal, or parotid gland uptake is referred to as the "panda pattern." Although uptake on the gallium-67 can occur in any inflammatory or neoplastic condition, it is fairly specific for sarcoid when it is positive in the lungs *(9)*. An angiotensin-converting enzyme (ACE) level is elevated in 56 to 85% of patients with sarcoid *(7)*. However, research shows that ACE levels are also elevated in other syndromes, such as liver disease, diabetes mellitus, hyperthyroidism, and systemic infection and is therefore not specific for sarcoidosis. Of note, the ACE level in sarcoid patients does tend to be higher, but a normal ACE level does not rule out the disease, nor does it provide prognostic information. Once sarcoid has been diagnosed by clinical and radiographic features and supported by histological features, additional tests are necessary to assess the extent of disease. A full neurological exam should be performed including a referral to an ophthalmologist for a complete eye exam. A baseline electrocardiogram should be documented, looking for the presence of rhythm or conduction abnormalities. Pulmonary function tests with spirometry and diffusion capacity for carbon monoxide should be performed. Pulmonary function tests usually show a pattern consistent with intrinsic restrictive disease including a reduced forced vital capacity, a normal or increased forced expiratory volume in 1 second to forced vital capacity ratio, reduced residual volume, reduced total lung capacity and decreased diffusion capacity for carbon monoxide. Of note, some patients with sarcoid also present with an obstructive pattern and markedly reduced forced expiratory volume in 1 second. These patients are often misdiagnosed with bronchitis or asthma. Serial labs including liver function tests (LFTs), complete blood count, basic metabolic panel including calcium levels, blood urea nitrogen, and creatinine should be documented again for future comparisons *(4)*. If neurosarcoidosis is of concern, in addition to the appropriate referral, a magnetic resonance imaging can be performed, which is sensitive but not specific for sarcoidosis. Recently, use of the positron emission tomography scan has identified patients with primary central nervous system involvement *(7)*.

Serial clinical exams remain the standard for monitoring and predicting the clinical course of patients afflicted by sarcoid. Surveillance should be most intense in the first 2 years to determine the need for treatment and likelihood of progression. Patients should be seen every 3 to 4 months if stage III or IV disease is present, and every 6 months if stages I or II is present. A full physical exam, chest radiograph, and spirometry should be performed at each visit in addition to more specific tests (e.g., electrocardiogram, calcium levels, or LFTs) depending on the individual clinical picture *(2)*.

TREATMENT

An incomplete understanding of the pathogenesis of sarcoidosis coupled with the heterogeneity of its clinical presentation and course has made the development of treatment guidelines a challenge to experts in the field. Systemic corticosteroids have been the mainstay of therapy for decades, and is still widely used today. A recent meta-analysis by the Cochrane group concluded that corticosteroids were of benefit for pulmonary sarcoid and there is usually an improvement in respiratory symptoms, chest radiograph, and pulmonary function tests in 6 to 24 months. Notably, it is common for symptoms to return with discontinuation of the steroids, and there is no evidence to date that corticosteroids change the long-term prognosis. For patients with asymptomatic disease and stage I disease, there is no evidence to support the need for corticosteroids. Many of these patients resolve spontaneously and therefore can be monitored closely for signs of progression *(6)*.

Although specific guidelines do not exist, it is usually recommended that corticosteroids be initiated for symptomatic or progressive stages II and III disease, neurosarcoidosis, ocular involvement, cardiac sarcoid, and significant hypercalcemia. The initial dose is usually 20 to 40 mg per day, although the dose may be higher in cases of ocular or neurological involvement. The patient should be monitored closely for 8 to 12 weeks after the initiation of steroids. If there are signs of clinical improvement, the corticosteroids can be tapered over the next 6 to 12 months. Conversely, if the patient does not demonstrate any clinical response, one should consider the following possible scenarios: the patient has already progressed to irreversible fibrosis, the dose is inadequate, the patient is not compliant, or the host has developed an intrinsic resistance to steroids. Inhaled steroids have been proposed as a potential treatment for pulmonary sarcoid. Most studies, however, have been inconclusive *(1)*.

Although symptoms of sarcoidosis may improve with systemic corticosteroids, this therapy is replete with potential risks and complications. Weight gain, hypertension, mood changes, hyperglycemia, osteoporosis, and immune suppression are just a few of the significant long-term side effects of steroid therapy. Diet and exercise should be encouraged in these patients. Calcium and vitamin D along with bisphosphonates are also recommended. A dual-energy X-ray scan every 2 years to monitor bone loss is also essential.

Given the multiple adverse side effects of corticosteroids, patients requiring persistent steroid therapy or are refractory to their use, should be considered for alternative medications, such as cytotoxic drugs or immunmodulators. The most commonly used cytotoxic medications, because of their efficacy and safety profile, are methotrexate and azathioprine. Methotrexate is generally well tolerated, although positive effects are often not seen for 6 months after the initiation of treatment and symptoms often return with its discontinuation. Methotrexate is particularly helpful with musculoskeletal symptoms and cutaneous sarcoid. Side effects are not uncommon, requiring very close monitoring of the patient while taking this medication. Bone marrow suppression with neutropenia can occur. Hypersensitivity pneumonitis, hepatitis, mucositis, and teratogenicity are all potential problems of methotrexate. Patients are advised to use contraception during treatment and for 6 months following the use of methotrexate *(3)*.

Azathioprine has also proven effective in the treatment of sarcoid in case studies. Like methotrexate, azathioprine should be considered a steroid, sparing medication for those with severe progressive disease who are dependent on corticosteroids. Major side effects include flu-like symptoms, nausea, bone marrow suppression, and carcinogenicity *(7)*. Blood counts including a complete blood count and LFTs should be monitored and treatment stopped if the white blood cell count drops to less than 3000/mm^3 or if the LFTs are five times the upper limit of normal. Chlorambucil can also be used in place of corticosteroids, however, this medication has fallen out of favor because of its more unfavorable side effect profile and carcinogenicity. Cyclophosphamide has also been considered for those sarcoid patients that are refractory to steroid treatment. Once again, its side effects, particularly placing a patient at increased risk for lymphoproliferative disorders and bladder cancer, has limited its use.

The immunomodulator medications work via the suppression of cytokines and inflammatory mediators, particularly TNF-α. The anti-malaria drugs, Chloroquine and Hydroxychloroquine, have shown some promising results. Hydroxychloroquine is generally better tolerated. It is particularly effective for sarcoid's disfiguring skin ailments *(1)*. Opthalmological examinations are necessary because of potential retinal toxicity of the anti-malaria drugs. Infliximab (Remicade®) also has anti-TNF-α activity and therefore has been used in the treatment of sarcoid in limited scenarios *(1)*. Pentoxifylline, another TNF-α inhibitor again has been used infrequently. Although all of the above immunomodulators show promising results for advanced sarcoid, further studies are required before definitive treatment guidelines are established.

Surgical treatment is the final option used in very limited circumstances. Lung transplants have been performed successfully on end-stage sarcoid. Sarcoid granulomas have been reported to develop in the lung allografts, although recurrence with clinical significance is minimal.

It is also important to recognize the various treatments for some of the individual organs affected by sarcoidosis. In the eye, for example, acute anterior uveitis usually responds to topical corticosteroids and cycloplegics. Although topical therapy is usually effective, optic neuritis requires systemic steroids and potentially surgical intervention. Lacrimal gland involvement, chorioretinitis, and retinal vasculitis all respond to oral corticosteroids. The treatment for cutaneous sarcoid depends on the type of skin lesions. For erythema nodosum, 6 to 8 weeks of nonsteroidal anti-inflammatory drugs alone are effective. The patient with lupus pernio most often requires systemic corticosteroids. Papules and plaques may respond to topical steroids or intralesion injections of triamcinolone monthly. Unlike pulmonary sarcoidosis in which mild or asymptomatic disease can be observed without intervention, the presence of neurosarcoidosis requires immediate treatment.

Unfortunately, little benefit has been shown for the use of medications in cardiac sarcoidosis. When medically indicated, pacemakers, automatic implantable cardioverter-defibrillators, cardiac resection, and even transplant are available. Finally, nephropathy secondary to hypercalcemia as seen in sarcoid generally responds to 10 to 20 mg per day of corticosteroids. Quinolones have also proven to be effective in the treatment of hypercalcemia. Patients should be instructed to eat a low-calcium diet and avoid excess vitamin D.

FUTURE DIRECTIONS

Although sarcoidosis was first described more than a century ago, and despite years of research, several important questions about this complex disease remain unanswered. The precise genetic and environmental predisposing factors have yet to be identified and the pathogenesis of granuloma formation is not completely defined. Moreover, prognostic markers for disease progression are often unreliable and the treatment is rarely curative, yet replete with adverse side effects. However, the future is bright. Researchers in immunology and molecular biology are currently addressing these mysteries and progress is being made. In time, we will advance our understanding of the pathogenesis of the disease, discover the causative agents, and improve our ability to diagnose and treat this perplexing condition. Until a cure is found, it is the role of the medical community to enhance the quality of life for those suffering from this condition and help patients with sarcoid maximize their functional capacity.

REFERENCES

1. Newman LS, Rose CS, Maier LA. Medical progress: sarcoidosis, N Engl J Med 1997;336: 1224–1234.
2. Statement on Sarcoidosis. Joint Statement of the American Thoracic Society (ATS), the European Respiratory Society (ERS) and the World Association of Sarcoidosis and other Granulomatous Disorders (WASOG) adopted by the ATS Board of Directors and by the ERS Executive Committee. Respir Crit Care Med 1999;160:736–755.
3. Martin WJ, Iannuzzi MC, Gail DB, Peavy HH. Future directions in sarcoid research. Am J Respir Crit Care Med 2004;170:567–571.
4. Thomas KW, Hunninghake GW. Sarcoidosis [see comment]. JAMA. 2003;289:3300–3303.

5. Judson M, Thompson BW, Rabin DL, et al. The diagnostic pathway to sarcoidosis. Chest 2003;123:406–412.
6. Baughman RP. Pulmonary Sarcoidosis. Clin Chest Med 2004;25:521–530.
7. Gullapalli D, Phillips II LH. Neurologic manifestations of sarcoidosis. Neurol Clin 2002;20:59–83.
8. Wu JL, Schiff KR. Sarcoidosis. Am Fam Physician 2004;70:312–322.
9. Roberts SD, Mirowski GW, Wilke D, Teague SD, Knox KS. Sarcoidosis. Part I: pulmonary manifestations. J Am Acad Dermatol 2004;51: 448–451.

18 Pneumonia

Mohamed Al-Darei and Matthew L. Mintz

CONTENTS
> CASE PRESENTATION
> KEY CLINICAL QUESTIONS
> LEARNING OBJECTIVES
> EPIDEMIOLOGY
> PATHOPHYSIOLOGY
> DIFFERENTIAL DIAGNOSIS
> DIAGNOSIS
> TREATMENT
> FUTURE DIRECTIONS
> SOURCES

CASE PRESENTATION

A 55-year-old male with a history of type 2 diabetes mellitus presents with dyspnea, high fever, chills, and productive cough with purulent sputum for 2 days duration. He denies hemoptysis. He has smoked two packs of cigarettes a day for the past 20 years and drinks six beers a day. On physical exam he appears acutely ill. His vital signs show a temperature of 39.8°C, pulse is 130 beats per minute, respiratory rate is 48 breaths per minute, blood pressure is 113/60, and oxygen saturation is 86% on room air. Lungs are dull to percussion and bronchial breath sound heard over the left lower lobe. Chest X-ray showed infiltrates in the left lower lobe.

KEY CLINICAL QUESTIONS

1. What are the most likely causative organisms of pneumonia in this patient?
2. What further diagnostic tests are recommended for diagnosis?

> From: *Current Clinical Practice: Disorders of the Respiratory Tract:
> Common Challenges in Primary Care*
> By: M. L. Mintz © Humana Press, Totowa, NJ

3. Can this patient be treated as an outpatient or should he be admitted?
4. What antibiotic agent would be recommended for this patient?
5. Assuming the diagnosis of community-acquired pneumonia (CAP), what preventive measures, if any, need to be taken with this patient to avoid future episodes?

LEARNING OBJECTIVES

1. Recognize the risk factors associated with CAP.
2. List the common and atypical pathogens causing pneumonia.
3. Recognize the common signs and symptoms of pneumonia, and discern the most appropriate tests necessary to make the diagnosis.
4. Understand how to determine whether a patient with pneumonia can be treated as an outpatient or should be admitted to the hospital.
5. Become familiar with guideline-based antimicrobial therapies for both the inpatient and outpatient treatment of pneumonia.

EPIDEMIOLOGY

The Infectious Diseases Society of America (IDSA) defines CAP as "an acute infection of the pulmonary parenchyma that is associated with at least some symptoms of acute infection, accompanied by acute infiltrate on chest X-ray or auscultatory findings consistent with pneumonia in a patient who is not hospitalized or residing in a long term care facility for 14 or more days before symptoms onset." Although pneumonia is a relatively common condition and often without major sequelae, it remains the leading cause of death from infection, the sixth leading cause of death in the United States, and the fourth leading cause of death in the elderly. There are approximately 4.5 million cases of pneumonia in the United States every year with 600,000 hospital admissions. It is estimated that approximately 10 million physician visits result from pneumonia, causing 64 million days of restricted activities. CAP is the most common type of pneumonia (71%). Of patients with CAP, 80% are treated successfully in the outpatient setting with mortality rate less than 1%. The death rate from CAP can be as high as 12% among the remaining 20% who require hospitalization. The oldest and the youngest members of the population have the highest attack rates. Twelve to eighteen cases per 1000 of pneumonia occur in the 0- to 4-year-old age group and 20 cases per 1000 in the 60-year and older group with an overall attack rate of 12 cases per 1000 persons per year. The cost of pneumonia management is estimated to be $9 billion and is mainly determined by the length of hospitalization.

Risk factors for CAP include chronic obstructive pulmonary disease (COPD), renal insufficiency, congestive heart failure (CHF), coronary artery disease, diabetes mellitus, malignancy, chronic neurological disease, and chronic liver disease. Studies have shown that there are independent risk factors for pneumonia, such as alcoholism, asthma, immunosuppression, institutionalization, and advanced age (>71). Aspiration is a major risk factor for pneumococcal infection. Dementia, seizure, CHF, and COPD all contribute to aspiration and consequently pneumococcal pneumonia. Another significant risk factor for pneumonia is living in overcrowded places, such as jails, homeless shelters, and nursing homes. AIDS and hematological malignancy are important risk factors for *Legionella* infection (Legionnaires' disease). Risk factors for specific pathogens are illustrated in Table 1.

PATHOPHYSIOLOGY

The lower respiratory tract is designed to effectively protect against pathogenic invasion. An infection occurs when the protective mechanisms are impaired or overwhelmed by pathogens. The most common pathway of lower respiratory infection occurs when organisms are aspirated from oropharyngeal secretions. Less common pathways of infections are hematogenous spread and inhalation of infected droplets. When the alveoli become overwhelmed by organisms that reach the lung parenchyma, a local inflammatory response is initiated. Inflammatory cells (white blood cells, lymphocytes, monocytes) and fluid penetrate the alveoli, which result in the consolidation of lungs. In addition, inflammatory mediators leak into the blood circulation, which explains the systemic response responsible for signs and symptoms of pneumonia.

Bacteria are responsible for 60 to 80% cases of CAP, whereas 15% of cases are related to viruses. *Streptococcus pneumoniae* is the most common cause of CAP requiring hospitalization. Among hospitalized patients with CAP, several studies concluded that *S. pneumoniae* was responsible for 9 to 50% of cases. The second most common causative organism of pneumonia is *Mycoplasma pneumoniae*, which accounts for approximately 15% of all CAP cases. It is transmitted person to person by respiratory droplets, and is associated with atypical pneumonia characterized by more gradual onset associated with headache, fatigue, myalgia, sore throat, and dry cough. *M. pneumoniae* is usually self-limited with low mortality rate and rarely requires hospitalization. *Chlamydia pneumoniae* and *Legionella pneumophila* are also associated with atypical pneumonia. *C. pneumoniae* is more common in older patients with comorbid diseases. Most cases of *C. pneumoniae* are self-limited but can lead to more severe cases requiring hospitalization with the mortality rate approaching 9%. *L. pneumophila* is transmitted by exposure to the organism in the environment. It inhabits fresh water, heating and cooling systems, and moist soil. It more often affects individuals with compromised immune system, renal or liver failure, malignancy, and diabetes. *L. pneumoplila* has the worst clinical course among the atypical pathogens with the highest mortality rate (14%). *Haemophilus influenzae* is more common in patients with COPD.

Table 1
Risk Factors for Specific Organisms Causing Community-Acquired Pneumonia

Organism	Risk factors
Streptococcus pneumoniae	Comorbid conditions
	Smoking
	Influenza virus
	Crowded places (prisons, shelters)
	Sickle cell disease
	Splenectomy
Drug-resistant *S. pneumoniae*	Advanced age (>65)
	Nursing home
	Alcoholism
	Recent use of antibiotics
	Recent hospitalization
	Day care center exposure
Haemophilus influenzae	Smoking
	Chronic obstructive pulmonary disease
	Influenza virus
Gram-negative *Enterobacteriaceae*	Older age
	Nursing home
	History of alcoholism
	Immunosuppression
	Recent antibiotic use
	Comorbid illness
Legionnaires' disease	AIDS
	Exposure to contaminated air-conditioning
	Hematological disease
	Renal failure
Pseudomonas aeruginosa	Bronchiectasis
	Cystic fibrosis
	Prolonged broad-spectrum antibiotics use
	Corticosteroid therapy
	Neutropenia
	Malnutrition
Anerobes	Aspiration
	Poor dental hygiene
	Airway obstruction
	History of alcoholism

Additionally, viruses have been implicated in CAP requiring hospitalization. Influenza virus is the most common cause of viral pneumonia and frequently leads to secondary bacterial pneumonia. It is thought that viral infection predispose to secondary bacterial infection by suppressing the immune system and

Table 2
Differential Diagnosis of Pneumonia

Upper respiratory tract infection
Sinusitis
Acute bronchitis
Acute exacerbation of chronic bronchitis
Pneumonia
Asthma
Congestive heart failure
Pulmonary embolism
Vasculitis
Pulmonary neoplasm

interfering with cilia's function to clear the organism. Respiratory syncytial virus is a common pathogen in the pediatric population with increasing frequency in adults, especially in nursing homes.

DIFFERENTIAL DIAGNOSIS

Distinguishing between pneumonia and acute bronchitis can be a challenging task. Patients with pneumonia present with high fever, chills, high respiratory rate, pleuritic chest pain, bloody sputum, crackles, and X-ray findings. In contrast, patients with bronchitis present with productive cough, but signs of consolidation are usually absent with normal chest X-ray. They may have low-grade fever but patients with bronchitis are most commonly afebrile. Tuberculosis can also present similar to CAP. They both present with malaise, anorexia, cough, fever, and night sweats. Other conditions that should be in the differential diagnosis include chronic pulmonary disease, atelectasis, lung abscess, pulmonary embolism, heart failure, and neoplasm (Table 2).

DIAGNOSIS

Clinical Presentation

CAP has been thought to present in two different clinical manifestations: typical and atypical. Typical CAP is associated with bacterial agents such as *S. pneumoniae* and *H. influenzae* (Table 3), and is characterized by sudden onset of fever, productive cough, pleuritic chest pain, and shortness of breath. Physical examination shows tachypnea (respiratory rate >20 breaths per minute), tachycardia, and signs of lung consolidations including dullness to percussion, increased fremitus, egophony, bronchial breath sounds, and crackles (Table 4).

In contrast, atypical CAP is caused by *C. pneumoniae*, *L. pneumophila*, and *M. pneumoniae* and present with more gradual onset of nonproductive cough and

Table 3
Community-Acquired Pneumonia Causative Organisms and Their Frequency

Pathogen	Frequency (%)
Bacteria	
Streptococcus pneumoniae	20–60
Haemophilus influenzae	3–10
Moraxella catarrhalis	<5
Staphylococcus aureus	3–5
Atypical bacteria	
Chlamydia	4–6
Mycoplasma	1–10
Legionella	0–15
Viruses	2–15
Unidentified pathogens	30–60

Table 4
Signs and Symptoms of Community-Acquired Pneumonia

Fever
Chills
Cough (dry or productive)
Pleuritic chest pain
Tachypnea
Dyspnea
Tachycardia
Diminished breath sound
Adventitious breath sounds (crackles, ronchi)
Hypoxemia

shortness of breath. Extrapulmonary manifestations (headache, myalgias, fatigue, and sore throat) are more prominent in the atypical form. Although this distinction of CAP has been used by physicians for a long time, it cannot be used to identify the etiological agent. Furthermore, presence of comorbid conditions and older age can influence the clinical manifestation of CAP. For example, signs and symptoms of CAP are less prominent in older patients who present more with altered mental status, general deterioration, decreased appetite, and increased falls. Because of the various manifestations of CAP, history and physical examination cannot make definitive diagnosis of pneumonia because of their low sensitivity and specificity. Therefore, evidence of new infiltrate on chest X-ray should be present to confirm the diagnosis.

Chest Radiograph

Chest X-ray is recommended for patients who present with symptoms suggestive of pneumonia. The American Thoracic Society (ATS) and IDSA require evidence of radiographic findings in their definition of pneumonia. Chest X-ray is more sensitive than physical examination for detecting pulmonary infiltrates; however, it is not 100% sensitive. In addition to its diagnostic value in detecting lung infiltrates, chest radiograph can be also helpful in assessing the other conditions, assessing the extent of the infection, identifying cavitations, and following up the response to therapy. The common perception that chest radiograph can identify the causative organism in no longer valid. A study was conducted in 1996 to compare *C. pneumonia* and pneumococcal pneumonia revealed no significant difference in the pattern, distribution, or extent between the two groups.

Laboratory Testing

According to ATS and IDSA guidelines, basic laboratory tests are unnecessary in patients without cardiopulmonary conditions who can be managed as outpatients. Patients with chronic heart or lung diseases require assessment of their oxygenation with the pulse oximetry. Patients who are candidates for admission as well as patients older than 65 years of age with comorbid conditions should have basic laboratory studies (complete blood count, chemistries, renal function, and liver function). Recent CAP recommendations suggest obtaining sputum culture in hospitalized patients; however, empirical therapy should not be delayed until the causative organism is identified. The findings of the culture should be used to narrow the antibiotic therapy and identify the drug-resistant bacteria. Furthermore, the IDSA and the ATS recommend blood cultures for hospitalized patients to help in identifying the causative organism and drug-resistant bacteria in bacteremic patients (4–18% of CAP patients develop bacteremia).

TREATMENT

The decision whether to hospitalize a patient with CAP or treat them as an outpatient is an important part in the management. More than 30% of hospitalized patients are low risk and can be managed outside the hospital. Some useful tools have been established to assess the severity of pneumonia and help in making the decision to admit the patient. The most commonly used model is the pneumonia severity index (PSI) (Fig.1). The PSI stratifies patients into five severity classes based on the mortality risk. The score of the PSI is based on information obtained from history and physical examination, chest radiograph findings, and laboratory studies. If the patient is 50 years old or younger, has no comorbid condition (neoplastic disease, liver disease, heart disease, CHF, cerebrovascular disease, or renal failure), has nonaltered mental status, and has stable vital signs, the patient is assigned to class I. Patients are assigned to subsequent

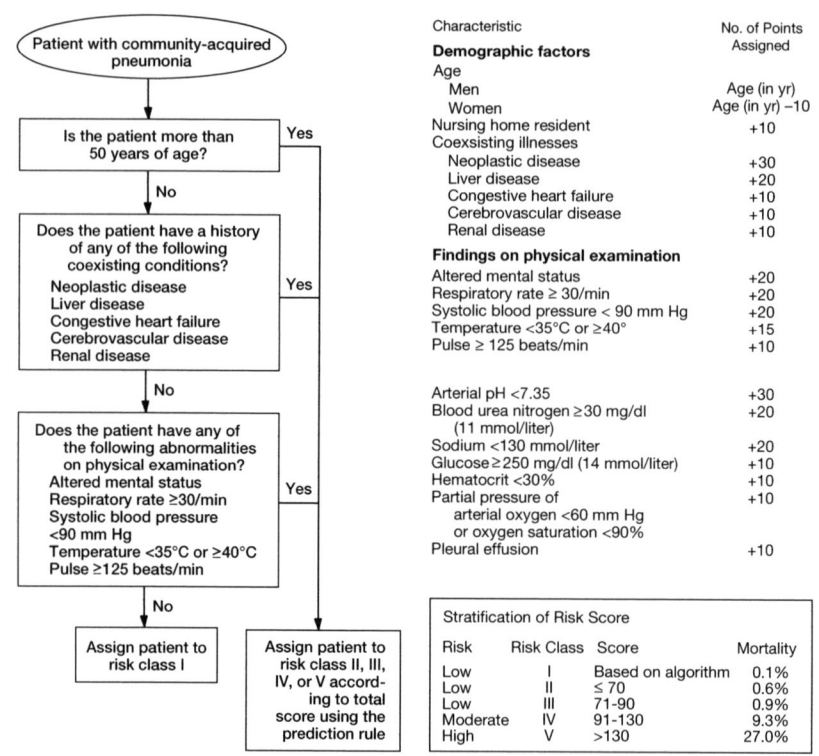

Fig. 1. The pneumonia severity index. The pneumonia severity index is used to determine a patient's risk of death. The total score is obtained by adding the points assigned for each additional applicable characteristic to the patient's age (in years for men or in years minus 10 for women). (Data have been adapted from Fine et al. with permission.)

categories of increasing severity based on the score obtained from PSI. The mortality risk in class I is 0.1% and approaching 27% in class V. According to the recommendations, classes I and II may not require hospitalization and can be managed as an outpatient. Class III may or may not require inpatient observation, and classes IV and V should be hospitalized. However, as with all prediction rules, clinical judgment is the critical in making decisions regarding whether or not to hospitalize a patient.

Treatment Principles

Treatment of pneumonia should be initiated as soon as the diagnosis is made, because delays in treatment are associated with increased morbidity and mortality. Because the CAP causative organism is often unknown at the time of presentation, the antimicrobial agent should be selected empirically based on the most likely pathogens. Factors that aid in choosing antibiotics include geographic distribution of pathogens, presence of comorbid diseases, and increased risk of drug-resistant streptococcal pneumonia (Table 1). In addition, factors related to the specific antimicrobial agent (tolerance, safety, cost, pharmacokinitics and pharmacodynamics, efficacy) should be considered.

Outpatient Treatment

According to the ATS, IDSA, and the Center for Disease Control and Prevention guidelines, recommended antibiotic for CAP patients in the outpatient setting includes macrolides, doxycycline, fluoroquinolones, or combination of β-lactam plus macrolide. Generally, macrolides are recommended as first-line therapy for patients with no comorbid diseases or risk for drug-resistant *S. pneumoniae*. The rational for these recommendations is that macrolides provide good coverage for common organisms, such as *S. pneumoniae*, as well as atypical pathogens, including *M. pneumoniae* and *C. pneumoniae*. Macrolide class includes the erythromycin and similar agents such as dirithromycin, and the extended spectrum macrolides, clarithromycin, and azithromycin. Azithromycin and clarithromycin are used more often than erythromycin because of their greater efficacy against *H. influenzae* with less gastrointestinal side effects. Doxycyclin is an acceptable alternative for patients who cannot tolerate macrolides. The use of fluroquinolones is not recommended for the treatment of CAP with no comorbid diseases and no recent antibiotic use to avoid the emergence of fluoroquinolone-resistant pathogens. Fluoroquinolones (gatifloxacin, gemifloxacin, levofloxacin, moxifloxacin) should be reserved for patients with comorbidities and recent antibiotic use because incidence of drug-resistant *S. pneumoniae* and enteric Gram-negative bacteria are higher in these patients. Telithromycin is a new class of medications similar to the macrolides, which has been approved to treat mild to moderate CAP if drug-resistant *S. pneumoniae* infection is suspected. In vitro studies have demonstrated the efficacy of telethromycin against *S. pneumoniae* resistant to macrolides, penicillins, and fluoroquinolones. It has similar efficacy against *H. influenzae* as the clarithromycin and azithromycin, with a low potential for resistance. The British Thoracic Society (BTS) guidelines recommend β-lactams (penicillins) as first-line option to treat CAP in outpatients because these agents are effective against *S. pneumoniae* and can be effective against most strains with low penicillin sensitivity if given in high doses. BTS guidelines do not place great significances on the empiric altreatment of patients infected with atypical pathogens. The rational is that the *M. pneumoniae* infection is self-limiting and affects the younger population more commonly, therefore setting a policy to empirically treat if it is considered unnecessary.

Inpatient Treatment

For patients who are admitted to the general wards, ATS, IDSA, and Centers for Disease Control and Prevention guidelines recommend combination of intravenous β-lactam and macrolide or monotherapy with fluoroquinolones because studies have demonstrated significant reduction in mortality rate and shorter hospital stays associated with these regimens as apposed to β-lactam therapy alone. BTS guidelines are similar to North American guidelines for inpatient antimicrobial selection. Patients who are admitted to the intensive care unit are thought to have more resistant organisms (*S. pneumoniae*, *Legionella* spp., *H. influenzae*, *Enterobacteriaceae*, *Staphylococcus aureus*, and *Pseudomonas* spp.). If intensive care unit patients are not at risk for *Pseudomonas*, combination of β-lactams and advanced macrolides or respiratory fleuroquinolones is recommended to ensure coverage for *S. pneumoniae* and *Legionella* species. If risk for *Pseudomonas* is present, β-lactams agents with effective coverage against this organism (piperacillin–tazobactam, imipenem, meropenem, and cefepime) are recommended. Once the causative organism is identified, therapy should be directed to the specific pathogen (Table 5).

Switching from intravenous to oral therapy should be considered once the patient's clinical condition has stabilized. The ATS suggests the use of Ramirez criteria for an early switch to oral therapy: improved cough and dyspnea, temperature of 37.8°C or less for at least 8 hours, normalized white blood cell count, oral intake with normal gastrointestinal function.

Few appropriately controlled studies have evaluated the optimal duration for the antimicrobial therapy in patients with CAP. The goal for the management of respiratory tract infections in general is to improve the clinical conditions and minimize the risk of antimicrobial resistance. To avoid resistance, the World Health Organization recommends using the most potent antimicrobial therapy for the shortest period required for effective results. Most CAP patients are treated for 7 to 10 days. Their clinical conditions begin to improve within 3 to 7 days. Patients who are not clinically stable may require longer duration of therapy, such as patients who are bacteremic with *S. aureus* pneumonia (increased risk with endocarditis), patients with meningitis, pseudomonia pneumonia, and patients infected with less common organisms.

After the patient is hospitalized, received the appropriate antibiotic therapy, and become clinically stable, the decision to discharge the patient should be considered. To be able to go home, patients should have stable vital signs, good oxygenation on room air, should be able to receive oral treatment, and have stable mental status (Table 6). In general, low-risk patients become clinically stable within 3 days. Moderate- and high-risk patients gain clinical stability in 4 and 6 days, respectively. Studies have shown that patients who are discharged while clinically unstable have a higher mortality rate and higher rate of re-admission.

Table 5
Recommended Therapy for Specific Pathogens

Organism	First-line therapy	Second-line therapy
Streptococcus pneumoniae penicillin-susceptible	Pencillin G, amoxicillin	Macrolide, telithromycin, cephalosporins, clindamycin, doxycyline, respiratory fluoroquinolone
S. pneumoniae penicillin-resistant	Cefotaxime, ceftriaxone, fluorquinolone, telithromycin	Vancomycin, linezolid
Haemophilus influenzae	Second- or third-generation cephalosporin, amoxicillin/clavulanate	Fluoroquinolone, azithromycin, clarithromycin
Legionella	Fluorquinolone, macrolide	Doxycyline
Moraxella pneumoniae/ Chlamydia pneumoniae	Macrolide	Fluorquinolone, telithromycin
Staphylococcus aureus methicillin-susceptible	Antistaphylococcus penicillin (nafcillin, dicloxacillin)	Cefazolin, clindamycin
S. aureus methicillin-resistent	Vancomycin, linezolid	
Pseudomonas aeruginosa	Antipseudomonal β-lactam (pipracillin, ticracillin) plus ciprofloxacin or aminoglycoside	Levofloxacin or ciprofloxacin plus aminoglycoside
Aspiration pneumonia (anerobes)	Clindamycin, β-lactam–β-lactamase inhibitor	Carbapenem
Enterobacteriaceae	Third-generation cephalosporin	β lactam β-lactamase inhibitor, fluoroquinolone, aztreonam

Prevention

There is higher frequency of CAP cases during influenza season related to secondary bacterial pneumonia complicating influenza as well as primary influenza pneumonia. Influenza vaccine has been proven to be effective in reducing the incidents of pneumonia cases during influenza outbreaks. Influenza vaccine is recommend for people who are at a higher risk of developing complications,

Table 6
Criteria for Discharge From the Hospital

Stable vital signs for 24 hours:
   Temperature less than 37.8°C
   Respiratory rate less than 24 breaths per minute
   Heart rate less than 100 beats per minute
   Systolic blood pressure more than 90 mmHg
   O_2 saturation more than 90% on room air
Ability to take oral medication
Ability to maintain enough hydration and nutrition
Normal mental status
Absence of other active clinical or psychosocial problems necessitating hospitalization

such as people older than 65 years, people who live in nursing homes, and people with chronic pulmonary or cerebrovasvular diseases. People who are likely to transmit the virus, such as health care providers, are also encouraged to receive the vaccine. Another vaccine that has contributed to the decline in pneumonia cases is pneumococcal vaccine. Recommendations for pneumococcal vaccine include patients aged 65 or older and patients less than 65 years old with chronic diseases such as CHF, COPD, diabetes mellitus, chronic liver disease, alcoholism, or asplenia. Cigarette smoking is considered an important contributor for pneumonia, so patients with history of pneumonia should be encouraged to quit smoking.

FUTURE DIRECTIONS

Given the significant morbidity and mortality of pneumonia, specifically CAP, this area continues to be a fertile ground for research. Controversy continues to exist regarding the best antibiotic regimen, especially as new agents continue to be developed. Telithromycin is a new type of macrolide with the potential to decrease resistance. If lower resistance and efficacy against drug-resistant *S. pneumoniae* continues to be seen, this agent may be recommended more frequently. Similarly, in acute exacerbations of bronchitis, one large randomized study showed superiority of moxifloxacin to standard therapy (amoxicillin, clarithromycin, or cefuroxime) in the occurrence of failure, new exacerbation, or any further antibiotic use. This has not yet been evaluated in CAP, but because the causative organisms are similar, moxifloxacin could potentially be considered early in CAP should future research show similar findings.

SOURCES

Anish EJ. Lower respiratory tract infection in adult outpatients. Clin Fam Prac 2004;6:75.
Boldt MD, Kiresuk T. Community acquired pneumonia in adults. Nurse Pract 2001;26:14–16, 19–24.
Dean NC, Bateman KA. Local guidelines for community acquired pneumonia: development, implementation, and outcome studies. Infect Dis Clin North Am 2004;18:975–991.
File TM. Streptococcus pneumoniae and community-acquired pneumonia: a cause for concern. Am J Med 2004;117:39–50.
File TM, Niederman MS. Antimicrobial therapy for community-acquired pneumonia. Infect Dis Clin North Am 2004;18:993–1016.
Fine MJ, Auble TE, Yealy DM, et al. A prediction rule to identify low-risk patients with community-acquired pneumonia. N Engl J Med 1997;336:243–250.
Gharib AM, Stern EJ. Radiology of pneumonia. Med Clin North Am 2001;85:1461–1490.
Halm EA, Teirstein AS. Management of community acquired pneumonia. N Engl J Med 2002;347:2039–2045.
Kleinpell RM, Elpern E. Community-acquired pneumonia: updated in assessment and management. Crit Care Nurs Q 2004;27:231–240.
Lim WS, Macfarlane JT. Importance of severity of illness assessment in management of low respiratory infection. Curr Opin Infect Dis 2004;17:121–125.
Mandell LA. Epidemiology and etiology of community acquired pneumonia. Infect Dis Clin North Am 2004;18:761–776.
Metlay JP, Fine MJ. Testing strategies in the initial management of patients with community-acquired pneumonia. Ann Intern Med 2003;138:109–118.
Niederman MS, Mandell LA, Anzueto A, et al. Guidelines for the management of adults with community-acquired pneumonia: diagnosis, assessment of severity, antimicrobial therapy, and prevention. Am J Respir Crit Care Med 2001;163:1730–1754.
Pimental L, Mcpherson SJ. Community-acquired pneumonia in the emergency department: a practical approach to diagnosis and management. Emerg Med Clin North 2003;21:395–420.
Ramirez JA. Community-acquired pneumonia in adults. Prim Care 2003;30:155–171.
Thibodeau KP, Viera AJ. Atypical pneumonia and challenges in community acquired pneumonia. Am Fam Physician 2004;69:1699–1706.
Wilson R, Allegra L, Huchon G, et al. Short-term and long-term outcomes of moxifloxacin compared to standard antibiotic treatment in acute exacerbations of chronic bronchitis. Chest 2004;125:953–964.

19 Bronchiolitis

Elizabeth A. Valois Asser, Alexander S. Asser, and Matthew L. Mintz

CONTENTS
> CASE PRESENTATIONS
> KEY CLINICAL QUESTIONS
> LEARNING OBJECTIVES
> EPIDEMIOLOGY
> PATHOPHYSIOLOGY
> DIAGNOSIS
> DIFFERENTIAL DIAGNOSIS
> PREVENTION
> TREATMENT
> REFERENCES

CASE PRESENTATIONS

Case 1

A 5-month-old boy presents with a 3-day history of cough, rhinorrhea, congestion, and fevers. Today his mother noticed he was breathing faster and taking in less formula than normal. His 4-year-old sister has a cold and he attends a local day care. On physical exam, the boy's temperature is 102.5°F, heart rate is 140 beats per minute, respiratory rate is 60 breaths per minute, and blood pressure is 90/50. His oxygen saturation is 95%. He appears alert and smiling but is tachypneic and coughing. He has subcostal and intercostal retractions. On auscultation of his lungs, wheezing is heard on both inspiration and expiration. A prolonged expiratory phase is also noted. The wheezing has a "wet" quality to it. The liver is palpated 2 cm below the costal margin.

> From: *Current Clinical Practice: Disorders of the Respiratory Tract:
> Common Challenges in Primary Care*
> By: M. L. Mintz © Humana Press, Totowa, NJ

Case 2

The mother of a 2-week-old infant is concerned because her son has had two episodes in which he "just stopped breathing." The episodes each lasted 20 to 30 seconds during which time he "became limp." She is now afraid to let her infant sleep alone and is calling the office for advice. She admits that she, her husband, and their two other children have a cold. The infant is not showing any upper respiratory symptoms at this time. Advice is given to go directly to the emergency department (ED). In the ED, the infant's vitals signs are within the normal range for age and the physical exam is also normal. The decision is made to admit for observation. Before the infant is brought up to a room, he has an apneic episode witnessed by the ED staff that lasts 1 minute and requires resuscitation. The infant is intubated and sent to the intensive care unit (ICU). An antigen detection test on a nasal swab aspirate reveals the most likely cause of this infant's apnea.

KEY CLINICAL QUESTIONS

1. At what point (case 1) should the physician be able to recognize that this patient may have more than just a cold?
2. How common is an infant with apnea (case 2) after the parents have a cold?
3. Is there a relationship between early respiratory inflammation and asthma?
4. How could either of these cases have been prevented?

LEARNING OBJECTIVES

1. Recognize the clinical presentations of bronchiolitis.
2. Understand the most common etiology of bronchiolitis.
3. List the risk factors contributing to the severity of the illness.
4. Understand the pathophysiology.
5. Identify patients with bronchiolitis and describe the clinical course of the disease.
6. Outline the treatment modalities and understand their effectiveness.
7. Describe the preventative measures currently used.

EPIDEMIOLOGY

Bronchiolitis is a very common respiratory disease in children younger than 2 years of age usually occurring during the winter months that results in narrowing or obstruction of the lower respiratory tract. Patients typically present with rhinorrhea, congestion, cough, wheezing, and low-grade fever. In more severe cases, patients will present with respiratory distress and require prompt hospitalization. Children rarely require the assistance of mechanical ventilation.

Bronchiolitis is usually caused by a viral infection. Although there are many causes of bronchiolitis (Table 1), the respiratory syncytial virus (RSV) is by far

Table 1
Causes of Bronchiolitis

- Respiratory syncytial virus (80%)
- Parainfluenza
- Adenovirus
- Rhinovirus
- Influenza virus
- Chlamydial pneumonia
- Source of viral infection is usually a family member with minor respiratory illness
- Older children and adults tolerate bronchiolar edema better than infants and do not acquire the clinical picture of bronchiolitis, even when the smaller airways of the respiratory tract are infected
- Fewer than 5% of recurrent attacks of clinical bronchiolitis are caused by viral infections

the most common pathogen isolated and is found in up to 80% of cases. RSV is a RNA paramyxovirus. It is unstable in the outside environment and is killed easily with soap and warm water. It may survive on hands and countertops for hours. Transmission of the infection is typically from a family member or caregiver who has an upper respiratory infection. Inoculation is usually through the conjunctiva or nasal mucosa via infected droplets in the air or on hands. Children usually shed the virus for 3 to 8 days but may be contagious for up to 4 weeks *(1)*. Previous infection with RSV does not convey immunity, and therefore it is possible to become infected again even in the same season, although symptoms may be less severe *(2)*.

Up to 50% of all children are infected with RSV each year and almost all are exposed to the virus by age 2 *(1)*. Although infection with RSV is relatively common, only a handful of children will develop bronchiolitis. Bronchiolitis is more common in children who are younger than 2 years of age. Although less common, bronchiolitis is also seen in the adult population. Risk factors for bronchiolitis include infants and children who are bottle fed, attend day care, have a family history of asthma, live with a mother who smokes, are premature, and have pre-existing lung or heart disease. Interestingly, the risk of developing bronchiolitis is lower in infants who attend day care than in infants of stay-at-home mothers who smoke.

Cases of bronchiolitis are seen throughout the year but occur as an epidemic each winter in the United States. The seasonal peak occurs usually occurs in the months of January and February but can occur anywhere from late December to early March *(3)*.

PATHOPHYSIOLOGY

In bronchiolitis, the virus penetrates the lower respiratory tract mucosa causing bronchoconstriction, inflammation, edema, and accumulation of mucous and cellular debris *(4)*. Resistance is inversely related to the fourth power of the radius of a circle. Therefore, a smaller airway produces an elevated resistance when compared with a larger airway. This is why older children and adults tolerate mucosal thickening better than younger children.

The mucous plugs that develop in the lower respiratory tract cause air trapping similar to a ball-valve effect. This leads to overinflation. When severe, these plugs completely block the smaller airways leading to absorption of air, and hence atelectasis. When widespread, this atelectasis leads to V-Q mismatch and hypoxia.

Case 1 illustrates a typical presentation of a child with bronchiolitis. There is usually a history of exposure to a caretaker or sibling with a cold within 1 week. Initially, mild to moderate upper respiratory symptoms predominate including cough, rhinorrhea, congestion, and sneezing. A fever to 101 to 102°F is not unusual. Gastrointestinal symptoms are mild or absent. Within 3 to 7 days, tachypnea and wheezing develop and can last for up to 1 week. Those who are more severely affected may have symptoms even longer.

A moderately affected child may present with a respiratory rate between 50 and 80 breaths per minute. Nasal flaring, use of accessory muscles, and hyperinflation will be noted on the physical exam. Wheezing is heard throughout the lung fields on inspiration and expiration and may have a wet quality to it. A prolonged expiratory phase may be noted. When air trapping occurs it is possible to palpate the spleen and liver just below the costal border. These children require close observation with frequent visits to the office and phone calls, or admission to the hospital.

Severely affected children present with fatigue, listlessness, dehydration, or hypoxia. Many cannot maintain the respiratory rate required for gas exchange. Often it is difficult to hear breath sounds because of poor aeration. These children require immediate medical attention.

Case 2 is a less common presentation of an infant with RSV. These infants are usually less than 1 month old with a history of exposure to a caretaker or sibling with a cold. Apnea is the presenting symptom. Episodes may respond to tactile stimulation. Infants require hospitalization and sometimes mechanical ventilation if the episodes of apnea are recurrent or prolonged. Upper respiratory symptoms and wheezing may be noted days later. Newborn infants have an immature respiratory center in the brain, but it is not completely understood how RSV modifies this center, leading to apnea *(5)*.

Only 2 to 3% of children who are hospitalized require mechanical ventilation. A higher proportion of these children have an underlying medical condition, such as heart disease, bronchopulmonary dysplasia, or an immunodeficiency. The mortality rate has improved from 37% to less than 4% in the last 30 years. The mortality rate for children with no comorbid condition is less than 1%. These children typically present with apnea, dehydration, and respiratory acidosis.

The association between bronchiolitis and the development of asthma remains unclear. The cause of asthma is multifactorial and it is likely that bronchiolitis plays a role in many patients. Children with a history of bronchiolitis were found to have increased reactivity of their airways compared with their peers at age 6. This did not persist through childhood *(6)*. However, those children with a family history of asthma, more severe symptoms on presentation with bronchiolitis, and repeated episodes of bronchiolitis are more likely to develop asthma. Therefore, bronchiolitis may lead to increased airway reactivity in the first decade of life but other factors appear to determine the persistence of this reactivity.

DIAGNOSIS

Beyond the physical exam, diagnostic tests are not indicated to diagnose bronchiolitis. If there is suspicion of a co-existing condition or an alternative diagnosis, the following tests may be useful.

Pulse Oximetery

Pulse oximetery is useful if hypoxia is suspected. It is not unusual for these infants to experience mucous plugs leading to hypoxia. If supplemental oxygen is required, the goal should be to maintain saturation levels between 90 and 94%.

Chest Radiograph

A chest radiograph is indicated if pneumonia, a chest mass, a foreign body, or heart failure are suspected. In bronchiolitis, the radiograph may show hyperinflation or scattered areas of atelectasis. This is can be misinterpreted as bacterial pneumonia.

Nasal Specimen

A nasal aspirate for antigen detection of RSV can be performed. It is useful if ribivirian is considered as a treatment option and for isolation purposes within the hospital. Influenza A and B and adenovirus can also be detected by this method.

Laboratory Studies

A complete blood count (CBC) and a blood culture should be considered if a bacterial infection such as pneumonia or sepsis are suspected. Sepsis is very rare.

**Table 2
Differential Diagnosis**

- Pneumonia
- Chronic lung disease
- Foreign body aspiration
- Asthma or reactive airway disease
- Gastroesophageal reflux disease
- Bronchopulmonary dysplasia
- Pertussis
- Congenital heart disease
- Heart failure
- Vascular rings

In bonchiolitis, a CBC is typically normal. If dehydration is suspected, a chemistry panel may serve as an adjunct to the physical exam. Determination of the blood gas is useful if the patient is very ill.

DIFFERENTIAL DIAGNOSIS

There are many other illnesses that may be confused with bronchiolitis (Table 2), the most common of which is asthma. Asthma should be suspected when wheezing is recurrent, there is a family history of asthma, the onset is without other upper respiratory symptoms, and there is clinical improvement after administration of a single dose of a bronchodilator. A chest radiograph will not differentiate asthma from bronchiolitis.

Bacterial pneumonia can accompany bronchiolitis. It can also present with wheezing. A prolonged fever, onset of fever after the first few days of an upper respiratory infection, and worsening respiratory symptoms may indicate pneumonia. Treatment consists of antibiotic therapy and oxygen if needed. A chest radiograph and a CBC may be helpful to differentiate pneumonia from bronchiolitis.

When children are able to manipulate small objects, they are at increased risk for aspiration. There are usually no upper respiratory symptoms. Auscultation reveals asymmetric breath sounds with less airflow to the side of the foreign body. Wheezing may also be heard. Chest radiograph may show hyperinflation secondary to a ball-valve effect or atelectasis if the obstruction is complete. The object should be removed as soon as possible.

Gastroesophageal reflux is very common in infants. Most infants tolerate the reflux well. They become symptomatic when the stomach contents enter the respiratory tract. This leads to chronic congestion and wheezing. There may be no episodes of "spitting up." Unlike bronchiolitis, onset is usually subacute and symptoms are typically prolonged, lasting months.

Pertussis rarely presents with wheezing. In pertussis, infants have paroxysms of cough that can end in a whoop as children attempt to catch their breath. Fever is uncommon. Apnea and cyanosis can occur. A deep nasal aspirate specimen for antibody testing and culture is diagnostic. Erythromycin is the treatment of choice.

Chlamydial infections also rarely present with wheezing. Presentation of pneumonia as a result of chlamydia is age-specific. Older children present with low-grade fever, cough, and headache. Infants less than 4 months old present with cough and tachypnea. Rales may be auscultated. Fever and wheezing are absent. The may be a history of conjunctivitis developing in the first 2 weeks of life. The chest radiograph resembles that of bronchiolitis and an elevated eosinophil count is seen on the CBC. In infants, isolation of *Chlamydia trachomatis* from the conjunctiva or nasopharynx is diagnostic. Treatment consists of 14 days of erythromycin.

Children with bronchopulmonary dysplasia have a history of lung injury, prematurity, or both. The alveoli are leaky, leading to accumulation of fluid in the smaller airways, which can lead to chronic wheezing. When infected with RSV, these infants are more likely to present with bronchiolitis. However, if there are no upper respiratory symptoms or no worsening of symptoms, they are unlikely to have bronchiolitis.

PREVENTION

General preventative measures are aimed at decreasing the exposure to agents that cause bronchiolitis. All infants between 6 and 24 months who are not allergic to eggs should receive the influenza vaccine. Young infants commonly contract respiratory infections from caretakers, whereas older infants can contract the disease from playmates and by sharing toys. Caretakers are encouraged to wash hands often with soap and warm water. Meticulous cleaning of countertops and toys will decrease of spread of most viral upper respiratory infections. If possible, avoidance of day-care facilities during the peak of the influenza and RSV season can decrease a child's risk of contracting the disease. Avoiding smoke exposure is also important. The risk of developing bronchiolitis is higher in infants of stay-at-home mothers who smoke than in those infants who attend day care.

Palivizumab is the currently the only agent available for the prevention of bronchiolitis caused by RSV. The RSV immune globulin currently is not in use. Palivizumab is a monoclonal antibody to the F glycoprotein of RSV. It is indicated for children with bronchopulmonary dysplasia or chronic lung disease, severe heart disease, and selected premature infants *(7)*. It has been found to decrease hospitalization in these patients by 45%. Palivizumab is administered once every 30 days with a total of five doses through the winter months, generally starting in November. The dose is 15 mg/kg administered intramuscularly. The

American Academy of Pediatrics recommends palivizumab for premature infants as follows *(2)*:

1. All infants born less than 28 weeks of gestation in their first 12 months of life.
2. All infants born 29 to 32 weeks of gestation up to 6 months of age. Once treatment is initiated, it should continue until the end of the RSV season.
3. Infants who are born 32 to 35 weeks gestation, are younger than 6 months of age at the start of the RSV season, and have two or more of the following risk factors: exposure to tobacco, child-care attendance, school-aged siblings, congenital abnormalities of the airways, or severe neuromuscular disease.

TREATMENT

The treatment for bronchiolitis is largely supportive. For children who cannot maintain extended feedings, offering frequent small amounts of liquids is suggested. Suctioning of nasal passages before feedings is helpful. Infants who are dehydrated should be admitted for intravenous hydration. It is very important to monitor fluid intake carefully. For infants who are hypoxic, cool humidified oxygen and an inclined position may prevent the need for mechanical ventilation. Oxygen saturation should be maintained between 90 and 94%. Mechanical ventilation is reserved for those in respiratory failure and in those with apnea.

Over-the-Counter Medications

Over-the-counter mediations containing antihistamines, decongestants, expectorants, and cough suppressants are not recommended for children with bronchiolitis. There is no evidence that they provide relief in even uncomplicated upper respiratory infections.

Antibiotics

Antibiotics provide no benefit to children with bronchiolitis. They are reserved only for a secondary bacterial infection, such as pneumonia or otitis media.

Bronchodilators

Bronchodilaters can be administered orally or by inhalation. They have been shown to provide a short period of symptomatic relief in some patients *(8)*; however, they have not been shown to decrease the rate of hospitalization, oxygen requirement, mechanical ventilation, the duration of hospital stay, or the duration of illness *(8–12)*. A trial of a bronchodilator can be tried. If there is no clinical improvement after one dose, the treatment should be discontinued.

Epinephrine

Racemic epinephrine may be somewhat helpful in some patients. As with bronchodilators, epinephrine appears to provide a period of symptomatic relief in some patients *(8)*. This period of relief is somewhat longer compared with bronchodilators. However, administration of epinephrine also has not been shown to change hospitalization rates, oxygen requirement, mechanical ventilation, the duration of hospital stay, or the duration of the illness *(8,13,14)*. Racemic epinephrine should be discontinued if there is no improvement after one treatment.

Corticosteroids

The use of corticosteroids in the treatment of bronchiolitis is controversial. There are a few studies that have shown the benefit of using steroids *(15–17)*. However, the majority of studies have shown no change in hospitalization rates, oxygen requirement, mechanical ventilation, the duration of hospital stay, or the duration of the illness *(18–21)*.

Ribivirin

Ribivirin is an antiviral agent that has good in vitro activity against RSV and is administered via inhalation. Its use remains controversial. The majority of studies with large sample sizes have shown no benefit *(22–24)*. The American Academy of Pediatrics recommends that ribivirin be use at the discretion of the physician based on the severity of the disease and comorbid conditions *(2,25)*. Select studies have shown that early ribivirin administration in patients with RSV may decrease long-term respiratory morbidity *(26)*.

Immunotherapy

RSV immune globulin and palivizumab have been closely studied to determine if administration during an episode of bronchiolitis caused by RSV infection improved morbidity or mortality. Neither has been shown to decrease the rate of hospitalization, oxygen requirement, mechanical ventilation, the duration of hospital stay, or the duration of illness if administered after infants became symptomatic *(27,28)*.

Surfactant

Surfactant may be useful for those patients who require mechanical ventilation. Several studies found that when surfactant was given early after mechanical ventilation, it decreased the oxygen requirement, improved the elimination of CO_2, shortened the time on the ventilator, and shortened the ICU stay *(29,30)*.

Heliox

Heliox may be useful for patients requiring mechanical ventilation. As with surfactant, several small studies have shown that heliox improves gas exchange and decreases length of stay in the ICU *(31)*.

Vaccine Development

Currently there is no vaccine available for the prevention of RSV. Efforts to develop a vaccine are ongoing.

REFERENCES

1. American Academy of Pediatrics. Respiratory syncytial virus. In: Pickering, LK, ed. Red Book 2003: The Report of the Committee on Infectious Diseases, 23th ed. American Academy of Pediatrics, Elk Grove Village, IL, 2003; pp. 523–524.
2. Henderson F, Collier A, Clyde W Jr, et al. Respiratory syncytial virus infections, reinfections and immunity. N Engl J Med 1979;300:530–534.
3. Anonymous. Respiratory syncytial virus activity—United States, 1999–2000 season. MMWR Morb Mortal Wkly Rep 2000;49:1091–1093.
4. Aherne W, Bird T, Court SD, et al. Pathological changes in virus infections of the lower respiratory tract in children. J Clin Pathol 1970;23:7–18.
5. Rayyan M, Naulaers G, Daniels H, et al. Characteristics of respiratory syncytial virus-related apnoea in three infants. Acta Paediatr 2004;93:847–849.
6. Martinez FD. Respiratory syncytial virus bronchiolitis and the pathogenesis of childhood asthma. Pediatr Infect Dis J 2003;22:S76–S82.
7. Committee on Infectious Diseases and Committee on Fetus and Newborn. Revised indications for the use of palivizumab and respiratory syncytial virus immune globulin intravenous for the prevention of respiratory syncytial virus infections. Pediatrics 2003;112:1442–1446.
8. Patel H, Platt RW, Pekeles GS, et al. A randomized, controlled trial of the effectiveness of nebulized therapy with epinephrine compared with albuterol and saline in infants hospitalized for acute viral bronchiolitis. J Pediatr 2002;141:818–824.
9. Kellner JD, Ohlsson A, Gadomski AM, Wang EE. Bronchodilators for bronchiolitis. Cochrane Database Syst Rev 2000;CD001266.
10. Patel H, Gouin S, Platt RW. Randomized, double-blind, placebo-controlled trial of oral albuterol in infants with mild-to-moderate acute viral bronchiolitis. J Pediatr 2003;142:509–514.
11. King VJ, Viswanathan M, Bordley WC, et al. Pharmacologic treatment of bronchiolitis in infants and children: a systematic review. Arch Pediatr Adolesc Med 2004;158:127.
12. Flores G, Horwitz RI. Efficacy of beta 2-agonists in bronchiolitis: a reappraisal and meta-analysis. Pediatrics 1997;100:233–239.
13. Sanchez I. A multicenter, randomized, double-blind, controlled trial of nebulized epinephrine in infants with acute bronciolitis. J Pediatr 2004;144:136–137.
14. Wainwright C, Altamirano L, Cheney M, et al. A multicenter, randomized, double-blind, controlled trial of nebulized epinephrine in infants with acute bronchiolitis. N Engl J Med 2003;349:27–35.
15. Schuh S. Efficacy of oral dexamethasone in outpatients with acute bronchiolitis. J Pediatr 2002;140:27–32.
16. Oral prednisolone in the acute management of children age 6 to 35 months with viral respiratory infection-induced lower airway disease: a randomized, placebo-controlled trial. J Pediatr 2003;143:725–730.
17. Garrison MM, Christakis DA, Harvey E, Cummings P, Davis RL. Systemic corticosteroids in infant bronchiolitis: a meta-analysis. Pediatrics 2000;105:E44.
18. Patel H, Platt R, Lozano JM, Wang EEL. Glucocorticoids for acute viral bronchiolitis in infants and young children. Cochrane Database Syst Rev 2004;3:CD004878.
19. Davison C. Efficacy of interventions for bronchiolitis in critically ill infants: a systematic review and meta-analysis. Pediatr Crit Care Med 2004;5:482–489.

20. Buckingham SC, Jafri HS, Bush AJ, et al. A randomized, double-blind, placebo-controlled trial of dexamethasone in severe respiratory syncytial virus (RSV) infection: effects on RSV quantity and clinical outcome. J Infect Dis 2002;185:1222–1228.
21. Cade A, Brownlee KG, Conway SP, et al. Randomised placebo controlled trial of nebulised corticosteroids in acute respiratory syncytial viral bronchiolitis. Arch Dis Child 2000;82: 126–130.
22. Moler F, Steinhart C, Ohmit S, et al. Effectiveness of ribavirin in otherwise well infants with respiratory syncytial virus-associated respiratory failure. J Pediatr 1996;128:422–428.
23. Meert K, Sarnaik A, Gelmini M, et al. Aerosolized ribavirin in mechanically ventilated children with respiratory syncytial virus lower respiratory tract disease: A prospective, double blind, randomized trial. Crit Care Med 1994;22:556–572.
24. Everard ML, Swarbrick A, Rigby AS, et al. The effect of ribavirin to treat previously healthy infants admitted with acute bronchiolitis on acute and chronic respiratory morbidity. Respir Med 2001;95:275–280.
25. Reassessment of the indications for ribavirin therapy in respiratory syncytial virus infections. American Academy of Pediatrics Committee on Infectious Diseases. Pediatrics 1996;97:137–140.
26. Edell D, Khoshoo V, Ross G, et al. Early ribavirin treatment of bronchiolitis: effect on long-term respiratory morbidity. Chest 2002;122:935–939.
27. Rodriguez WJ, Gruber WC, Groothius JR, et al. Respiratory syncytial virus immune globulin treatment of RSV lower respiratory tract infection in previously healthy children. Pediatrics 1997;100:937–942.
28. Saez-Llorens X, Moreno MT, Ramilo O, et al. Safety and pharmacokinetics of palivizumab therapy in children hospitalized with respiratory syncytial virus infection. Pediatr Infect Dis J 2004;23:707–712.
29. Luchetti M. Multicenter, randomized, controlled study of porcine surfactant in severe respiratory syncytial virus-induced respiratory failure. Pediatr Crit Care Med 2002;3:261–268.
30. Tibby SM, Hatherill M, Wright SM, et al. Exogenous surfactant supplementation in infants with respiratory syncytial virus bronichiolitis. Am J Respir Crit Care Med 2000;162:1251–1256.
31. Martinón-Torres F. Heliox therapy in infants with acute bronchiolitis. Pediatrics 2002;109: 68–73.

IV Non-Airway Disorders That Present With Respiratory Symptoms

20 Obstructive Sleep Apnea

Vikram Bakhru and Matthew L. Mintz

CONTENTS
>   CASE PRESENTATION
>   KEY CLINICAL QUESTIONS
>   LEARNING OBJECTIVES
>   EPIDEMIOLOGY
>   PATHOPHYSIOLOGY
>   DIAGNOSIS
>   TREATMENT OPTIONS
>   REFERENCES

CASE PRESENTATION

A 61-year-old obese male presents to a new primary medical doctor for a regular check-up with continued complaints of fatigue and drowsiness. The patient reports he often falls asleep during the day while watching television and recently fell asleep while driving. The patient's wife comments she has noticed her husband snores loudly. The patient's past medical history is significant for hypertension diagnosed 7 years ago and a cholecystectomy performed 15 years ago.

KEY CLINICAL QUESTIONS

1. At what point should this patient be considered for a work-up for obstructive sleep apnea (OSA)?
2. How does sleep apnea differ from other sleep syndromes?
3. What are the main causes of OSA and why are some patients more predisposed to sleep apnea?
4. Are there any long-term sequellae associated with chronic OSA?
5. What are the appropriate diagnostic procedures and treatments for OSA?

> From: *Current Clinical Practice: Disorders of the Respiratory Tract:*
> *Common Challenges in Primary Care*
> By: M. L. Mintz © Humana Press, Totowa, NJ

LEARNING OBJECTIVES

1. Identify the main signs and symptoms of OSA.
2. Understand the pathophysiology behind OSA.
3. Create a differential diagnosis for a patient with suspected OSA.
4. Utilize appropriate diagnostic interventions for patients with signs or symptoms suggestive of OSA.
5. Become familiar with currently available treatment options for patients with OSA.

EPIDEMIOLOGY

Sleep apnea is defined as a cessation of breathing during sleep. Sleep apnea can be caused centrally from the brain, by anatomical obstruction, or have a mixed pattern. OSA, which is characterized by interruptions in breathing caused by intermittent complete or partial obstruction of the airway is the most common form of sleep apnea and is the focus of this chapter. Patients with OSA must have at least 10 apneic (cessation of breath for >10 seconds) or hypopneic (reduction of airflow and thus oxygenation) episodes per sleep hour. This causes sleep interruptions that lead to symptoms of excessive daytime sleepiness (EDS), and is associated with many chronic conditions.

The identification of individuals with OSA depends on a number of selection criteria, which can differ among clinicians. Varying opinions on what constitutes OSA and one's own experience in recognizing classic signs and symptoms of sleep apnea lead to inconsistent reporting *(1)*. In evaluating the prevalence of sleep apnea, it is useful to consider the results of four large prevalence studies, all of which used similar methods in gathering and analyzing data. For those adults with an average body mass index of 25 to 28 kg/m^2, it is suspected that 1 in 5 white adults suffer from mild sleep apnea, and 1 in 15 suffer from moderate disease *(2–6)*. It is estimated that sleep apnea syndrome affects nearly 5% of adults in Western countries *(6)*. Three factors generally accepted as important to the development of sleep apnea include baseline obesity, older age, and the presence of snoring *(6)*.

Data from the Wisconsin Sleep Cohort study indicates that individuals with mild sleep apnea will progress to moderate or severe disease with a sixfold risk if a 10% weight gain occurs *(7)*. Obesity as a factor for the development of sleep apnea is especially significant in circumstances in which the airway narrowing is perhaps in part because of excess soft tissue in the oropharynx *(8)*. Some studies that show a correlation between neck circumference and prevalence of sleep apnea only support this theory. Some literature suggest men have a higher prevalence of sleep apnea than women, often citing hormonal causes as an explanation for the varying prevalence *(1)*. Furthermore, postmenopausal women are more frequently affected with sleep apnea than premenopausal women *(6)*. It is suspected that hormone replacement therapy may alleviate this difference in prevalence among women *(9)*.

The correlation between age and the prevalence of sleep apnea is vague. Several studies show an increase in prevalence with increasing age, whereas others show a limited correlation after age 65. Overall, the literature demonstrates conflicting reports on age as a factor in the development of sleep apnea *(1)*. Although data is limited on the prevalence of sleep apnea in non-white populations, great variability does not exist among different ethnicities *(10–13)*.

EDS is the most common presenting symptom among patients with sleep apnea *(1)*. Precise quantification of sleepiness is difficult given the variable descriptions provided by patients. In assessing patients for sleep apnea, the challenge for the clinician exists in determining when further evaluation is necessary. Given the high correlation between motor vehicle accidents and patients with sleep apnea, it can be argued that such quantification should be less important than the presence or absence of daytime sleepiness *(14,15)*.

The causal relationship between EDS and sleep apnea results from the fragmentation of the affected patient's sleep. Such fragmentation is associated with central nervous system arousal during each apneic episode *(1)*. Arousal from sleep is further evidenced by such objective measures as transient blood pressure or heart rate elevations. Despite the alterations in vital signs during sleep, patients with sleep apnea do not typically demonstrate any change on the electroencephalogram *(16)*.

The complexity of recognizing sleep apnea is further evidenced by reports of patients diagnosed with sleep apnea but who did not present with EDS. It is therefore important for the clinician to consider as many factors, subjective and objective, in evaluating a patient who may have sleep apnea. For example, the correlation between snoring and sleep apnea is significant despite the subjective nature of snoring. It is important to note that additional factors, such as snoring, may have their own independent correlations with EDS *(17)*.

PATHOPHYSIOLOGY

The classic pattern of sleep is inclusive of rapid eye movement (REM) sleep, one of several stages during the normal sleep cycle. During REM sleep, elevations in heart rate and blood pressure are commonly seen, whereas non-REM sleep is typified by decreased sympathetic outflow and lower heart rate and blood pressure. This continual modulation during the sleep stages is disturbed in patients with OSA, which results in a loss of homeostasis *(18)*.

Craniofacial abnormalities are partly to blame in terms of the anatomical differences in patients with sleep apnea. Specifically, these include macroglossia, retroagnathia, and acromegaly *(19)*. Despite the seemingly clear linkage of these abnormalities to the pathophysiology of OSA, only a small percentage of sleep apnea patients are characterized as having these craniofacial abnormalities. Therefore, it is likely that other factors are largely responsible for causing sleep apnea in most affected patients *(1)*. Specifically, atonia of the pharyngeal dilator muscles and the presence of excess nonadipose soft tissue in the pharyngeal space are most likely the major contributing factors for disease in patients with sleep apnea *(1)*. In affected patients, high levels of electromyographic activity are seen during wakeful hours with significantly less activity seen during sleeping hours. This suggests a compensatory mechanism in affected patients during wakeful hours that is absent when the patient falls asleep. It is specifically the loss of this compensatory mechanism that results in brief periods of apnea *(20,21)*.

The accumulation of apneic episodes results in a temporary state of hypercapnia and hypoxemia. The body's response to the abnormal acid–base balance is provided by a series of chemoreceptors, the most significant of which are located in the carotid bodies (located in the internal carotid arteries) *(1)*. The response of the carotid bodies is primarily determined by the serum oxygen tension *(22)*. By contrast, serum carbon dioxide tension is primarily monitored by the brainstem central chemoreceptors *(23)*. The healthy individual will experience a blunted response by these receptors during sleep as compared with wakefulness (quantification of the gas tensions seen during sleep in the normal patient are on the order of an increase of partial pressure of carbon dioxide by 2 to 6 mmHg and a decrease in oxygen saturation of up to 2%) *(24)*. Thus, the effect in a patient with sleep apnea is all the more critical and results in an inadequately compensated acid–base balance irregularity.

There are several medical conditions that are comorbid with OSA, and causative associations are currently under investigation. Cardiovascular disease is common in patients with OSA *(1)*. Hypertension has been documented in patients with OSA, and may be a consequence of the disease *(25)*. There have also been associations with OSA and arrhythmias, myocardial infarctions, and stroke. Cardiomyopathy can be caused by OSA, and reverses with successful treatment. Patients with both chronic obstructive pulmonary disease and OSA are predisposed to severe nighttime oxygen desaturations, and this may lead to persistent pulmonary hypertension and right-sided heart failure. Finally, psychosocial problems can affect patients with OSA. Affected patients often have depression, irritability, and impaired concentration *(1)*.

DIAGNOSIS

Confirming the diagnosis of OSA generally requires a sleep study. However, clinical history is extremely important. Patients with symptoms or who are at risk of having sleep apnea (Table 1) should first be asked whether or not they snore.

Table 1
Symptoms and Signs of Patients at Risk for Sleep Apnea

Symptoms

- Chronic, loud snoring
- Gasping or choking episodes during sleep
- Excessive daytime sleepiness (expecially drowsy driving)
- Automobile or work-related accidents as a result of fatigue
- Personality changes or cognitive difficulties related to fatigue

Signs

- Obesity, especially nuchal obesity (neck size ≥17 inches in males, ≥16 inches in females)
- Systemic hypertension
- Nasopharyngeal narrowing
- Pulmonary hypertension
- Cor pulmonale (rarely)

From ref. *12*.

Clinicians should further define if this occurs frequently, if the snoring is loud, and if it is affected by sleeping position (lying on back or side). Because patients are not aware of their own snoring in most cases, it is important to query their sleeping partners. Additionally, clinicians should ask about EDS. Finally, if there is a sleeping partner, the clinician should inquire whether or not the partner observes any apneic episodes during the night. If any of these questions are positive, further work-up with an objective test should be considered.

In order to make a diagnosis of sleep apnea, a clinician may decide to request one or more objective tests. The gold standard for diagnosing sleep apnea is in-laboratory polysomnography. Another method frequently used to diagnose sleep apnea is nocturnal pulse oximetry. A third method employed by clinicians is morphometric examinations of the head and neck. Although such examination is often more cost-effective and does not require valuable bed space in sleep laboratories, the imprecise, operator-dependent nature of this test makes it unreliable as the sole mechanism in determining sleep apnea. Furthermore, nocturnal pulse oximetry is also a less specific test, whereby a negative result will still require polysomnography to confirm the negative result. Despite the high expense and scarcity of bed space in the sleep lab, high clinical suspicion should always result in appropriate diagnostic testing to avoid the long-term negative consequences on the health of a patient with sleep apnea *(1)*.

In-laboratory polysomnography or sleep study measures the number and severity of apneas (cessations of airflow) and/or hypopneas (reductions in airflow) that cause sleep disruption. These are measured in events per hour and are referred to as the apnea–hypopnea index or respiratory disturbance index. Apneas or hypopneas that last at least 10 seconds are considered clinically significant. Most apneas or hypopneas last between 20 and 30 seconds and can sometime last more than 1 minute. Episodes usually resolve when the patient is slightly aroused, although the patient is usually not aware of this. Apnea–hypopnea or respiratory disturbance indexes higher than 20 are considered a sign of significant disease warranting treatment. However, patients with fewer than five events per hour may also benefit from treatment if they have significant symptoms or comorbid conditions. In addition, some patients can have several hundred episodes per night.

TREATMENT OPTIONS

The goal of treatment of OSA is to eliminate apnea and hypopnea, reduce snoring and arousal, and ultimately improve sleep and eliminate symptoms and conditions attributed to sleep disturbance, as well as reduce risk of adverse events such as involvement in motor vehicle collisions. The various treatments available for reducing the degree of sleep apnea are limited to a few options (Table 2).

The first option is weight loss, because a high degree of clinical improvement is seen with a 10% reduction in body weight *(26)*. The literature demonstrates that the correlation between amount of weight lost and the degree of sleep apnea is inversely related to one another. However, it should be noted that such reductions in weight do not result in a complete cure of the sleep apnea but rather only improvements in the severity of disease *(6)*.

The most studied treatment, continuous positive airway pressure (CPAP), is widely considered to be the most effective therapy for the treatment of sleep apnea *(1)*. There is significant evidence that CPAP improves upper airway flow and reduces the daytime symptoms in patients. Other studies have demonstrated that CPAP improves mood and functional status, and can decrease the incidence of motor vehicle collisions. This form of treatment often compensates for the pathophysiological consequences of sleep-disordered breathing discussed earlier. Some studies suggest that daytime symptoms are an important determining factor in the effectiveness of CPAP, and the absence of such symptoms may be less of an indication for CPAP therapy. Although CPAP is still an effective option, it has been show to have minimal effect on improving sleep apnea-induced change in blood pressure in those patients who do not show daytime symptoms *(27)*.

The CPAP unit is a machine containing a fan that delivers pressurized air to the patient's nostrils and thus acts as a pneumatic splint that keeps the airway

Table 2
Treatment of Sleep Apnea

Modification of behavioral factors

- Weight loss (including exercise regime)
- Avoidance of alcohol and sedatives before sleep
- Avoidance of supine sleep position

Nasal CPAP

- Noninvasive
- Very effective
- Patient adherence variable

Oral/dental devices

- May be useful in mild to moderate cases
- Not uniformly effective

Surgical procedures (UPPP, nasal surgery, tonsillectomy, LAUP, maxillofacial surgery, tracheostomy)

- Invasive
- Not uniformly effective
- May carry risk
- Repeat sleep study is necessary after each procedure

CPAP, continuous positive airway pressure; UPPP, uvulopalatopharyngoplasty; LAUP, laser-assisted uvulopalatoplasty.

open. CPAP does not correct the disorder, and must be used by the patient each evening. CPAP machine pressure settings are best determined in the sleep lab during a sleep study. Once the diagnosis is confirmed, a trial of CPAP is usually observed while the patient is sleeping in the lab. During this study, adjustments are made to the CPAP pressure setting, and reductions of apnea and hypopnea are documented. Once therapy is initiated, patients should be re-evaluated periodically because pressure requirements can change over time.

Despite the high efficacy of CPAP, its universal use in the treatment of sleep apnea is inhibited by patient intolerance or refusal secondary to discomfort caused by the CPAP apparatus. The most common complaint made by patients after initiating CPAP treatment is excessive nasal congestion. In-line heated humidification and the use of moisturizing creams or corticosteroids have been shown in some patients to make therapy tolerable *(1)*.

Surgical treatment options for OSA are not as widely used because of a lack of data supporting this treatment modality as being highly effective. One example of a commonly performed procedure is uvulopalatopharyngoplasty, a procedure that only shows improvement in a small portion of patients *(28)*. This finding suggests that several anatomical features contribute to sleep·apnea. Objective data from imaging studies and airway pressure measurements indicate that the two areas most susceptible to collapse are the spaces behind the soft palate and tongue base *(29,30)*. Notably, despite initial perceived improvements postsurgically, there is concern for permanent improvement in the patient with sleep apnea. As a result, it is recommended that polysomnography be repeated within 4 to 6 months after the surgical procedure *(1)*.

Finally, mandibular devices can be used as an alternative to the previous treatment options. As discussed previously, retrognathia is one of the contributing factors in the development of sleep apnea. Therefore, mandibular devices function to reduce retroglossal airway collapse by inducing mandibular protrusion in those patients needing such anatomical adjustment. Such devices are most useful in patients with mild disease or nonapneic snoring, and improvement in daytime symptoms has been noted with the consistent use of mandibular devices *(31,32)*.

REFERENCES

1. Caples SM, Gami AS, Somers VK. Obstructive sleep apnea. Ann Intern Med 2005;142:187–197.
2. Bixler EO, Vgontzas AN, Lin HM, et al. Prevalence of sleep-disordered breathing in women: effects of gender. Am J Respir Crit Care Med. 2001;163:608–613.
3. Bixler EO, Vgontzas AN, Ten Have T, Tyson K, Kales A. Effects of age on sleep apnea in men: I. Prevalence and severity. Am J Respir Crit Care Med 1998;157:144–148.
4. Duran J, Esnaola S, Rubio R, Iztueta A. Obstructive sleep apnea-hypopnea and related clinical features in a population-based sample of subjects aged 30 to 70 yr. Am J Respir Crit Care Med 2001;163:685–689.
5. Young T, Palta M, Dempsey J, Skatrud J, Weber S, Badr S. The occurrence of sleep-disordered breathing among middle-aged adults. N Engl J Med 1993;328:1230–1235.
6. Young T, Peppard PE, Gottlieb DJ. Epidemiology of obstructive sleep apnea: a population health perspective. Am J Respir Crit Care Med 2002;165:1217–1239.
7. Peppard PE, Young T, Palta M, Dempsey J, Skatrud J. Longitudinal study of moderate weight change and sleep-disordered breathing. JAMA 2000;284:3015–3021.
8. Davies RJ, Ali NJ, Stradling JR. Neck circumference and other clinical features in the diagnosis of the obstructive sleep apnea syndrome. Thorax 1992;47:101–105.
9. Shahar E, Redline S, Young T, et al. Hormone replacement therapy and sleep-disordered breathing. Am J Respir Crit Care Med 2003;167:1186–1192.
10. Kim J, In K, Kim J, et al. Prevalence of sleep disordered breathing in middle-aged Korean men and women. Am J Respir Crit Care Med 2004;170:1108–1113.
11. Redline S, Tishler PV, Hans MG, Tosteson TD, Strohl KP, Spry K. Racial differences in sleep-disordered breathing in African-Americans and Caucasians. Am J Respir Crit Care Med 1997;155:186–192.
12. National Institutes of Health. Sleep apenea: is your patient at risk? National Institutes of Health National Heart, Lung, and Blood Institute, Bethesda, MD, 1995, NIH publication no. 95-3803.
13. Udwadia ZF, Doshi AV, Lonkar SG, Singh CI. Prevalence of sleep-disordered breathing and sleep apnea in middle-aged urban Indian men. Am J Respir Crit Care Med 2004;169:168–173.

14. Barbe, Pericas J, Munoz A, Findley L. Automobile accidents in patients with sleep apnea syndrome. An epidemiological and mechanistic study. Am J Respir Crit Care Med 1998;158:18–22.
15. Teran-Santos J, Jimenez-Gomez A, Cordero-Guevara J. The association between sleep apnea and the risk of traffic accidents. Cooperative Group Burgos-Santander. N Engl J Med 1999;340:847–851.
16. Martin SE, Wraith PK, Deary IJ, Douglas NJ. The effect of nonvisible sleep fragmentation on daytime function. Am J Respir Crit Care Med 1997;155:1596–1601.
17. Gottlieb DJ, Yao Q, Redline S, Ali T, Mahowald MW. Does snoring predict sleepiness independently of apnea and hypopnea frequency? Am J Respir Crit Care Med 2000;162:1512–1517.
18. Somers VK, Dyken ME, Skinner JL. Autonomic and hemodynamic responses and interactions during the Mueller maneuver in humans. J Auton Nerv Syst. 1993;44:253–259.
19. Veasey SC, Panckeri KA, Hoffman EA, Pack AI, Hendricks JC. The effects of serotonin antagonists in an animal model of sleep-disordered breathing. Am J Respir Crit Care Med 1996;153:776–786.
20. Fogel RB, Malhotra A, Pillar G, et al. Genioglossal activation in patients with obstructive sleep apnea versus control subjects. Mechanisms of muscle control. Am J Respir Crit Care Med 2001;164:2025–2030.
21. Mezzanotte WS, Tangel DJ, White DP. Waking genioglossal electromyogram in sleep apnea patients versus normal controls (a neuromuscular compensatory mechanism). J Clin Invest 1992;89:1571–1579.
22. Lugliani R, Whipp BJ, Seard C, Wasserman K. Effect of bilateral carotid body resection on ventilatory control at rest and during exercise in man. N Engl J Med 1971;285:1105–1111.
23. Gelfand R, Lambertsen CJ. Dynamic respiratory response to abrupt change of inspired CO_2 at normal and high PO_2. J Appl Physiol 1973;35:903–913.
24. Douglas NJ, White DP, Pickett CK, Weil JV, Zwillich CW. Respiration during sleep in normal man. Thorax 1982;37:840–844.
25. Peppard PE, Young T, Palta M, Skatrud J. Prospective study of the association between sleep-disordered breathing and hypertension. N Engl J Med 2000; 342:1378–1384.
26. Smith PL, Gold AR, Meyers DA, Haponik EF, Bleecker ER. Weight loss in mildly to moderately obese patients with obstructive sleep apnea. Ann Intern Med 1985;103:850–855.
27. Barbe F, Mayoralas LR, Duran J, et al. Treatment with continuous positive airway pressure is not effective in patients with sleep apnea but no daytime sleepiness. A randomized, controlled trial. Ann Intern Med 2001;134:1015–1023.
28. Sher AE, Schechtman KB, Piccirillo JF. The efficacy of surgical modifications of the upper airway in adults with obstructive sleep apnea syndrome. Sleep 1996;19:156–177.
29. Shepard JW Jr, Thawley SE. Localization of upper airway collapse during sleep in patients with obstructive sleep apnea. Am Rev Respir Dis 1990;141:1350–1355.
30. Trudo FJ, Gefter WB, Welch KC, Gupta KB, Maislin G, Schwab RJ. State-related changes in upper airway caliber and surrounding soft-tissue structures in normal subjects. Am J Respir Crit Care Med 1998;158:1259–1270.
31. Gotsopoulos H, Chen C, Qian J, Cistulli PA. Oral appliance therapy improves symptoms in obstructive sleep apnea: a randomized, controlled trial. Am J Respir Crit Care Med 2002;166:743–748.
32. Mehta A, Qian J, Petocz P, Darendeliler MA, Cistulli PA. A randomized, controlled study of a mandibular advancement splint for obstructive sleep apnea. Am J Respir Crit Care Med 2001;163:1457–1461.

21　Obesity

Rebecca Chatterjee and Matthew L. Mintz

CONTENTS

    CASE PRESENTATION
    KEY CLINICAL QUESTIONS
    LEARNING OBJECTIVES
    EPIDEMIOLOGY
    PATHOPHYSIOLOGY
    DIAGNOSIS AND DIFFERENTIAL DIAGNOSIS
    TREATMENT
    FUTURE AREAS OF STUDY
    REFERENCES

CASE PRESENTATION

A 45-year-old woman with past medical history significant for mild hypertension and dyslipidemia presents for an annual exam. She is concerned about dyspnea on exertion, occurring when she walks up stairs or more than a few blocks. This has been occurring for about 2 years. She denies any chest pain, nausea, vomiting, or diaphoresis. She denies any dyspnea at rest. She has no known pulmonary disease. She does not smoke and has no history of allergic rhinitis. She has had no recent illness. Her vitals signs are stable. Her O_2 saturation is 99% on room air, and between 97 and 99% with ambulation around the office. Her body mass index (BMI) is 31 kg/m². Physical exam is within normal limits, except for obesity. Besides encouraging her to lose weight, her physician reassures her that her heart and lung exams are normal.

From: *Current Clinical Practice: Disorders of the Respiratory Tract:
Common Challenges in Primary Care*
By: M. L. Mintz © Humana Press, Totowa, NJ

KEY CLINICAL QUESTIONS

1. Is obesity enough to cause this patient's respiratory symptoms, or is further work-up required?
2. What is the diagnostic work-up for the obese patient who presents with dyspnea on exertion?
3. How does obesity cause respiratory problems?

LEARNING OBJECTIVES

1. Understand the relationship between obesity and respiratory symptoms and disease.
2. Learn the diagnostic work-up for obese patients presenting with respiratory symptoms.
3. Learn the treatment and management plan for obese patients presenting with respiratory symptoms.

EPIDEMIOLOGY

The obesity epidemic is a continual challenge for health care professionals. About 97 million Americans are either overweight or obese. It is well known that obesity is a risk factor in the development of many diseases, such as hypertension, diabetes, and hyperlipidemia. Its role in the metabolic syndrome and development of coronary artery disease is well-established *(1)*.

Obesity has also been associated with respiratory diseases such as obstructive sleep apnea (OSA) and obesity hypoventilation syndrome (OHS). OHS is characterized by daytime elevation of the $PaCO_2$. Patients have symptoms such as dyspnea, headaches, hyersomnolence, and sleep arousals. It is usually seen in extremely obese individuals and can cause hypoxia as well as pulmonary hypertension. OSA, caused by upper airway obstruction, results in airflow reduction during sleep.

Obesity, independent of pulmonary disease, can affect pulmonary gas exchange, oxygenation of the blood, and work of breathing. It also affects ventilatory drive and pattern of breathing. Obese patients are at increased risk for complications such as pneumonia, hypoxemia, atelectasis, and pulmonary embolism *(2)*.

Many obese patients complain of exertional dyspnea and have genuine abnormalities in lung function. This chapter focuses on the pulmonary abnormalities associated with simple obesity.

PATHOPHYSIOLOGY

Compliance

Lung compliance is defined as the change volume per unit change in pressure. It is a measure of the lung's elastic properties. Simple obesity can decrease chest wall compliance by 92% of predicted normal values *(3)*. The suggested mechanism for a decrease in chest wall compliance is the excess adipose tissue on the thoracic cage *(2)*, however, there is some controversy to this statement because as more accurate measurements of compliance are used, such as the pulse airflow technique, chest wall compliance is found to be relatively normal in simple obesity, even in morbidly obese patients *(2)*.

Resistance

Resistance to airflow is another obstacle the respiratory muscles must overcome. Airway resistance is defined as the change in pressure over the change in airflow. Obesity is associated with increases in airway and respiratory system resistance, in part because of the reduction in lung volume (at lower volumes airflow resistance increases). After correcting for lung volume, specific airway conductance may be reduced to 50 to 70% of normal. Because the forced expiratory volume in 1 second to forced vital capacity (FEV_1:FVC) ratio is normal, indicating that there is no airway obstruction, the source of the increased airway resistance in obesity appears to lie in lung tissue and small airways rather than in the large airways *(2)*.

Spirometry and Lung Volumes

The most common lung volume abnormality in simple obesity is a decrease the expiratory reserve volume (ERV), defined as the maximum volume of air that can be expired from the functional residual capacity (FRC). The ERV can be decreased to an average of 60% normal predicted values, and is inversely proportional to the BMI *(1)*. As ERV decreases, residual volume increases. This is often so marked that the FRC approaches the residual volume. The cause of this abnormality is the displacement of the diaphragm into the chest by the obese abdomen. Consequently, the lung bases are often underventilated *(2)*. Other lung volumes are usually preserved but can be affected, especially in extremely obese individuals. These include a decrease in total lung capacity, which is the volume found in lungs on maximum inspiration. The FRC may also be decreased. These values tend to remain normal until BMI exceeds 45 kg/m^2 *(1)*.

An association between distribution of fat and abnormalities in lung function has been described in the literature. Upper body fat has been found to correlate with lung abnormalities more so than lower body fat *(4–6)*.

The FEV_1:FVC ratio is usually normal in obese subjects, unless they are morbidly obese *(1)*.

Ventilatory Drive

Work of breathing is increased in uncomplicated obesity *(3,7)*. As a result, the respiratory drive is also increased. This is not reflected in normal tests of ventilatory drive, such as ventilatory response to inhalation of carbon dioxide. These tests actually show a reduction of ventilatory drive of about 40% in uncomplicated obesity. These tests are not accurate because they do not factor in respiratory muscle mechanics and respiratory muscles. A better marker of respiratory drive is the mouth occlusion pressure, which reflects neurogenic drive to respiratory muscles. In simple obesity, the mouth occlusion pressure is two times normal and increased normally with CO_2 inhalation. Another marker of respiratory drive is the diaphragmatic electromyogram response to CO_2, which is also about two times normal in simple obesity. Therefore, obese patients tend to have an increase ventilatory drive, which corresponds to their increase work of breathing *(2)*.

Pattern of Breathing

The respiratory rate of obese patients is about 40% higher than normal weight subjects at rest *(2)*. This is accomplished by shortening the inspiratory and expiratory time, but the ratio of inspiratory to total breath time is normal. Measurements of tidal volumes are normal in obese patients at rest and during maximal exercise. However, when normalized to body weight, the tidal volume shows a decrease of 50% at rest and 33% during maximal exercise *(2)*.

Gas Exchange

In the majority of cases, obese patients are not hypoxic or have mild hypoxia in the supine position *(8)*. This hypoxemia is caused by a ventilation perfusion mismatch because of underventilated lung bases, seen primarily in obese individuals with compromised lung volumes. Obese individuals not suffering from OHS are usually eucapnic *(2)*.

Exercise Capacity

Obese individuals consume 25% more oxygen at rest than normal weight individuals *(9,10)*. The oxygen consumption also increases during exercise. The extra work needed to move the body is responsible for the increase in oxygen consumption. Minute ventilation, respiratory rate, and heart rate are also higher during exercise that normal weight individuals *(10)*.

Obesity and Asthma

The association between obesity and asthma is frequently mentioned in current literature. Ronmark et al. found that BMI was a significant risk factor for the incidence of asthma independent of gender and allergic status in adults in northern Sweden *(11)*. Another study of nearly 86,000 adults followed for 5 years showed a linear relationship between BMI and the risk of developing asthma *(12)*. However, as mentioned earlier, a patient is usually morbidly obese before

Table 1
Causes of Dyspnea in an Obese Patient

- Obstructive airway disease
- Cardiac disease
- Interstitial lung disease
- Neuromuscular disease
- Obesity-related dyspnea
- Pulmonary vascular disease
- Gastroesophageal reflux disease

one sees airflow obstruction on spirometry, so it is still questionable whether there is a true association between obesity and asthma. Some studies have been based on patient reports of dyspnea or the use of inhaled β-agonists, rather than objective evidence of airflow obstruction. When data from 16,171 participants in the National Health and Nutrition Examination Survey III were analyzed, obesity was an independent risk factor for dyspnea, but not for airflow obstruction (from www.uptodate.com).

DIAGNOSIS AND DIFFERENTIAL DIAGNOSIS

The differential diagnosis for dyspnea in the obese patient is broad (Table 1). The diagnosis should focus on a thorough history of physical exam. The timing of dyspnea, precipitating factors, and associated symptoms should be evaluated. A history of dyspnea after a period of weight gain and an absence of prior pulmonary disease, smoking, or allergic symptoms may indicate obesity-related dyspnea. Physical exam should be focused on pulmonary, cardiac, and neuromuscular systems. If any evidence of other causes of dypnea (as seen in Table 1) is found, the work-up should proceed accordingly. If no other cause can be found and spirometry is normal, or shows changes that may be related to obesity (as mentioned previously), a diagnosis of obesity-related dyspnea should be considered.

TREATMENT

Weight loss is the obvious treatment for obesity-related pulmonary complications. A reduction of 80 lbs results in a 75% increase in ERV, 25% increase in residual volume and FRC, and a 10% increase in maximum voluntary ventilation. As a result there is increased ventilation of lung bases, and improved oxygenation *(2)*.

Respiratory muscle strength may improve with weight loss *(2)*.

Weight loss has been shown to improve most obesity-related illnesses. One study looked at the association between weight loss and improvement of obesity-related illnesses in 500 patients following gastric banding surgery and found that 81.8% of patients had improvement in asthma and 33% had improvement in sleep apnea *(13)*.

FUTURE AREAS OF STUDY

As in the case presented here, obesity affects nearly every organ system. Therefore, future studies need to focus on the primary prevention of obesity. With regard to obesity-related pulmonary complications, studies should focus on improvement of dyspnea in obese patients with a normal $FEV_1:FVC$ ratio after weight loss or weight loss surgery.

REFERENCES

1. Tzelepis GE, McCool FD. The lungs and chest wall disease. In: Murray, Nadel, eds. Textbook of Respiratory Medicine, 4th Ed. W. B. Saunders, Philadelphia, PA, 2005, pp. 2326–2328.
2. Koenig S. Pulmonary complications of obesity. Am J Med Sci 2001;321:249–279.
3. Sharp JT, Henry JP, Sweany SK, et al. The total work of breathing in normal and obese men. J Clin Invest 1964;43:728–739.
4. Enzi G, Baggio B, Vianello A, et al. Respiratory disturbances in visceral obesity. Int J Obesity 1990;14:26.
5. Muls E, Vryens C, Michels A, et al. The effects of abdominal fat distribution measured by computed tomography on the respiratory system of non-smoking obese women. Int J Obesity 1990;14(suppl):136.
6. Collins LC, Hoberty P, Walker J, et al. The effect of body fat distribution on pulmonary function tests. Chest 1995;107:1298–1302.
7. Kress J, Pohlman A, Alverdy J, Hall J. The impact of morbid obesity on oxygen cost of breathing at rest. Am J Respir Crit Care Med 1999;160:883–886.
8. Douglas FG, Chong PY. Influence of obesity on peripheral airway patency. J Appl Physiol 1972;33:559–563.
9. Bosman AR, Goldman HI. The oxygen cost and work of breathing in normal and obese subjects. S Afr J Lab Clin Med 1961;7:62–67.
10. Salvadori A, Fanari P, Mazza P, et al. Work capacity and cardiopulmonary adaption of the obese subject during exercise testing. Chest 1992;101:674–679.
11. Ronmark E, Anderson C, Nystrom L, et al. Obesity increases the risk of incident asthma among adults. Eur Respir J 2005;25:282–288.
12. Camargo CA Jr, Weiss ST, Zhang S, et al. Prospective study of body mass index, weight change, and risk of adult-onset asthma in women. Arch Intern Med 1999;159:2582–2588.
13. Spivak H, Hewitt MF, Onn A, Half EE. Weight loss and improvement of obesity-related illness in 500 U. patients following laparoscopic adjustable gstric banding procedure. Am J Surg 2005;189:27–32.

22 Vocal Cord Dysfunction

Amy Humfeld and Matthew L. Mintz

CONTENTS

>   CASE PRESENTATION
>   KEY CLINICAL QUESTIONS
>   LEARNING OBJECTIVES
>   BACKGROUND
>   PATHOPHYSIOLOGY
>   ETIOLOGY
>   DIAGNOSIS
>   DIFFERENTIAL DIAGNOSIS
>   TREATMENT
>   CASE RESOLUTION
>   FUTURE DIRECTIONS
>   REFERENCES

CASE PRESENTATION

A 22-year-old Caucasian female who recently moved to the area presents for an emergency room visit follow-up. Over the weekend, she developed sudden difficulty breathing while grocery shopping. She describes chest tightness with wheezing and says that her voice sounded funny when she tried to call for help. The store manager called 911 and she was rushed to the local emergency room. Upon arrival, however, her wheezing had stopped and she was breathing comfortably. She states that all of her lab work was normal but is not sure what tests were performed and did not bring her paperwork with her. After further questioning, she states that she has had several episodes like this in the past year including four severe episodes that required emergency room visits. She was diagnosed with asthma last year as a result of these episodes and was prescribed budesonide and albuterol. She uses the albuterol on occasion when her wheezing is severe but is not sure whether either of the inhalers really help.

From: *Current Clinical Practice: Disorders of the Respiratory Tract:
Common Challenges in Primary Care*
By: M. L. Mintz © Humana Press, Totowa, NJ

She states that she is otherwise in good health and takes no other medication. There is no family history of asthma or other respiratory problems. She does not smoke and drinks occasionally.

On exam, vital signs were: temperature, 37.2°C; heart rate, 80 beats per minute; respiration, 20 breaths per minute; blood pressure, 118/78; and oxygen saturation, 99% on room air. She is a well-nourished/well-developed female of average build in no respiratory distress. Her neurological, head, ears, eyes, nose, throat, neck, heart, chest, and abdominal exams are within normal limits.

KEY CLINICAL QUESTIONS

1. What diagnostic tests, if any, should be ordered for this patient?
2. Is this case presentation atypical for asthma?
3. Are there non-airway disorders that can present with similar respiratory symptoms?

LEARNING OBJECTIVES

1. Understand the definition and pathophysiology of vocal cord dysfunction (VCD).
2. Broaden the differential diagnosis of a patient with dyspnea and wheezing.
3. Learn how to differentiate VCD from asthma.
4. Learn common diagnostic procedures for VCD.
5. Learn both acute and long-term management of VCD.

BACKGROUND

VCD was first described in the medical literature in the 1980s *(1)*. It has since become a significant differential diagnosis among patients with upper respiratory symptoms. It is especially important for primary care physicians to recognize VCD because it is most commonly mistaken for asthma, leading to improper treatment including use of corticosteroids, hospitalization, even intubation *(2)*. The prevalence in the population is difficult to determine because of misdiagnosis as asthma as well as co-existence with asthma. One military study showed that 15% of patients with exertional dyspnea or suspected asthma had VCD *(3)*. Another study of adult patients with seemingly intractable asthma showed that 10% actually had VCD instead of asthma, and an additional 30% had VCD co-existing with asthma *(2)*. It is therefore important to learn how to distinguish the two diagnoses and how to properly work-up and treat VCD.

PATHOPHYSIOLOGY

The larynx is an area in the anterior neck region that is often divided into the supraglottis, the glottis, and the subglottis (*see* Fig. 1A). The glottis is the region

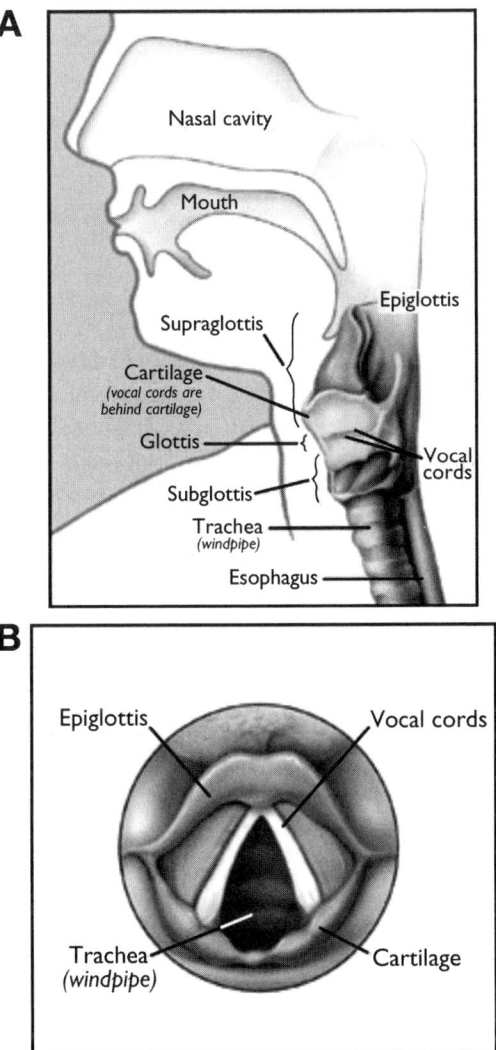

Fig 1. (**A**) The larynx, divided into the supraglottic, glottic, and subglottic regions. (**B**) A superior view of the vocal cords.

that contains two opposing muscles known as the vocal cords (*see* Fig. 1B). The larynx is therefore the area for voice production but is also critical in breathing and swallowing.

The glottic opening between the vocal cords normally varies with breathing. Vocal cord movement is controlled by a number of muscles within the larynx. The thyroarytenoid, cricoarytenoid lateralis, interarytenoid, and aryepiglottic muscles cause the vocal cords to come together, whereas the posterior cricoarytenoid muscle is responsible for glottic opening. Normally, the glottic opening widens during inspiration. Paradoxical narrowing of the glottic structures during inspiration defines VCD.

ETIOLOGY

The etiology of VCD is not clear, although a number of theories exist. One such theory suggests that local inflammation of the vocal cords leads to autonomic dysfunction, which in turn causes vocal cord hyperactivity, much like bronchial hyperresponsiveness is thought to be a cause of asthma (4). It is generally believed that the cause of VCD can be divided into two categories: psychological or nonpsychological. Nonpsychological causes are far less common but include neurological disorders and gastroesophageal reflux disease (GERD). Neurological disorders, such as brain stem compression, upper motor neuron injuries, and movement disorders, have rarely been associated with VCD (5). A careful neurological exam is therefore important in the work-up and a computed tomography or magnetic resonance imaging scan may be useful if questions remain. The association between GERD and VCD is not clear, although it is important to assess a patient with possible VCD for signs of reflux (5).

Much research has been done on the association between psychological disorders and VCD. In fact, when VCD was initially described in the early 1980s, it was considered to be a conversion disorder (1). The patients described in this seminal paper were young females who had any of a variety of psychiatric problems including depression, obsessive-compulsive disorder, borderline personality disorder, and somatization disorder. One study also linked VCD with a childhood history of sexual abuse (6). Further studies have since shown that a true conversion disorder with an underlying subconscious conflict is not always seen. The link between the psyche, and VCD, however, remains today. It is now thought that emotional stress is a major trigger for psychological VCD (5), which has important implications when discussing appropriate treatment options.

DIAGNOSIS

Understanding the pathophysiology of paradoxical vocal cord movement helps to explain common patient presentations of this disorder. Patients can have acute onset of shortness of breath, cough, chest tightness, voice change (such as hoarseness), and wheezing, especially on inspiration (7). Both children and adults can be affected, although it is reported in the literature most often in young adult females (8).

Given the presenting symptoms, it is not surprising that VCD is often misdiagnosed as asthma. Further complicating the clinical picture is that the two can also co-exist. There may be subtle differences on history and physical examina-

Table 1
Differences Between Vocal Cord Dysfunction and Asthma

Laboratory test/study	Vocal cord dysfunction	Asthma
Chest X-ray	Normal	Hyperinflation, peribronchial cuffing
Pulmonary function testing: 1. Flow volume loops 2. Forced expiratory volume in 1 second (FEV_1) 3. Peak expiratory flow 4. FEV1:forced vital capacity (FVC)	1. Flattening of inspiratory flow–volume loop 2. Normal 3. Normal 4. Normal	1. Obstructive pattern 2. Decreased 3. Decreased 4. Decreased
Arterial oxygen saturation	Normal	Decreased
Alveolar–arterial gradient	Normal	Increased
Peripheral eosinophil count	Normal	Increased

tion that can assist in further work-up. Patients will VCD not only have a quick onset of symptoms, but also usually a quick resolution as well. VCD is most commonly symptomatic during the day, unlike asthma, which frequently produces nighttime cough. Patients with VCD may be able to hold their breath despite symptoms and cough does not tend to worsen the wheezing *(7)*. The physical examination during asymptomatic periods in those with VCD is often nonremarkable. If the patient is symptomatic, the wheezing may be high-pitched and loudest over the larynx, but this is not always true, and often the wheezing is indistinguishable from that of a patient with asthma. Despite their symptoms, patients with VCD will often have a normal oxygen saturation and a normal alveolar–arterial gradient *(5)*. Furthermore, a chest X-ray in a patient with VCD is often normal, lacking the hyperventilation and peribronchial cuffing often associated with asthma. Pulmonary function testing can also be useful in distinguishing VCD from asthma, especially if the test is performed while the patient is symptomatic. The classic patient with VCD will have flattening of the inspiratory flow-volume loop, whereas a patient with asthma will have more profound effects on the expiratory portion of the loop *(5)*. Table 1 summarizes some of the differences between VCD and asthma.

A careful history and physical examination is important in diagnosing VCD, although additional studies are needed. Because of the respiratory symptoms, a chest X-ray may be performed along with pulmonary function tests. Although these may be helpful as shown above, they may still be equivocal regarding the diagnosis. The gold standard for diagnosing VCD is direct visualization of the vocal cords via laryngoscopy. The classic finding indicating VCD is closure of the anterior two-thirds of the glottis upon inspiration with a remaining diamond-shaped "chink," or space, in the posterior glottis. There is variability in this finding including complete glottic closure during inspiration and closure during expiration as well as inspiration *(5)*. Given that VCD is episodic, some physicians attempt to provoke symptoms with exercise or methacholine *(8)*. An experienced laryngoscopist is needed to avoid mistaking the gag reflex induced by insertion of the laryngoscope for true VCD *(7)*. A small percentage of patients with VCD may also have concurrent laryngeal abnormalities including laryngomalacia, vocal cord nodules, and subglottic stenosis, further showing the importance of always performing laryngoscopy and not to simply diagnosis VCD based on symptoms alone *(9)*.

DIFFERENTIAL DIAGNOSIS

Although VCD is most commonly misdiagnosed as asthma, it is important to be familiar with a variety of other diagnoses in the differential (*see* Table 2). The complete clinical picture can help distinguish VCD from diagnoses such as angioedema (in which swelling of the face often occurs), anaphylaxis (in which urticaria and vital sign instability can occur), and croup (in which a child may have cold-like symptoms as well as fever). Chest X-rays can help distinguish VCD from foreign body aspiration.

TREATMENT

Acute management of VCD includes reassurance to help calm the patient's anxiety. Creating a quiet, calm environment and explaining the patient's normal oxygen saturation, for example, may help ease fears of suffocation *(5)*. Panting may be a useful technique because it activates the posterior cricoarytenoid muscle, therefore widening the space between the vocal cords. Also, making an "s" sound on expiration may be a useful way to divert the patient's attention from the attack *(2)*. Heliox (70–80% helium, 20–30% oxygen) has also been used successfully in acute attacks of VCD. Helium is less dense than nitrogen, therefore decreasing the turbulence across the narrowed glottic opening, which in turn reduces the symptoms of VCD *(2)*. Sedatives, such as diazepam, have been used in extremely anxious patients. It may acutely help with anxiety, thereby stopping the attack, but long-term use is not encouraged *(2)*.

Appropriate long-term management of VCD is dependent on the etiology of the disorder. The minority of patients who have VCD as a result of neurological problems or GERD will benefit from the treatment of their primary disorder. All

Table 2
Differential Diagnosis of Vocal Cord Dysfunction

- Asthma
- Anaphylaxis
- Angioedema
- Exercise-induced bronchospasm
- Foreign body aspiration
- Traumatic injury
- Croup
- Epiglottitis
- Upper respiratory infection in presence of subglottic stenosis or laryngomalacia

patients with VCD, however, and especially those with psychological VCD, will benefit from education about the disorder. It may be helpful to have the patient visualize the paradoxical vocal cord movement during laryngoscopy in an attempt to help them understand the mechanics of their disorder (2). Although patients may have concurrent asthma, many have simply been misdiagnosed and overmedicated. Unless asthma can be documented with the appropriate testing (such as pulmonary function tests [PFTs]), the patient's asthma medication should be discontinued (2).

The mainstays of VCD management include speech therapy, which can train a patient to abort an attack once it occurs, and psychological counseling, which may help a patient avoid attacks all together. Patients should be reassured that VCD is a real diagnosis, and although is may have psychological components, it is certainly not "all in their head." Speech therapy attempts to divert the patient's attention away from the larynx and focuses on diaphragmatic and "wide-open throat" breathing (5). Typically, three to four sessions with a trained professional are adequate to train the patient in these breathing exercises (2). One way a primary care physician can find a speech therapist trained in VCD therapy is through the American Speech–Language–Hearing Association (www.asha.org). Psychological treatment is important to address life issues that may be triggering VCD. Each patient will require an individualized approach. Therapies can range from yoga and hypnosis, which may help to decrease stress, to psychological counseling, which allows a patient to discuss issues in greater detail. The long-term prognosis for VCD is thought to be quite good for patients who receive appropriate speech and psychological therapies and who avoid unnecessary use of β-agonists and corticosteroids (10), although data is lacking on the amount of improvement possible with particular therapies. Table 3 summarizes the approaches to acute and long-term management of VCD.

Table 3
Acute and Long-Term Management of VCD

Acute management of VCD	Long-term management of VCD
Calm environment with reassurance	Speech therapy: • diaphragmatic breathing • "wide-open mouth breathing"
Panting	Psychological therapy • yoga • hypnosis • biofeedback • pharmacotherapy • psychotherapy
Making an "s" sound on expiration	Discontinuation of asthma medication if no documented asthma
Heliox (70–80% helium/20–30% oxygen)	
Sedatives (to be used sparingly)	

VCD, vocal cord dysfunction.

CASE RESOLUTION

Because the validity of the patient's asthma diagnosis is questioned and there is concern for VCD, a chest X-ray and PFTs are ordered and the patient is referred to an experienced laryngoscopist. Further questioning shows that the patient has been very stressed lately over starting her new job and moving away from home for the first time. The patient returns to your office 1 week later with all of her results. Her chest X-ray and PFTs are all within normal limits. The laryngoscopy report states that the vocal cords appear normal, but after an exercise challenge, the vocal cords are seen to paradoxically adduct during inspiration. The patient has therefore been given the diagnosis of VCD. Also, given that there is no documented diagnosis of asthma, the patient's budesonide and albuterol are discontinued. At the recommendation of the otolaryngologist, appointments are made for speech therapy and the patient enters counseling to address her anxiety surrounding her recent life changes. The patient follows up in her primary care physician's office in 3 months, having been attack-free in this time period.

FUTURE DIRECTIONS

VCD is becoming an increasingly important diagnosis to consider, especially given the unnecessary treatment and medical costs that can result if the disorder is misdiagnosed as asthma. Although the current management seems to help many patients, studies are still needed to provide data on long-term prognosis.

The National Jewish Medical and Research Center has been at the forefront of research for this particular disorder and offers information for patients and physicians through its website: http://www.nationaljewish.org/diseases/dt1.html.

By increasing awareness of VCD, patients will hopefully receive appropriate treatment in a timely manner, and research will continue to investigate current therapies and well as those on the horizon.

REFERENCES

1. Christopher KL, Wood RP, Eckert RC, et. al. Vocal-cord dysfunction presenting as asthma. N Engl J Med 1983:308:1566–1570.
2. Brugman SM, Simons SM. Vocal cord dysfunction; don't mistake it for asthma. Phys Sports Med 1998:26:63–75.
3. Morris MJ, Deal LE, Bean DR, Grbach VX, Morgan JA. Vocal cord dysfunction in patients with exertional dyspnea. Chest 1999;116:1676–1682.
4. Ayres JG, Gabbott PLA. Vocal cord dysfunction and laryngeal hyperresponsiveness: a function of altered autonomic balance? Thorax 2002;57:284–285.
5. Bahrainwala AH, Simon MR. Wheezing and vocal cord dysfunction mimicking asthma. Curr Opin Pulm Med 2001;7:8–13.
6. Freedman MR, Rosenbery SJ, Schmaling KB. Childhood sexual abuse in patients with paradoxical vocal cord dysfunction. J Nerv Ment Dis 1991;179:295–298.
7. Wood RP, Milgrom H. Vocal cord dysfunction. J All Clin Immunol 1996;98:481–485.
8. Parker JM, Guerrero ML. Airway function in women: bronchial hyperresponsiveness, cough, and vocal cord dysfunction. Clin Chest Med 2004;25:321–330.
9. Patel NJ, Jorgensen C, Kuhn J, Merati AL. Concurrent laryngeal abnormalities in patients with paradoxical vocal cord dysfunction. Otolaryngol Head Neck Surg 2004;130:686–689.
10. Poirier MP, Pancioli AM, DiGiulio GA. Vocal cord dysfunction presenting as acute asthma in a pediatric patient. Pediatr Emerg Care 1996;12:213–214.

23 Pulmonary Embolism

Eric Wollins and Matthew L. Mintz

CONTENTS
- CASE PRESENTATION
- KEY CLINICAL QUESTIONS
- LEARNING OBJECTIVES
- EPIDEMIOLOGY
- PATHOPHYSIOLOGY
- CLINICAL MANIFESTATIONS
- DIFFERENTIAL DIAGNOSIS
- DIAGNOSIS
- TREATMENT
- FUTURE DIRECTIONS
- REFERENCES

CASE PRESENTATION

A 65-year-old obese male with a past medical history of prostate cancer and a recent left hip fracture presents to the emergency department after experiencing progressive shortness of breath with an inability to ambulate and perform his activities of daily living. Two weeks prior the patient noticed the onset of dyspnea on exertion and left lower extremity pain and swelling that he attributed to his recent injury. In the emergency department, the patient's vital signs were temperature, 38.1°C; blood pressure, 110/64; pulse, 114 beats per minute; respiratory rate, 30 breaths per minute; and oxygen saturation on room air, 90%. Physical exam disclosed a tachypneic gentleman in mild respiratory distress with tachycardia, a clear lung exam, and a tender, swollen left calf. Chest radiograph showed an elevated right hemidiaphragm without infiltrates or effusions and an electrocardiogram revealed sinus tachycardia without evidence of ischemia.

From: *Current Clinical Practice: Disorders of the Respiratory Tract: Common Challenges in Primary Care*
By: M. L. Mintz © Humana Press, Totowa, NJ

KEY CLINICAL QUESTIONS

1. Given the patient's risk factors, clinical presentation, and physical findings, what should the next step be in evaluation of this patient for pulmonary embolism (PE)?
2. What are the various diagnostic tests available for PE, and how should they be chosen?
3. Assuming the evaluation confirms the diagnosis of PE, how should the patient be treated and managed?
4. Can PE be managed as an outpatient, and when does this patient need to be admitted to the hospital?

LEARNING OBJECTIVES

1. Understand the spectrum and pathogenesis of venous thromboembolic disease.
2. Recognize the wide variety of clinical presentation of PE.
3. Become familiar with the appropriate diagnostic work-up of PE.
4. Become familiar with the appropriate management, both inpatient and outpatient, for the treatment of PE.

EPIDEMIOLOGY

Published studies estimate that 600,000 episodes of PE occur yearly in the United States, 60,000 to 200,000 cases of which result in death. However, the true incidence of PE mortality is actually believed to be even higher because autopsy studies suggest that the antemortem diagnosis of PE is frequently missed. The 3-month and 1-year mortality rate after PE has been reported to be as high as 17 and 24%, respectively *(1)*. Data from the 1990 PIOPED study demonstrated that 1% of hospitalized patients suffer an acute PE. However, 16 years after this study, acute PE continues to remain a leading cause of death in hospitalized patients with an estimated incidence 1 in 1000 on general medicine wards *(1–6)*.

PATHOPHYSIOLOGY

Deep vein thrombosis (DVT) and PE should be considered as part of the same process, venous thromboembolic disease (VTE). The pathogenesis of venous thrombosis involves three factors, coined as "Virchow's Triad," which has remained the primary mechanism to explain the development of VTE since the 19th century. Virchow identified three factors that lead to the pathogenesis of venous thrombosis including stasis of blood, local trauma to the intimal layer of vessel walls, and hypercoagulability. Venous stasis or obstruction will inhibit the clearance and dilution of activated coagulation factors leading to a procoagulant state. Damage to vessel walls prevents the endothelium from inhibiting coagulation and initiating local fibinolysis, whereas a hypercoagulable state, either from congenital or inherited thrombophilia, promotes coagulation *(7)*. When one or more of the triad constituents is present, a platelet nidus will form and continue to grow as the result of the additional recruitment of platelets and fibrin. As the nidus enlarges, it may partially or totally occlude the vein and then dislodge and embolize more proximally.

The most clinically important PEs originate at sites of decreased flow, such as the valve cusps or bifurcations of the proximal deep veins the lower extremities. Autopsy data shows that 65 to 90% of PE arise from within veins of the lower extremities including the popliteal, femoral, and iliac. Although uncommon, pulmonary emboli may also originate in the pelvic, renal, upper extremities, or right heart chambers. However, it is important to note that patients with PE may have no leg symptoms or findings at the time of diagnosis. In fact, in the landmark PIOPED study, less than 30% of patients with PE had the signs or symptoms of lower extremity venous thrombosis *(1)*. Furthermore, additional research has demonstrated that the risk of developing a PE with a proximal DVT is approximately 30 to 50% *(2,7)*.

The lower extremity thrombi that dislodge and propagate proximally can enter the right-sided heart chambers and into the pulmonary circulation. Small thrombi tend to travel through the right heart and past the pulmonic valve and into pulmonary circulation to more distal regions of the lungs where they are capable of occluding the smaller vessels in the periphery. This development can lead to serious complications that stem from the reduction in the cross-sectional area of the pulmonary vascular bed and resulting increase in the pulmonary vascular resistance. Increased alveolar dead space, a redistribution of blood flow, and impaired gas exchange ensue and can cause a reflex bronchconstriction that may lead to pulmonary edema, decreased pulmonary compliance, and an increase in right ventricular afterload. On the other hand, the larger thrombi or massive emboli may lodge at the bifurcation of the main pulmonary artery or at the lobar branches and lead to hemodynamic compromise and cardiogenic shock.

At least one established risk factor is present in approximately 75% of patients who develop a DVT or PE *(8)*. The risk factors for VTE are diverse and may be further subdivided into primary (or inherited) and secondary (or acquired). It is important to recognize that there is a complex balance between coagulation and anticoagulation and that this balance can be easily altered by numerous acquired disease states. Also, there are a number of inherited thrombophilias, such as factor V Leiden (protein C resistance), prothrombin gene *20210A* mutation, and deficiencies in protein C and S that predispose patients to hypercoagulable states and subsequent venous thromboses. It has been estimated that the inherited thrombophilas can be identified in 24 to 37% of patients with DVT and in the majority of patients with familial thrombosis *(9,10)*. One of the most common inherited defects that predispose to the development of blood clots in people of northern European ancestry is factor V Leiden defect, which is a point mutation (arginine is substituted for glutamine) on the factor V gene that leads to the resistance of degradation by protein C. This mutation has been reported to be the most common cause of thrombophilia, occurring in approximately 5% of the general population, and is identified in approximately 50% of individuals with recurrent VTE *(3,11)*.

Secondary risk factors include a long list of acute or chronic comorbidities such as obesity, malignancy, postoperative states, trauma, nephrotic syndrome, and congestive heart failure (Table 1). Other secondary risk factors include increasing age, prolonged immobility, estrogenic medications (oral contraceptive pills and hormone replacement therapy), hyperhomocysteinemia, and disease states that alter the blood's viscosity, such as polycythemia vera and Waldenstroms macroglobulinemia. VTE, especially PE, is also common in pregnancy and has been estimated to occur in 1 out of every 2000 women and is the leading cause of pregnancy-related mortality in the United States *(12)*.

Malignancy is also a well-recognized risk factor for VTE as the result of the production of thrombin and procoagulants from neoplastic cells. All forms of cancer, both active and those in remission, are believed to predispose patients to VTE. Neoplasms most commonly associated with PE include pancreatic cancer, bronchogenic carcinoma, and cancer of the colon, stomach, and breast. Additionally, several studies have evaluated the incidence and relationship of a diagnosis of an unsuspecting cancer after a first episode of idiopathic VTE. Such studies have demonstrated a 10 to 20% chance of developing cancer over the 2-year period after the index VTE. This area, including the need to initiate an extensive diagnostic evaluation for a malignancy, continues to remains controversial *(13,14)*.

In 1954, Homan first described several cases of travel-related DVT including air travel *(15)*. Initial studies suggested that prolonged travel more than 4 hours duration is associated with an increased in risk for VTE, even in patients without any of the other well-known risk factors. More recent studies suggest that the risk for acquiring travel-related VTE is higher for those individuals who travel for more than 6 hours in duration or more than 3500 miles *(16)*.

CLINCAL MANIFESTATIONS

The clinical manifestations of PE are so diverse, with a variety of nonspecific signs and symptoms, that the diagnosis is often missed. Classically, a patient with an acute PE can present with a sudden onset of shortness of breath and pleuritic chest pain with or without hemoptysis. However, patients may vary in their presentation from no obvious symptoms to progressive dyspnea or a sudden onset of air hunger. The most common symptoms of PE in the PIOPED study were dyspnea (73%), pleuritic chest pain (66%), cough (37%), and hemoptysis (13%) *(1)*. Patients may also present with atypical symptoms including seizures,

Table 1
Venous Thromboembolic Risk Factors

Inherited thrombophilia

Antithrombin III deficiency
Protein C and S deficiency
Factor V leiden (protein C resistance)
Prothrombin gene *20210A* mutation
Hyperhomocysteinemia
Dysfibrinogenemia
Disorders of plasmin generation

Acquired (transient)

Intensive care unit admission
Respiratory failure
Pneumonia
Infection
In-dwelling central venous catheters
Heparin-induced thrombocytopenia and thrombosis
Hyperhomocysteinemia
Medications: thalidomide, oral contraceptive, estrogen replacement therapy
Nephrotic syndrome
Postoperative trauma/burns
Pregnancy
Prolonged immobilization (bed rest, travel)
Obesity
Bone fractures
Surgery with more than 30 minutes of anesthesia

Acquired (permanent)

Over age 40
Malignancy (myeloproliferative disorders)
Alterations in blood viscosity (polycythemia, sickle cell, Waldenstrom's)
Antiphospholipid syndrome antibodies (lupus anticoagulant, anticardiolipin antibody)
Prior history of deep vein thrombosis or pulmonary embolism
Stroke
Heart failure
Chronic lung disease
Active collagen vascular disorder
Inflammatory disorder (inflammatory bowel disorder)
Varicose veins
Nephrotic syndrome

syncope, fever, productive cough, wheezing, mental status changes, and new onset atrial fibrillation.

Physical exam findings in patients with PE may be broad and varied and can range from the nonspecific findings of decreased breath sounds and low-grade fever to the extreme signs of impending shock, such as poor perfusion, tachycardia, and tachypnea. Whereas the presence of dyspnea, syncope, or cyanosis, is believed to be indicative of a diagnosis of a massive PE, the symptoms of pleuritic chest pain, cough, or hemoptysis are suggestive of a small embolism near the lung's pleura. Other physical exam findings include signs of right ventricular dysfunction and pulmonary hypertension (palpable impulse over the second left interspace, elevated jugular venous distention, loud P2, right ventricular S3 gallop, and a left sternal border systolic murmur consistent with tricuspid regurgitation), decreased excursion of hemithorax, palpable or audible friction rub, palpable chest wall tenderness, and audible crackles or wheezes over area of embolization. The most common physical signs in the PIOPED study included tachypnea (70%), adventitious breath sounds including crackles (51%), tachycardia (30%), a fourth heart sound (24%), and accentuated pulmonic component of the second heart sound (23%) *(1)*.

DIFFERENTIAL DIAGNOSIS

The differential diagnosis of PE is remarkably diverse and may mimic other disorders, especially common cardiopulmonary illnesses (*see* Table 2). PE may be considered in any condition that encompasses chest pain, shortness of breath, cough, wheezing, or syncope. An acute PE can be mistaken for an exacerbation of a chest wall syndrome, such as pleurisy or costochondritis. However, it is important to recognize that PE may also have a chest wall tenderness component and that clinical response to nonsteroidal anti-inflammatory drugs, which is the treatment for choice for costochondritis, does not rule out an underlying PE. Furthermore, pleurisy may be indistinguishable from PE. Although both may produce pleuritic chest pain, a PE is more likely to produce tachycardia, tachypnea, and a widened alveolar–arterial gradient. Underlying infectious diseases of the lung including pneumonia are often difficult to distinguish from PE. Patients with PE present with a low-grade fever, productive cough of purulent sputum, shortness of breath, and sometimes a chest X-ray (CXR) finding suspicious for an infiltrate. However, the time course may provide some clue because the onset of a PE is more abrupt.

DIAGNOSIS

The majority of preventable deaths associated with PE can be ascribed to a missed diagnosis rather than to a failure of treatment *(17)*. It has been estimated that the diagnosis of PE is missed in approximately 400,000 patients in the United

Table 2
Differential Diagnosis of Pulmonary Embolism

Anemia
Angina/acute myocardial infarction
Aortic stenosis
Atypical emboli (fat, air, tumor)
Aortic dissection
Atrial fibrillation
Cardiogenic shock
Congestive heart failure
Chronic obstructive pulmonary disease
Cocaine use
Drug reaction
Intoxication
Metabolic disorder
Mitral stenosis
Myocardial ischemia
Musculoskeletal disorders (chest contusion, rib fracture, costochondritis)
Myocarditis
Pleurisy
Pneumothorax
Pneumomediastinum
Pneumonia
Panic attack/anxiety disorder
Pericardial disease
Syncope
Sepsis
Shock

States per year, of which 100,000 deaths may have been prevented with the proper diagnosis and treatment. Most patients succumb to an acute PE within the first few hours of the event if prompt recognition and treatment is not immediately instituted. Because the diagnosis of PE can be elusive, even when considered by the most astute clinician, it should be actively sought in patients with respiratory symptoms that are unexplained by an alternative diagnosis. Because the detection of a PE hinges on clinical suspicion, the evaluation process begins with a careful history and physical and thorough assessment of the patient's underlying comorbidities, risk factors, and family history.

Basic laboratory studies including a complete blood count and comprehensive metabolic and coagulation studies are usually nonspecific in PE, although may assist in the diagnosis of an alternative disorder. An arterial blood gas is useful and characteristically reveals hypoxemia, hypocapnia, and respiratory alkalosis. It is important to recognize that a normal arterial blood gas test does not rule out the diagnosis of PE and cannot be accurately used to differentiate between patients suspected of having a PE and those in whom a more thorough diagnostic evaluation is not warranted.

D-dimer is a degradation product of crosslinked fibrin within circulating plasma that can be easily measured. The use of D-dimer tests in recent years has added to the noninvasive evaluation process of patients with suspected PE presenting to the emergency room. It is a highly sensitive but nonspecific screening test for suspected VTE. Although D-dimer values may be elevated in almost all patients with VTE, it is also elevated in patients with advanced age, myocardial infarction, pneumonia, heart failure, or inflammatory states or underlying malignancy. As a result, because of its lack of specificity, its role is limited in ruling out embolic disease. Depending on the modality in which it is measured, D-dimers miss approximately 10% of PEs, whereas only 30% of patients with positive D-dimer findings have a confirmatory diagnosis of PE. A D-dimer can be helpful when the result is negative in a patient with a low to moderate pretest probability of thrombus and a negative ventilation–perfusion (V/Q) scan. As a result, D-dimer alone is not recommended in establishing a definitive diagnosis in patients suspected to have a PE. It is, however, useful when used in conjunction a V/Q scan, computed tomography (CT) scan, or a clinical prediction rule.

Electrocardiogram (EKG) should be incorporated into the evaluation of patients with a suspected PE. The most common EKG abnormalities associated with PE include tachycardia without specific ST-T wave changes. Neither finding is sensitive or specific enough to aid in the diagnosis of a PE. Classic but uncommon EKG changes associated with PE include new onset atrial fibrillation, right-bundle branch block, and S1-Q3-T3 pattern. Data from the PIOPED study demonstrated that EKGs were abnormal in 70% of patients, although none were specific or sensitive (1).

CXR is a typical initial imaging study for any patient with respiratory complaints. In patients with PE, the CXR is commonly normal. However, in later stages, a CXR may have radiographic features including dilatation of the pulmonary vessels, an area of oligemia (Westermark's sign), a peripheral wedge-shaped density (Hampton's hump), or an elevated hemi-diaphragm. Other radiographic findings, such as atelectasis, pleural effusions, and cardiomegaly, are neither sensitive nor specific for PE (1). A CXR alone is insufficient to confirm the diagnosis of PE, however, it may assist in demonstrating alternative diagnoses for the patient's respiratory complaints.

V/Q scanning has long been the first-line study in the evaluation of patients with suspected PE. Defects in radiotracer uptake from ventilated and perfused areas of the lungs are reported as normal or having a low, intermediate, or high probability of embolus. Patients with normal or near normal V/Q scans and a low clinical suspicion have a very low incidence of PE, whereas high-probability V/Q scans are strongly associated with diagnosis of PE. One gray area of V/Q scanning occurs when the result is indeterminant (low or intermediate probability) in a patient in whom the clinical suspicion is high. Given the high clinical suspicion, such patients may require additional investigation with a CT scan. It is also important to recognize that in patients with underlying chronic obstructive pulmonary disease or congestive heart failure, a V/Q scan may be of limited utility because they are difficult to interpret in these setting. Because a V/Q scan will most likely be nondiagnostic in this setting, such patients should instead proceed directly to a CT scan as the initial diagnostic imaging modality for the evaluation of PE.

PE may occasionally be seen on a conventional contrast-enhanced CT scan; however, such a finding is usually dependent on on the timing of the intravenous contrast bolus within the pulmonary vasculature. Spiral CT scanning (also known as helical CT) was introduced in the early 1990s and involves an X-ray beam and a coupled array of detectors rotating continuously in a spiral manner. This novel technique results in a reduction in examination time (allowing for imaging of the entire thorax in a single breath) compared with conventional CT scanning. Compared with conventional CT scans, helical CT scanning utilizes faster and more powerful computers and technology to acquire multiple transverse and thinner slices.

Spiral CT allows for direct visualization of the main, lobar, and segmental pulmonary emboli as small as 2 mm. The features diagnostic of PE include a central intravascular filling defect within the vessel lumen, eccentric tracking of contrast material around a filling defect, and complete vascular occlusion that may cause parenchyma oligemia, and hemorrhage with ground glass attenuation. In worst case scenarios, infarction may be identified and represented by a peripheral wedged-shaped pleural-based opacification. The major advantages of helical CT over conventional CT include a higher degree of lesion detection, better lesion characterization, reduction in contrast volumes, and minimization of artifacts. The sensitivity and specificity of spiral CT in the detection for PE has been reported to be 53 to 100% and 78 to 96%, respectively. The negative predicted value is 81 to 100%, and the positive predictive value is 60 to 100% for detecting emboli in segmental or larger arteries.

Because the differential diagnosis for a patient presenting with a suspected PE is broad, CT scanning also affords the potential advantage of identifying other disease states that mimic PE (e.g., lung tumors, pleural disease), nonvascular structures, parenchymal abnormalities, and alternative diagnoses when a PE is, in fact, not present. The disadvantages of CT scanning include interobserver disagreement and technically poor quality exams as the result of artifact from respiratory or cardiac motion that may produce false filling defects. Additionally, CT scanning is expensive and limited to patients without an allergy to contrast or renal insufficiency.

However, spiral CT scans are extremely useful in the work-up of a suspected PE. The current use of CT scanning in the evaluation of PE is determined by its availability and varies by institution. At some institutions, the gold standard may be to proceed directly to a CT scan of the chest in patients with a moderate to high clinical suspicion. At other institutions, a patient may first have a V/Q scan and then proceed to a CT scan when such tests are nondiagnostic. Given the limitations of V/Q scanning, it is no surprise that spiral CT scanning has gained popularity because it can actually visualize the clot, whereas V/Q scanning only displays the secondary effects of the pulmonary emboli within the pulmonary vasculature bed.

Pulmonary angiogram, which is the injection of iodinated contrast into the patient's pulmonary vasculature with subsequent images, remains the gold standard in the diagnosis of PE. A positive result consists of a filling defect or sharp cutoff of an affected artery, whereas a negative angiography finding excludes clinically relevant PE. However, because this procedure is invasive, risky, and requires the expertise of the interventional radiology department for interpretation, its utility is often limited. Angiography is thus reserved for a small group of patients in whom the diagnosis of embolism cannot be established by less invasive means.

Because most clinically relevant pulmonary emboli originate in the lower extremities, it is often necessary to screen for a DVT in a patient being evaluated for a PE. This is especially true in patients with a negative CT or nondiagnostic V/Q scan with a high clinical suspicion. Color-flow doppler imaging and compression ultrasonography are highly accurate with a sensitivity and specificity of more than 95% for the detection of proximal DVT in symptomatic patients *(7)*. It is estimated that ultrasound is positive in 10 to 20% of all patients without leg symptoms or signs who undergo evaluation and approximately 50% of patients with proven PE *(17)*. As a result, normal lower extremity dopplers do not rule out the presence of a PE especially if the suspicion is high.

In a stable patient with minimal or no risk factors, normal alveolar–arterial gradient, and negative D-dimer result, a PE appears to be an unlikely diagnosis. However, because of the variation in which patients present, this is not always the scenario. As a result, evidence-based algorithms and clinical prediction rules have been proposed as a means of providing an objective basis for the clinical assessment of the probability of PE. These rules involve gathering data that can be easily acquired in the outpatient setting or within the emergency room that then allows a clinician to standardize the diagnostic process and categorize patients into low-, intermediate-, and high-probability cohorts. The oldest and most used decision rule is the Wells clinical prediction rule for PE, which uses a point system based on the clinical features and the likelihood of diagnoses other than PE *(18)*. Using the Wells system in combination with other data, such as D-dimer results, have been shown to improve the accuracy in diagnosing PE. Other prediction rules have been devised and tested, although no consensus has emerged on the best clinical prediction rule for PE.

TREATMENT

The treatment for a PE is the same as that for a DVT and includes immediate and full anticoagulation with one of the intravenous or subcutaneous heparins, along with the simultaneous administration of the oral vitamin K antagonist, warfarin. Whereas some patients with DVT may be safely managed as outpatients, because of the potential for rapid clinical deterioration in patients with PE, inpatient hospitalization is recommended and advised.

In general, outpatient treatment of PE remains controversial as the result of sparse data evaluating the efficacy and safety of treating PE in the ambulatory setting. To date, there are no large studies validating the treatment of a PE as an outpatient. The data that is available is limited by the few trials and small numbers in each. One prospective study of 108 patients with PE who were treated as outpatients suggested that ambulatory management of PE was safe and feasible *(19)*. Despite this and other small studies demonstrating some promise in the outpatient management of PE, this approach is not yet widely practiced. In general, if considering outpatient therapy, good candidates include those who are low risk (i.e., no history of bleeding diathesis or renal dysfunction) and those who are relatively young, compliant, responsible, and capable of treating themselves at home. Such patients should also be hemodynamic stable with a good cardiopulmonary reserve and without impairment of gas exchange.

Because of the high morbidity and mortality associated with PE, diagnostic investigations should not take precedence over empiric anticoagulation in patients with scenarios highly suspicious for PE. Clinicians treating patients with PE must remain diligent about strictly monitoring for hemodynamic instability including the need for vasopressor therapy for advanced airway management. Therefore, given the acuity in which the clinical status of a patient with a PE may worsen, clinicians must have a low threshold for transferring patients to the intensive care setting.

Heparins

Anticoagulation remains the mainstay of treatment of PE with the goals of stopping clot propagation, preventing recurrence, and halting the development of pulmonary hypertension. Traditionally, unfractionated heparin (UH) has been most commonly used to treat PE, although in the last several years numerous studies have demonstrated that low-molecular-weight heparin (LMWH) is as safe and effective in treating both DVT and PE.

UNFRACTIONATED HEPARIN

UH prevents the conversion of fibrinogen to fibrin through the activation of antithrombin III (ATIII) and inhibition of factors XIIa, XIa, IXa, and Xa. As a result, heparin does not dissolve the existing venous embolism, but rather prevents additional thrombi from forming. Treatment with UH is based on body weight with dose titration based on the activated partial thromboplastin time (PTT) to 1.5 to 2.5 times the baseline control value. There are several weight-based heparin nomograms that can assist clinicians achieve and manage anticoagulation with UH. UH is typically stopped after approximately 5 days and when the international normalization ratio (INR) of prothrombin clotting time has exceed 2.0 for 2 consecutive days while on the combined therapy of heparin and warfarin.

LOW-MOLECULAR-WEIGHT HEPARINS

LMWHs are novel heparins that have greatly simplified the management of DVT and PE and represents a significant advancement in the treatment of VTE. This class of heparin has been widely studied and has proven to be at least as effective as UH in treating VTE. As with UH, vitamin K antagonists, such as warfarin, are started concomitantly with LMWHs for the treatment of VTE. LMWH offers numerous advantages over UH including superior bioavailability, fixed dosing schedule, and a lower incidence of heparin-induced thrombocytopenia. Furthermore, because LMWH primarily inhibits factor Xa and does not elevate the PTT, laboratory studies are not necessary to determine the adequacy of anticoagulation as with UH. Thus, LWMH appears to be a safe and cost-effective option, revolutionizing the outpatient management of DVT in patients who are without significant comorbidities such as renal failure or at high risk for a bleeding diathesis..

Vitamin K Antagonist

Warfarin (Coumadin®) is the drug of choice for long-term anticoagulation to prevent clot recurrence. Warfarin's mechanism of action is based in the inhibition of the vitamin K-dependent clotting factors including factors II, VII, IX, and X. Based on numerous studies, the starting dose of warfarin is typically 5 mg orally per day titrating the dose approximately every 3 days to achieve an INR between 2.0 and 3.0. The peak effect of warfarin is reported to occur about 36–72 hours after the first dose, however, "true anticoagulation" does not occur until approximately day 5 when there is a complete depletion of the coagulation factor (factor II or thrombin) with the longest half-life. As a result, at least 5 days of heparin is required as overlap and until the INR has reached therapeutic range for at least 2 consecutive days. Recently, numerous studies have investigated the risks and benefits of a warfarin starting dose of 10 mg daily as well as maintaining patients at a lower INR value between 1.5 and 2.0. However, until there is additional data that is equivocally convincing of the benefits of these changes, the anticoagulation with Coumadin should be initiated at a dose of 5 mg daily with a goal INR value between 2.0 and 3.0.

Thrombolysis

In contrast to the anticoagulant therapies, thrombolytic therapy works by actually dissolving fresh clots and restoring vessel patency. The indications for thrombolytics such as tissue plasminogen activator, altepase, urokinase, and streptokinase include patients who are hemodynamical unstable or have right heart dysfunction with poor cardiopulmonary reserve. It is estimated that less than 10% of patients with documented PE receive thrombolytics *(14)*. Because thrombolytics are not without adverse effects, including risk for major hemorrhage, it is limited for use in those patients with documented massive PE and hemodynamic instability.

Inferior Vena Caval Filters

The use of a mechanic barrier such as an inferior vena caval (IVC) filters is indicated in patients with a strong contraindication to anticoagulation, such as those patients with hemorrhagic stroke or active bleeding or in patients with recurrent PEs despite prolonged anticoagulation. Vena caval barriers only prevent additional emboli from further advancing through the circulatory and pulmonary systems. IVC filters do not halt the thrombotic process and are not considered first-line therapy in the management of acute PE. One study demonstrated that placement of an IVC filter was associated with a lower 12-day rate of PE, but a higher rate of DVT recurrence and no difference in survival at 2 years *(20)*.

Embolectomy

Embolectomy may be considered in those patients who are not candidates for anticoagulation and are acutely unstable or in those in whom thrombolysis is contraindicated or unsuccessful. As a result of the high mortality risk associated with this invasive procedure, it is an option that is only considered in the most unstable and moribund patients.

Duration of Therapy

The optimal duration and intensity of anticoagulation after a PE remains uncertain and is an area of continuous research and debate. Warfarin is typically continued for at least 3 months in patients with their first thrombotic event in the setting of a reversible risk factor, such as recent surgery or trauma. However, research demonstrates that treatment of 6 months duration prevents more recurrences in patients after their first PE *(21)*. In the absence of an identifiable risk factor, the first thrombotic episode is usually treated for a minimum of 6 months. Patients with recurrent VTE events or in whom there is an irreversible risk factor, such as one of the thrombophilias, often require long-term and potentially indefinite anticoagulation.

Pulmonary Embolism: Prophylaxis

Fatal PE has been recognized as one of the most common preventable causes of in-hospital death. As a result, all inpatients and outpatients with significant risk factors and comorbidities should have a thorough risk assessment to determine the need for pharmacological or nonpharmacological prophylaxis. It has been recommended that the specific regimen or type of heparin appears to be less important than ensuring that all patients, especially those who are hospitalized, are properly risk stratified and begun on appropriate prophylaxis if warranted. Pharmacological prophylaxis in a medical patient without renal failure includes either low-dose UH at a dose of 5000 IU subcutaneously every 8 or 12 hours or Enoxaparin at a dose of 40 mg subcutaneously daily. There are also a number of nonpharmacological measures to prevent VTE disease, including early mobilization and the use of mechanical devices to prevent clot formation.

Nonpharmacological Mechanical Devices

Graded or graduated elastic compression stockings (30–40 mmHg gradient) are useful in patients at the lowest risk for VTE or those who are at high risk for a VTE event when anticoagulation is not desirable. Furthermore, these stockings have been associated with a 50% reduction of postphlebitic syndrome *(22)*. Intermittent pneumatic compression devices are also a useful adjunct to anticoagulation and an alternative when anticoagulation is contraindicated. It has been proposed that these devices may assist in increasing the endogenous fibrinolysis via stimulation of the vascular endothelial wall *(23)*.

Hypercoagulable Work-Up

Although approximately 30% of patients will have a DVT or PE secondary to a thrombophilia, numerous retrospective studies have suggested that not every patient should have a thorough and costly evaluation to determine the precise thrombophilia. There is no clear evidence to suggest that screening all or even selected patients for thrombophilia improve long-term outcomes. Despite the lack of evidence and prospective studies to guide the decision making about when to evaluate patients for thrombophilias, it has been suggested that an extensive evaluation is recommended in those patients who are strongly thrombophilic, such as patients who have had recurrent thrombosis or have a positive family history or are under the age of 50 with an idiopathic thrombotic episode. If a thrombophilia is being investigated, it is important to recognize that ATIII and proteins C and S levels can be depressed during acute thrombotic events. Also, assays for these proteins may also be misleadingly low if they are measured after the initiation of heparin, which decreases the ATIII levels, or Coumadin, which decreases the protein C and S levels.

FUTURE DIRECTIONS

Areas of future research and investigation include the following:

- Fondaparinux: a heparin pentasaccharide that is one of the first of a new class of synthetic factor Xa inhibitors that catalyzes factor Xa inactivation by ATIII without inhibiting thrombin is currently being evaluated for the treatment of PE. This drug has a higher affinity for binding to ATIII than UH or LMWH, thus causing a conformational change in ATIII that increases the ability of ATII to inactivate factor Xa. Currently, fondaparinux is approved by the Food and Drug Administration for the prophylaxis of DVT in patients undergoing surgery for hip fracture or hip/knee replacement. Advantages of fondaparinux include a fixed, once daily subcutaneous dosing without the need for monitoring and an inability to interact with platelets or platelet factor 4 thus causing heparin-induced thrombocytopenia and thrombosis. A recent trial of once-daily fondaparinux was found to be as effective and safe as intravenous UH in the initial treatment of hemodynamically stable patients with PE *(24)*. Additional studies are currently ongoing comparing fondaparinux with LMWH.
- Ximelagatran: a novel oral direct thrombin inhibitor that is rapidly absorbed and converted to its active form, melagatran. This drug has a favorable pharmokinetic profile and is administered at a fixed oral dose of 24 mg twice daily without monitoring of coagulation (PT/PTT) has recently been studied both for the postoperative prevention of VTE and for the treatment of DVT. One recent study demonstrated that long-term treatment with ximelagatran was superior to placebo for the prevention of recurrent VTE and did not require monitoring of coagulation or adjustments in the dose *(25)*. Unlike warfarin, ximelagatran has not been reported to have any clinically relevant interactions with food or with drugs metabolized by the cytochrome P-450 system. To date, the most notable adverse effect appears to be a transient elevation in the alanine aminotransferase level.
- VTE and cancer: numerous small studies have indicated an association between VTE and a subsequent diagnosis of cancer. This area remains debatable and controversial. Additional studies are ongoing to determine if a thorough evaluation beyond age-related screening is warranted in such patients after their first VTE event.

REFERENCES

1. The PIOPED investigators. Value of the ventilation/perfusion scan in acute pulmonary embolism. Results of the prospective investigation of pulmonary embolism diagnosis (PIOPED). JAMA 1990;263:2753–2759.

2. Kim V, Spandorfer J. Epidemiology of venous thromboembolic disease. Emerg Med Clin North Am 2001;19:839–859.
3. Moser KM, Fedullo PF, LittleJohn JK, et al. Frequent asymptomatic pulmonary embolism in patients with deep venous thrombosis. JAMA 1994;271:223–225.
4. Meignan M, Rosso J, Gauthier H, et al. Systematic lung scans reveals a high frequency of silent pulmonary embolism in patients with deep venous thrombosis. Arch Intern Med 2000;160:159–164.
5. Goldhaber SZ, Visani L, De Rosa M. Acute pulmonary embolism: clinical outcomes in the International Cooperative Pulmonary Embolism Registry (ICOPER). Lancet 1999;353: 1386–1389.
6. American Public Health Association. Deep vein thrombosis: advancing awareness to protect patient lives. Public Health Leadership Conference on Deep-Vein Thombosis, Washington, DC. Feb 26, 2003.
7. Bates S, Ginsberg J. Treatment of deep-vein thrombosis. N Engl J Med. 2004;351:268–277.
8. Ramzi D, Leeper K. DVT and pulmonary embolism: part 1. Diagnosis. Am Fam Physician 2004;69:2829–2836.
9. Mateo J, Oliver A, Borrell M, et al. Laboratory evaluation and clinical characteristics of 2,132 consecutive unselected patients with venous thromboembolism—results of the Spanish Multicentric Study on Thrombophilia (EMET-Study). Thomb Haemost 1997;77:444–451.
10. Bauer KA. The thrombophilas: well defined risk factors with uncertain therapeutic implications. Ann Inter Med 2001;135:367–373.
11. Simioni P, Prandoni P, Lensing AWA, et al. The risk of recurrent venous Thromboembolism in patients with A, Arg506→Gln mutation in the gene for factor V. N Engl J Med 1997;336:399–403.
12. Kaunitz AM, Hughes JM, Grimes DA, et al. Causes of maternal mortality in the USA. Obstet Gynecol 1985;65:605–610.
13. Martinelli I. Risk factors in venous thromboembolism. Thromb Haemost 2001;86:395–403.
14. Sorenson HT, Mellemkjar L, Steffensen FH, et al. The risk of a diagnosis of cancer after primary deep venous thrombosis or pulmonary embolism. N Engl J Med 1998;338:1169–1173.
15. Homans J. Thrombosis of the deep vein due to prolonged sitting. N Engl J Med 1954;250: 148–150.
16. Lapostelle F, Surget V, Borron SW, et al. Severe pulmonary embolism associated with air travel. N Eng J Med 2001;345:779–783.
17. Fedullo P, Tapson V. The evaluation of pulmonary embolism. N Engl J Med. 2003;349:1247–1256.
18. Wells PS, Anderson DR, Rodger M, et al. Derivation of a simple clinical model to categorize patients' probability of pulmonary embolism: increasing the models utility with the SimpliRed D-Dimer. Thromb Haemost 2000;83:416–420.
19. Kovacs MJ, Anderson D, Morrow B, et al. Outpatient treatment of pulmonary embolisin with dalteparin. Thromb Haemost. 2000;83:209–211.
20. Decousus H, Leizorovicz A, Parent F, et al. A clinical trial of vena caval filters in the prevention of pulmonary embolism in patients with proximal deep-vein thrombosis. N Engl J Med 1998;338:409–415.
21. Schulmna S, Rhedin A, Lindmarker P, et al. A comparison of six weeks with six months of oral anticoagulation therapy after a first episode of venous Thromboembolism. N Engl J Med 1995;332:1661–1665.
22. Brandjes DP, Buller HR, Heijboer H, et al. Randomized trail of effect of compression stockings in patients with symptomatic proximal-vein thrombosis. Lancet 1997;349:759–762.

23. Kessler CM, Hirsch DR, Jacobs H, et al. Intermittent pneumatic compression in chronic venous insufficiency favorably affects fibrinolytic potential and platelet activation. Blood Coagul Fibrinolysis 1996;7:437–446.
24. The Matisse Investigators. Subcutaneous fondaparinux versus intravenous unfractionated heparin in the initial treatment of pulmonary embolism. N Engl J Med 2003;349:1695–1702.
25. Schulman S, Wåhlander K, Lundström T, et al. Secondary prevention of venous thromboembolism with the oral direct thrombin inhibitor ximelagatran. N Engl J Med 2003;349:1713–1721.

24 Hemoptysis

Samantha McIntosh and Matthew L. Mintz

CONTENTS
> CASE PRESENTATIONS
> KEY CLINICAL QUESTIONS
> LEARNING OBJECTIVES
> EPIDEMIOLOGY
> PATHOPHYSIOLOGY
> DIFFERENTIAL DIAGNOSIS
> DIAGNOSIS
> TREATMENT/MANAGEMENT
> REFERENCES

CASE PRESENTATIONS

Case 1

A 27-year-old man presents to the community health clinic with a complaint of cough for the past 3 weeks. It is productive of yellow sputum that has become streaked with dark blood in the past week. He has had low-grade fevers with sweats, dyspnea on exertion, and generalized weakness progressive over the same period of time. His past medical history is unremarkable, and he takes no medications except for recent use of an over-the-counter cough suppressant. He immigrated to the United States from Ethiopia 2 years ago to attend graduate school and travels back to Ethiopia twice per year. He does not smoke cigarettes.

On physical exam, his temperature is 100.5°F, pulse is 90 beats per minute, blood pressure is 120/80, and respiratory rate is 22 breaths per minute. There are decreased breath sounds in the right chest, and chest radiograph reveals an infiltrate with a cavitation in the right upper lobe.

> From: *Current Clinical Practice: Disorders of the Respiratory Tract:*
> *Common Challenges in Primary Care*
> By: M. L. Mintz © Humana Press, Totowa, NJ

Case 2

A 40-year-old man with history of bronchiectasis is hospitalized and on intravenous antibiotics for fevers and purulent sputum production. On hospital day 2, the intern is called to his bedside because he has coughed up approximately 100 cc of dark blood with clots, but is not expectorating any further blood at the time of evaluation.

On physical exam, he is afebrile with a pulse of 90 beats per minute, a blood pressure of 120/80, respiratory rate of 24 breaths per minute, and pulse oximetry of 94% on 2 L oxygen via nasal cannula. He appears to be in mild respiratory distress. He has bilateral crackles on chest exam; the remainder of his exam is normal.

KEY CLINICAL QUESTIONS

1. What are the causes of hemoptysis in these two patients? How might the differential diagnosis differ based on the clinical scenarios?
2. What should be the next step in the management of these patients?
3. When can the primary care clinician manage hemoptysis expectantly and when are specialists need to assist with diagnosis and management?
4. What are the treatment options in either scenario?

LEARNING OBJECTIVES

1. Become familiar with the vast differential diagnosis of hemoptysis.
2. Recognize massive hemoptysis and the need for aggressive management.
3. Understand the evaluation and management of massive and stable hemoptysis.

EPIDEMIOLOGY

In the United States, the causes of hemoptysis vary according to the specific population studied, but in one recent review at a tertiary referral center the top causes were bronchitis (18%), pneumonia (16%), bronchiectasis (20%), and lung cancer (19%). Bronchiectasis was the major cause of severe hemoptysis, whereas bronchitis and lung cancer were the causes of mild bleeding. Tuberculosis (TB) used to be a major cause of hemoptysis in this country, but its incidence has decreased in more recent studies *(1)*. The most common cause worldwide is infection with the lung fluke (paragonimiasis).

PATHOPHYSIOLOGY

Hemoptysis, defined as expectoration of blood from below the vocal cords, is a symptom that may accompany a variety of diseases of the airways or lung parenchyma. The amount of blood seen can vary widely, from flecks or streaks in the sputum to expectoration of large amounts of gross blood without any sputum. Blood is a powerful airway irritant and thus can contribute significantly toward respiratory symtoms. Most hemoptysis is in small amounts and although alarming to the patient, is not life threatening *(2)*. Massive hemoptysis, exceeding 600 cc of blood in a 24-hour period, requires urgent or emergent action to secure the patient's airway and maintain hemodynamic stability.

The lung is supplied by two separate circulatory systems: the vast majority of the blood traversing the lungs is supplied by the low-pressure pulmonary arteries; a small amount is supplied by the systemic-pressure bronchial arteries that typically arise from the aorta or occasionally the intercostal arteries. Although the bronchial arteries carry only a small fraction of the pulmonary blood flow, they supply blood to the airways, and are a much more important source of hemoptysis than the pulmonary arteries. In massive hemoptysis, 90% of bleeds have a bronchial arterial source.

When considering the various etiologies of hemoptysis, it is easiest to categorize the location of potential sources of bleeding. The main sources of blood are directly from the airway, from the lung and thoracic parenchyma, iatrogenic sources, and idiopathic causes of bleeding (Table 1).

Airway sources include bronchitis, bronciectasis, neoplasms of the airway, vascular-bronchial fistula, and airway foreign bodies. Bronchitis, either acute or an acute exacerbation of chronic bronchitis, is the most common cause of blood in the sputum. This is usually because of viral or bacterial infection of the airways that is self-limited and does not usually require antibiotics. Hemoptysis in this condition usually appears as blood streaking on top of purulent sputum. Bronchiectasis is a pathological dilatation of the bronchi owing to breakdown of the bronchial walls; the bronchial circulation also becomes dilated and tortuous. It is usually caused by scarring after an acute or recurrent infection and is commonly seen with cystic fibrosis and in areas of old TB involvement. Patients may present with a long history of cough with copious purulent sputum. The hemoptysis is often minimal, although it may be massive *(3)*.

There are several neoplasms involving the airways that can cause hemoptysis: primary bronchogenic carcinoma, metatstatic cancer, carcinoid, and Kaposi's sarcoma (KS). Primary bronchogenic carcinoma often occurs in older smokers. Tumors that commonly metastasize to the lungs and may cause hemoptysis include breast, colon, renal cell carcinoma, and malignant melanoma. Bronchial carcinoid is a very vascular tumor that may be seen in young nonsmokers. KS may involve the airways or lung parenchyma and can be a cause of hemoptysis in patients with AIDS.

Aortic aneurysms in the thorax can fistulize with the left tracheobroncial tree formings a vascular-bronchial fistula. This is a rare but potentially fatal cause of massive hemoptysis. Finally, a foreign body in the airway or broncholithiasis can erode into a vessel and cause bleeding.

Table 1
Causes of Hemoptysis

Airway sources

Bronchitis
Bronchiectasis
Neoplasms
- Primary bronchogenic carcinoma
- Metastatic disease involving the bronchial tree
- Bronchial carcinoid
- Kaposi's sarcoma

Vascular–bronchial fistula
Foreign body

Parenchymal sources

Infections
- Tuberculosis
- Pneumonia
- Mycetomas/aspergilloma
- Lung abscess
    Parasitic infections
    Pulmonary embolus with lung infarction

Inflammatory conditions
- Wegener's granulomatosis
- Goodpasture's syndrome
- Pneumonitis because of systemic lupus erythematosis
- Idiopathic pulmonary hemosiderosis

Increased pulmonary capillary pressure
Pulmonary arterio-venous malformations
Thoracic endometriosis
Drugs/toxins

Iatrogenic causes

Tracheostomy
Percutaneous or transbronchial lung biopsy
Perforation from pulmonary artery catheterization
Idiopathic hemoptysis

Parenchymal sources of hemoptysis include pulmonary infections, pulmonary embolism, inflammatory disorders of the lung, as well as several other miscellaneous causes. Pulmonary infections causing hemoptysis include TB, pneuomonia, lung absecesses, aspergillous, and parastic infections. Pulmonary TB is one of the most common causes of hemoptysis in the United States. Hemoptysis occurs when TB infection cavitates in the lung parenchyma, and is usually scant. Sudden rupture of a Rasmussen's aneurysm (a weakened pulmonary artery that ruptures into an adjacent cavity) can cause massive hemorrhage. Bacterial pneumonias can occasionally cause hemoptysis. Gram-negative pneumonias are more common in the elderly and institutionalized patients and may present with "currant jelly sputum," a mixture of blood and pus (especially *Klebsiella*). *Staph aureus* causes pneumonia in patients who have had preceding influenza infection and can cause cavitating lung infection with "salmon-pink" bloody sputum. Hemoptysis occurs in 50 to 85% of aspergillomas and may be massive. The fungus ball forms in a pre-existing lung cavity (such as an old TB scar) and may erode into a vessel. Invasive parenchymal Aspergillus and Mucor infections can also cause bleeding. Anaerobic organisms are the most common pathogens in lung abscesses that complicate aspiration pneumonia. Abscess can also result from septic emboli, as in tricuspid endocarditis in intravenous drug abusers. Paragonimiasis (infection with the lung fluke), although rarely seen in the United States, is the most common cause of hemoptysis worldwide.

Other parenchymal conditions causing hemoptysis include pulmonary embolism, which causes bleeding from infarction to lung tissue, and certain inflammatory conditions of the lung. Wegener's granulomatosis is a vasculitis that affects the upper respiratory tract and sinuses, lung parenchyma, and kidney. Hemoptysis arises from cavitary nodules caused by granulomatous vasculitis. Goodpasture's syndrome is an auto-immune disease that causes intermittent pulmonary bleeding (may be a severe hemorrhage) and glomerulonephritis owing to the formation of anti-glomerular basement membrane antibodies and deposition of immunoglobulin G and C3 in the glomerular and alveolar basement membranes. Other inflammatory causes of hemoptysis include pneumonitis secondary to systemic lupus erythematosis and idiopathic pulmonary hemosiderosis, a rare condition leading to intermittent pulmonary hemorrhage.

Mitral stenosis, which is now uncommon because rheumatic heart disease has become less common, is a thoracic cause of hemoptysis because of increased pulmonary capillary pressure. The stenotic mitral valve leads to back pressure in the pulmonary veins. This causes blood to flow from the pulmonary capillaries into the bronchial veins, leading to submucosal bronchial varices that may eventually rupture. Another vascular cause of hemoptysis is pulmonary arterio-venous malformations, such as hereditary hemorrhagic telangiectasia, or Osler-Weber-Rendu syndrome. Endometriosis can also involve the lung parenchyma (and less commonly the airways). In this case, hemoptysis and chest pain are coincident with menses. Finally, certain drugs and toxins can affect the lung parenchyma, leading to hemoptysis. Solvents, penicillamine, and other toxins can be a cause of hemoptysis. Smoking free-base cocaine ("crack") is associated with diffuse alveolar hemorrhage through an unknown mechanism, possibly direct toxicity of the inhaled substance to alveolar epithelial cells *(4)*.

Complications from many common procedures can result in hemoptysis. A tracheostomy tube can erode into the innominate artery if placed too low, resulting in a tracheo-innominate fistula and potentially life-threatening hemoptysis. Hemoptysis complicates 5 to 10% of percutaneous lung biopsies, and about 2% of transbrochial and endobronchial biopsies. Bleeding in these cases is usually small and self-limited. Hemoptysis can be a result of the perforation of the pulmonary artery by a pulmonary arterial catheter, which carries more than 50% mortality.

Finally, up to 30% of patients with hemoptysis have no identifiable cause even after thorough evaluation and diagnostic studies including high-resolution computed tomography (CT) scan and bronchoscopy. Most of these patients have a good prognosis with resolution of the bleeding within 6 months of evaluation.

DIFFERENTIAL DIAGNOSIS

The differential diagnosis of hemoptysis is very broad, although a small number of conditions account for the vast majority of cases. Initial work-up includes a thorough history and physical exam along with chest radiograph and relevant lab tests.

When evaluating a patient with the complaint of "coughing up blood," it is important to keep in mind that bleeding from the nose, upper airway, or even the upper gastrointestinal tract might mimic or be misinterpreted as hemoptysis. True hemoptysis originates from below the vocal cords.

DIAGNOSIS

Given the broad causes of hemoptysis, diagnosis will often be made clinically. Thus, a thorough history and physical exam are necessary. During the history, practitioners should pay special attention to prior lung, cardiac, or renal disease; tobacco history; illicit drug use; travel history; use of anticoagulants; or a history of bleeding disorder. On physical examination, one should pay special attention to the upper airway (telangectasias may be seen in the mucous membranes, crusting of the nasal passages may suggest Wegener's); clubbing (nonspecific finding that may be seen in many chronic lung diseases); and adventitious heart sounds (mitral stenosis murmur, loud P2 in pulmonary hypertension). A chest radiograph should be done as part of every evaluation of hemoptysis. Appropriated laboratory studies will follow from a careful history and physical exam. This might include a complete blood count, white blood cell (to evaluate for infection), and platelet count; prothrombin and partial thromboplastin times; urinalysis and measure of renal function (blood urea nitrogen and creatinine); and sputum sample for acid fast bacilli, bacterial, and fungal cultures. If Wegener's granulomatosis is suspected, the cytoplasmic anti-neutrophilic cytoplasmic antibody is both 90% sensitive and specific for this entity. Check for anti- glomerular basement membrane antibodies if Goodpasture's syndrome is suspected.

Fiberoptic Bronchoscopy and High-Resolution Chest CT

If the previously mentioned studies are suggestive of bronchitis or other diseases likely to resolve, the patient can be treated for that disease appropriately with no further tests and observed for recurrence of hemoptysis. However, if the history does not suggest a disease that would likely resolve or if the patient has risk factors or a history suspicious for cancer, further work-up should be done using bronchoscopy and/or high-resolution CT (HRCT). Generally, fiberoptic bronchoscopy (FOB) and HRCT are considered to be complementary studies: each supplies unique information and is the preferred study for different sets of diseases *(5)*. There is currently no firm data to support the use of one study before the other. Bronchoscopy is better at detecting bronchitis and subtle mucosal abnormalities (such as KS lesions); additionally, it allows for biopsy of any lesion seen. HRCT is better at detecting more peripheral neoplasms, bronchiectasis, and aspergillomas. The particular clinical situation, X-ray findings, and risk factors of the individual patient should guide which study is done first; however, many patients will have both studies done as part of the work-up.

TREATMENT/MANAGEMENT

In treatment and management of hemoptysis, the first differentiating factor is whether or not hemoptysis is minor or massive. If massive, management is the primary focus, because it is a life-threatening condition. If hemoptysis is minor, then management focuses on treating the underlying condition as well as further working up hemoptysis suggestive of neoplasm *(6)*.

Minor Hemoptysis

Because minor hemoptysis is not life-threatening, clinicians should focus on the specific cause of the hemoptysis, administer appropriate treatment, and make sure to rule out any serious underlying disease, such as malignancy *(6)*. As mentioned, a chest radiograph should be done as part of every evaluation of hemoptysis. If the chest radiograph is normal, and history is consistent with mild disease such as bronchitis, then appropriate treatment (cough suppressant, antibiotics, supportive care) can be administered with close observation and follow-up. Sputum cytology and purified protein derivative can be considered in patients at risk for tuberculosis. FOB in patients with minor hemoptysis and a normal chest radiograph is controversial, and should be considered on a case-by-case basis. Some suggest that FOB should be considered in all smokers older than 40 years of age, given their high risk for lung cancer. In several studies, lung cancer was found in 3 to 6% of patients with minor hemoptysis and normal or nonlocalizing chest radiographs *(7–9)*.

If the chest radiograph is abnormal, further evaluation is guided by the specific findings and clinical correlation. Lesions suspicious of cancer should be worked up appropriately, including sputum cytology, needle aspiration, bronchoscopy, and biopsy.

Massive Hemoptysis

Massive hemoptysis is defined as expectoration of more than 600 cc of blood in a 24-hour period *(10)*. The initial management depends on the patient's clinical status. If oxygenation is compromised or the bleeding is brisk, the patient should be intubated for airway protection. A large (8.0 mm or larger) endotracheal (ET) tube should be used to prevent occlusion of the tube by clots and so that rigid or FOB can be performed through the ET tube. If the bleeding is brisk enough to cause hemodynamic instability, crystalloid fluids, or packed red blood cells, platelets or fresh-frozen plasma (if indicated for an underlying coagulopathy) should be administered.

After hemodynamic stabilization and establishment of a secure airway, the most important element in the management of massive hemoptysis is localization of the site of bleeding. Therapeutic steps, such as bronchoscopic electrocautery or balloon tamponade, arterial embolization, or surgery, require knowledge of the bleeding site. When bleeding is brisk and ongoing, techniques exist to protect the nonbleeding lung from spillage of blood, preventing asphyxiation. The simplest is to place the patient in the lateral decubitus position with the bleeding side down. Selective intubation, in which a single lumen ET tube is placed into the mainstem bronchus of the nonbleeding lung, can be done. Selective intubation can also be done with a double-lumen ET tube, but positioning these tubes, maintaining a patent airway, and passing a bronchoscope through a double-lumen tube can be difficult.

Bronchoscopic techniques may be effective to manage massive hemoptysis, so bronchoscopy should be performed early in these cases *(11)*. Even if the bleeding has abated, the site may still be visualized if bronchoscopy is done within 24 hours. Also, a self-limited "sentinel" bleed may precede a massive pulmonary hemorrhage. Rigid bronchoscopy (done in the operating room under general anesthesia) offers better visualization and suctioning if the bleeding is ongoing, but FOB can see more distal lesions in the lung segments.

If a lesion is visualized, laser therapy and electrocautery may be used through the scope. Topical application of epinephrine, vasopressin, or thrombin may also be administered. Balloon tamponade of the bleeding site involves inflation of a balloon catheter in the bronchus leading to the bleeding site. The balloon is left inflated for 24 to 48 hours, after which the balloon is deflated and the patient is observed for rebleeding.

Pulmonary arteriography may be performed after bronchoscopy in the patient who is continuing to bleed rapidly, or electively after the patient has been stabilized. Usually arteriography suggests the bleeding site by the presence of a tortuous, hypervascularized area (e.g., in bronchiectasis). It is rare for the bleeding to be fast enough to see extravasation of contrast from the vessel. Theraputic embolization of the culprit vessel can be performed during angiography. Embolization stops the bleeding 85% of the time, but rebleeding will occur (up to 1 year later) in 10 to 20% of patients *(12)*. Arteriography should be performed by an experienced interventionalist. Usually the bronchial arteries are evaluated first by arteriography; other systemic arteries may be evaluated if a bleeding source is not identified in the bronchial circulation. The anterior spinal artery arises from the bronchial artery in 5% of the population, so canulation of the bronchial artery or proximal embolization carries the rare (<1%) risk of blocking flow to the anterior spinal cord, resulting in paraplegia *(13)*.

SURGERY

All patients with massive hemoptysis require surgical consultation, even if surgery is not used *(14)*. Surgery is usually reserved when angiographic and bronchoscopic intervention fails. There is a 30 to 40% operative mortality when used to treat acute, life-threatening massive hemoptysis. Surgery is contraindicated in certain conditions such as carcinoma invading the heart, mediastimum, and trachea; as well as in poor operative candidates who would be unlikely to survive surgery, such as patients with end-stage chronic obstructive pulmonary disease or heart failure. Certain conditions are more ammenable to surgery, including massive hemoptysis owing to chest injuries, arteriovenous malformations, aortic aneurysm, hydatid cyst, bronchial adenoma, fungal lesion refractory to other therapies, and iatrogenic pulmonary rupture. Clinicians must also consider the surgical capabilities at their particular institution.

REFERENCES

1. Santiago S, Tobias J, Williams A. A reappraisal of the causes of hemoptysis. Arch Intern Med 1991;151:2449–2451.
2. Hirshberg B, Biran I, Glazer M, Kramer M. Hemoptysis: etiology, evaluation, and outcome in a tertiary referral hospital. Chest 1997;112:440–444.
3. Barker A. Medical progress: bronchiectasis. N Engl J Med 2002;346: 1383–1393.
4. Specks U. Diffuse alveolar hemorhage syndromes. Curr Opin Rheumatol 2001;12:12–17.
5. Set PA, Flower CD, Smith IE, Twentyman OP, Shneerson JM. Hemoptysis: comparative study of the role of CT and fiberoptic bronchoscopy. Radiology 1993;189:677–680.
6. Johnson JL. Manifestations of hemoptysis. Postgrad Med 2002;112:101–113.
7. Lederle FA, Nichol KL, Parenti CM. Bronchoscopy to evaluate hemoptysis in older men with nonsuspicious chest roentgenograms. Chest 1989;95:1043–1047.
8. O'Neil KM, Lazarus AA. Hemoptysis: indications for bronchoscopy. Arch Intern Med 1991;151:171–174.

9. Poe RH, Israel RH, Marin MG, et al. Utility of fiberoptic bronchoscopy in patients with hemoptysis and a nonlocalizing chest roentgenogram. Chest 1988;93:70–75.
10. Lordan JL, Gascoigne A, Corris PA. Assessment and management of massive haemoptysis. Thorax 2003;58:814–819.
11. Haponik EF, Chin R. Hemoptysis: clinicians' perspectives. Chest 1990;97:469–475.
12. White RI Jr. Bronchial artery embolotherapy for control of acute hemoptysis: analysis of outcome. Chest 1999;115:912–915.
13. Wong M, Szkup P, Hopley M. Percutaneous embolotherapy for life-threatening hemoptysis. Chest 2002;121:95–102.
14. Corder R. Hemoptysis. Emerg Med Clin N Am 2003;21:421–435.

25 Gastroesophageal Reflux Disease, Cough, and Asthma

Niral Shah and Matthew L. Mintz

CONTENTS
>   CASE PRESENTATION
>   KEY CLINICAL QUESTIONS
>   LEARNING OBJECTIVES
>   BACKGROUND
>   PATHOPHYSIOLOGY
>   DIAGNOSIS AND TREATMENT
>   COST-EFFECTIVENESS
>   SUMMARY
>   REFERENCES

CASE PRESENTATION

A 54-year-old female with history of asthma presents with ongoing asthma not responsive to therapy. She complains of persistent coughing and wheezing that occurs on a weekly basis. Over the last year, she has suffered from one attack that required hospitalization. When asked further about her symptoms, she states that she can feel her attacks coming and that they often start with coughing spells and a slight uneasiness in her chest. From previous visits, her therapy has been maximized to a long-acting β-agonist and inhaled corticosteroid combination.

KEY CLINICAL QUESTIONS

1. Does gastroesophogeal reflux induce pulmonary symptoms such as cough?
2. What is the proper algorithm to evaluate and treat patients with chronic cough?
3. Does the treatment of reflux improve asthma symptoms?

From: *Current Clinical Practice: Disorders of the Respiratory Tract:
Common Challenges in Primary Care*
By: M. L. Mintz © Humana Press, Totowa, NJ

LEARNING OBJECTIVES

1. Understand the relationship between cough and reflux, and how this may help in the diagnosis and management of asthma and other respiratory disorders.
2. Recognize how a patient with asthma and gastroesophogeal reflux disease (GERD) may present.
3. Utilize treatment algorithms for the diagnosis and management of GERD-associated cough.

BACKGROUND

GERD is the regurgitation of the stomach contents into the esophagus or possibly the pharynx. When the contents of the regurgitated materials, the reflux, enter the pharynx, it can be occasionally aspirated into the trachea and lead to pulmonary symptoms such as coughing and wheezing.

Patients with pulmonary disease, such as asthma, also present with similar symptoms of coughing or wheezing. These symptoms are often associated solely to the underlying pulmonary disease. In difficult-to-control patients, it is essential to recall that other disease processes, such as GERD, can also affect airway responsiveness. For instance, the three most common causes of chronic cough are postnasal drip, asthma, and GERD. Physicians must keep these etiologies in mind when evaluating patients with pulmonary symptoms whose therapies are refractory to the initial therapy approach.

There have been many studies showing the association between GERD and pulmonary disease *(1)*. It has been suggested that GERD often influences asthma symptoms, as supported by various clinical trials. The most prevalent presenting symptom of asthma affected by reflux is cough (Table 1). Studies have also shown that patients with GERD can present with symptoms as minor as cough or wheezing, which may originally be confused with uncontrolled pulmonary disease *(2)*.

PATHOPHYSIOLOGY

Sontag showed that GERD occurs in about 60 to 80% of adults who have asthma *(2)*. Although patients with asthma and GERD often present with both respiratory and gastrointestinal (GI) symptoms, quite often, the GI symptoms are their only presenting symptom (Fig. 1).

A question that often arises in this area is the primum relationship between asthma and GERD. In other words, does GERD cause cough or does cough cause GERD? GERD and asthma have been known to co-exist for decades, but not until recently has it been so well-researched and defined. There have been more than 200 studies showing the relationship between GERD and asthma in adults and in children. Numerous studies also suggest that the GERD–asthma relationship

Table 1
Respiratory Symptoms of Gastroesophageal
Reflux Disease in Patients With Asthma

Respiratory symptoms	
Cough	47%
Bronchitis	35%
Asthma/wheezing	16%
Pneumonitis	16%
Hemoptysis	13%
Intermittent dyspnea	13%
Hoarseness	12%

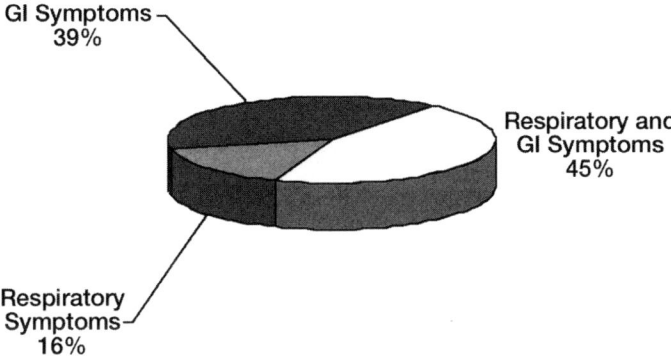

Fig. 1. Presenting symptoms for gastroesophageal reflux disease in asthma patients.

is a self-propagating situation in which continuous acid exposure causes further pulmonary symptoms that exacerbate GERD (Fig. 2).

Physicians should have a high suspicion for GERD in patients with asthma who are difficult to control and refractory to standard therapy. Often they do not present with classic symptoms of reflux disease but rather subtle symptoms that would otherwise go unnoticed. Richter reports that in 24% of patients with difficult-to-control asthma, a diagnosis of GERD was missed (1). Another study of a population referred for repairs of hiatal hernias reported that patients with asthma presented in various ways: 39% had classic reflux symptoms, 45% had reflux and respiratory symptoms, and 16% had respiratory symptoms only (3).

Two possible mechanisms that may cause GERD and cough are described in a review article by Sontag (2): the activation of GERD induced vagal reflex arc from the esophagus to the lung or microaspiration of gastric contents into the lung resulting in mucosal reactions. First, the vagal mediated reflex theory stems

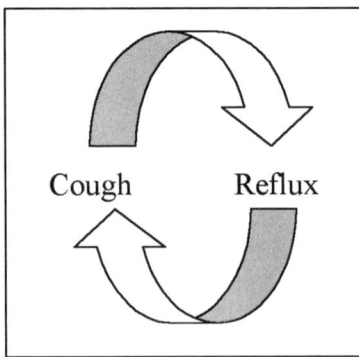

Fig. 2. Relationship of cough and reflux.

from the idea that the GI tract and respiratory tree are derived from the same embryonic ridge, and, therefore, have similar vagal connections. Mansfield et al. also showed that acid esophageal infusions increase airway resistance, which rapidly reverse when reflux symptoms were treated and relieved (4). Another study by Davis et al. suggested that other factors were necessary for GERD to exacerbate asthma: reflux of gastric acid into the esophagus, an acid-sensitive esophagus, and a low nocturnal threshold for bronchoconstrictive stimuli (5).

Sontag's second theory, the microaspiration theory, stems from the idea that acid material trickling into the trachea may cause bronchospasms. This idea was confirmed by Tuchman et al. when they instilled acid in the esophagus and measured lung resistance in animals models (6). This study showed that rather than reflux alone causing airway responsiveness, microaspiration is a much more likely mechanism to explain bronchospasm.

It important to also review how asthma can contribute to the worsening of GERD symptoms. Reflux symptoms are often dependent on the lower esophageal sphincter (LES) tone, which acts as a barrier to prevent gastric juices from entering the esophagus and causing heartburn. Patients with uncontrolled asthma may suffer from coughing and wheezing episodes, which in turn can change intra-esophageal and intrathoracic pressures leading to lower LES tone, and thus allowing reflux to enter the esophagus. Additionally, drugs that may be used to treat asthma may also lower the LES pressure, thereby worsening reflux.

The exacerbation of GERD is purportedly caused by various factors in regard to asthma. Factors that promote GERD include bronchodilators, and it is suggested that bronchodilator therapy relaxes the LES and increases the risk of reflux (7). However, other studies indicate that reflux was not related and not a result of bronchodilator therapy. It has been shown that the prevalence of cough and wheezing at night is much greater in asthmatics with reflux than those patients who suffer from asthma alone *(2)*. After therapy with acid suppression agents, nighttime asthma symptoms improved significantly according to Goodall et al. *(8)*.

Two final causes that affect the GERD–asthma relationship are overeating and hiatal hernias. Overeating, which may cause postprandial reflux, can worsen bronchoconstriction and asthma symptoms. Finally, hiatal hernias in asthmatic subjects were shown to be related to more serious esophagitis.

By keeping these theories in mind, it is clear that GERD can trigger asthma, and asthma can trigger GERD. Therefore, the relevant clinical question becomes whether or not a patient with well-controlled asthma will have decreased incidence of GERD and whether or not a patient with well-controlled reflux symptoms will experience decreased asthma exacerbations.

DIAGNOSIS AND TREATMENT

The theory behind treating GERD in a patient with asthma is that it will decrease the patient's respiratory symptoms. The three most common causes of cough, as stated earlier, are postnasal drip, asthma, and GERD *(9)*. Postnasal drip can often be ruled out by taking an extensive history and asthma can be diagnosed with a methylcholine challenge test. Finally, previous studies have shown that 24-hour pH monitoring is the gold standard for diagnosing GERD.

By keeping these diagnostic tests in mind, when a physician is faced with a patient with a chronic cough, a logical approach would be to take an extensive history, refer for a methylcholine challenge test, and finally send the patient for 24-hour pH monitoring. However, when keeping a patient's comfort and invasiveness of tests in mind, a second approach would include the use of proton pump inhibitors (PPIs). Studies by Ours et al. have demonstrated that proper acid suppression therapy can be used in place of 24-hour pH monitoring when symptoms are followed over time *(10)*.

With the overlap of GERD and asthma, acid suppression therapy may be a logical first step in the treatment of difficult-to-control asthma. When a trial of PPIs is initiated, physicians should keep in mind that a proper dose should be started to adequately suppress acid reflux that may be exacerbating asthma symptoms. Harding et al. have shown increasing responsiveness of patient symptoms with longer duration of acid suppression therapy *(11)*. Similar studies reported showed a 30% reduction of asthma symptoms after 1 month of PPI therapy, a 43% reduction at 2 months, and a 57% reduction at 3 months *(1)* (Fig. 3). Ours et al. concluded that empirical treatment with 2 weeks of high-dose PPI in patients with chronic cough in which postnasal drip and asthma have been ruled out, represents a first step to treatment *(10)*.

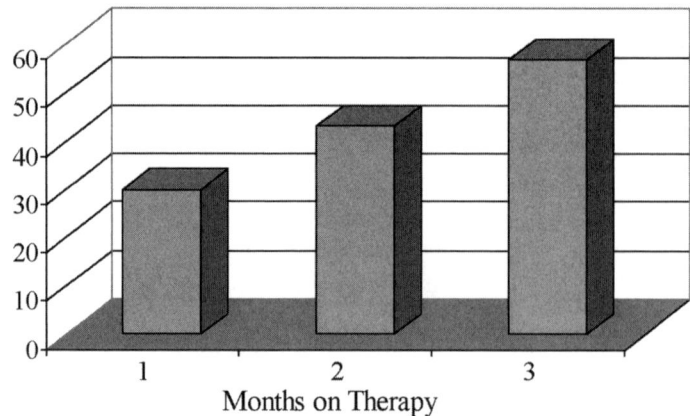

Fig. 3. Reduction of symptoms during months of therapy with proton pump inhibitors.

Despite these findings, there will be patients who fail acid suppression therapy and continue to have difficult-to-control asthma. These patients may be candidates for surgical antireflux therapy, which includes Nissen fundiplication. Studies by Sontag et al. have shown that Nissen antireflux surgery doubled LES pressure, and, consequently improved asthma and reflux symptoms *(12)*.

COST-EFFECTIVENESS

With constant pressures to evaluate patients properly and in a cost-effective manner, it is important to utilize the most sensitive yet efficient management strategy. As studied extensively by O'Connor et al. *(13)*, who performed 11 different strategies for treating reflux that may be exacerbating asthma, the most cost-effective diagnostic approach is to start with 3 months of PPI therapy, followed by 24-hour pH testing in nonresponders. O'Connor presented multiple strategies, including (a) pH testing, followed by incremental PPI therapy if pH testing was positive; (b) incremental PPI therapy, followed by pH testing in nonresponders; and (c) incremental PPI therapy alone.

Through all these treatment arms, the most cost-effective approach was the initiation of PPI therapy in patients with suspected GERD with concomitant asthma, followed by pH testing only in nonresponders *(13)*. However, with the availability of new PPI therapies and over-the-counter options since 1999, further studies would be necessary to define this relationship further.

SUMMARY

There is a close, proven relationship between gastroesophageal reflux and asthma symptoms, such as a persistent cough. This entity should be considered when patients present with difficult-to-control asthma, especially if they possess concomitant GI reflux symptoms. The two theories relating GERD to asthma include the activation of a vagal reflex arc from the esophagus to the lung, or the microaspiration of gastric contents into the lung resulting in bronchial reactions.

A proper algorithm would include a thorough history to rule out other causes, such as postnasal drip or improperly treated asthma. Then, if GERD is considered, a trial of acid suppression therapy with PPIs may be a reasonable first step in the treatment of difficult-to-control asthma. Finally, only if the patient does not respond to PPI therapy, esophageal pH monitoring should be considered.

REFERENCES

1. Richter JE. Gastroesophageal reflux disease and asthma: the two are directly related. Am J Med 2000;108:153S–158S.
2. Sontag SJ. Gastroesophageal reflux disease and asthma. J Clin Gastroenterol 2000;30:S9–S30.
3. Urschel HC Jr, Paulson DL. Gastroesophageal reflux and hiatal hernia. Complications and therapy. J Thorac Cardiovasc Surg 1967; 53:21–32.
4. Mansfield LE, Hameister HH, Spaulding HS, Smith NJ, Glab N. The role of the vague nerve in airway narrowing caused by intraesophageal hydrochloric acid provocation and esophageal distention. Ann Allergy 1981;47:431–434.
5. Davis RS, Larsen GL, Grunstein MM. Respiratory response to intraesophageal acid infusion in asthmatic children during sleep. J Allergy Clin Immunol 1983;72:393–398.
6. Tuchman DN, Boyle JT, Pack AI, et al. Comparison of airway responses following tracheal or esophageal acidification in the cat. Gastroenterology 1984;87:872–881.
7. DiMarino AJ Jr, Cohen S. Effect of an oral beta2-adrenergic agonist on lower esophageal sphincter pressure in normals and in patients with achalasia. Dig Dis Sci 198227:1063–1066.
8. Goodall RJ, Earis JE, Cooper DN, Bernstein A, Temple JG. Relationship between asthma and gastro-oesophageal reflux. Thorax 1981;36:116–121.
9. Smyrnios NA, Irwin RS, Curley FJ, French CL. From a prospective study of chronic cough: diagnostic and therapeutic aspects in older adults. Arch Intern Med 1998;158:1222–1228.
10. Ours TM, Kavuru MS, Schilz RJ, Richter JE. A prospective evaluation of esophageal testing and a double-blind, randomized study of omeprazole in a diagnostic and therapeutic algorithm for chronic cough. Am J Gastroenterol 1999;94:3131–3138.
11. Harding SM, Richter JE, Guzzo MR, et al. Asthma and gastroesophageal reflux: acid suppressive therapy improves asthma outcome. Am J Med 1996;100:395–405.
12. Sontag SJ, O'Connell S, Khandelwal S, et al. Asthmatics with gastroesophageal reflux: long term results of a randomized trial of medical and surgical antireflux therapies. Am J Gastroenterol 2003;98:987–999.
13. O'Connor JF, Singer ME, Richter JE. The cost-effectiveness of strategies to assess gastroesophageal reflux as an exacerbating factor in asthma. Am J Gastroenterol 1999;94:1472–1480.

Index

A

Abscess
  hemoptysis, 311
  lung
    hemoptysis, 310
ACE. *See* Angiotensinogen converting enzyme (ACE)
Acquired immunodeficiency syndrome (AIDS)
  Mycobacterium avium complex, 7
  Pneumococcus carinii pneumonia, 7
  tuberculosis, 7
ACT. *See* Asthma control test (ACT)
Acute bronchitis
  adult acute cough, 162
Acute cough, 159–170, 176
  case presentation, 159, 160
  child, 163–165
    diagnosis, 166, 167
  cost, 160, 161
  differential diagnosis, 161–165
  future, 170
  pathophysiology, 161
  physical exam, 166, 167
  treatment, 167–169, 169f
Acute nephritic syndrome, 80
Acute poststreptococcal glomerulonephritis (APG), 80
Acute rheumatic fever
  pharyngitis, 79
Adenocarcinoma
  lungs, 207–211
Adrenergic agents
  short-acting
    adult asthma, 141
Adult acute cough, 162, 163
Adult asthma, 131–145
  acute exacerbations, 141, 142
  case presentation, 131
  diagnosis, 135–137, 136t
  differential diagnosis, 134, 135t
  epidemiology, 132
  future, 144, 145
  monitoring, 137–139
  pathogenesis, 132–134
  therapy, 139–144, 139t
Adult chronic cough
  causes, 178–181
Adult croup, 108
  complications, 110
Adventitious (extra) breath sounds, 8
African Americans
  sarcoidosis, 228
Afrin
  sinusitis, 72
AIDS. *See* Acquired immunodeficiency syndrome (AIDS)
Aircraft personnel
  sarcoidosis, 223
Airway
  conducting
    anatomy, 12
  inflammation
    cellular mechanisms, 118f
    deaths, 118t
    pediatric asthma, 117, 118
  obstruction
    croup, 110
    upper, 7, 22f, 23
  wall remodeling
    airflow limitation, 134t
Albuterol
  adult asthma, 141
  pediatric asthma, 126
Alcohol, 7
  laryngitis/hoarseness, 92, 95
Allergen avoidance, 40t
Allergen-specific serum IgE
  allergic rhinitis, 38
Allergic rhinitis, 31–44
  asthma, 44
  case presentation, 31
  diagnosis, 36–39
  differential diagnosis, 35, 36, 36t
  epidemiology, 32, 33
  future, 44
  pathophysiology, 33–35
  patient history, 37t
  proposed reclassification, 33t
  treatment, 39–44, 43t

Allergic shiners, 37
Alveolar-capillary membrane
 gas diffusion across, 15
Alveoli, 13
Ambulatory monitoring of peak flow, 20
Aminophylline
 adult asthma, 144
Amoxicillin
 pharyngitis, 84
Amoxicillin-clavulanate potassium
 pharyngitis, 84
Amyloidosis
 laryngitis/hoarseness, 95
Aneurysms
 aortic
  hemoptysis, 309
Angiotensinogen converting enzyme (ACE)
 inhibitors
  adult chronic cough, 180
  sarcoidosis, 230
Animal dander
 allergen avoidance, 40t
Ankylosing spondylitis, 7
Anorexia
 sarcoidosis, 224
Anterior rhinoscopy
 allergic rhinitis, 36
Anterior uveitis
 sarcoidosis, 226
Antibiotics
 bronchiolitis, 256
 chronic obstructive pulmonary disease, 200
Anticholinergics
 adult asthma, 141
 non-allergic rhinitis, 58
Antihistamines
 allergic rhinitis, 39–41
 non-allergic rhinitis, 58
Antileukotrienes
 non-allergic rhinitis, 60
Antioxidants
 chronic obstructive pulmonary disease, 201
Anxiety
 laryngitis/hoarseness, 95
Aorta
 hemoptysis, 309

Aortic aneurysms
 hemoptysis, 309
APG. *See* Acute poststreptococcal glomerulonephritis (APG)
Arcanobacterium haemolyticum
 pharyngitis, 81, 82
Argentaffin cells, 208
Arrhythmias
 obstructive sleep apnea, 266
Arterial blood gas, 10
 pulmonary embolism, 295, 296
Asbestos, 6
 lung cancer, 209
Aspergillomas
 hemoptysis, 311
Aspergillous infection
 hemoptysis, 310
Aspiration. *See also* Foreign body aspiration
 community-acquired pneumonia, 237
Asthma, 7, 8, 320. *See also* Pediatric asthma
 adult chronic cough, 178, 179
 bronchiolitis, 253, 254
 bronchoprovocation hyperresponsiveness, 20
 child chronic cough, 182
 chronic cough, 178
 classification, 138t
 GERD, 318, 319, 321
 obesity, 276, 277
 vocal cord dysfunction, 282, 283, 283t
Asthma control test (ACT), 137, 140f
Atopic dermatitis
 rhinitis, 55
Atopy
 adult asthma, 133
Auscultation, 8
Azelastine
 allergic rhinitis, 41
 non-allergic rhinitis, 58
Azathioprine
 sarcoidosis, 232
Azithromycin
 pneumonia, 243

B

Bacterial pneumonia
 bronchiolitis, 254
 hemoptysis, 311

Bacterial rhinosinusitis
   adult acute cough, 162
Bacterial tracheitis, 107
Balloon tamponade
   hemoptysis, 314
Beclomethasone
   non-allergic rhinitis, 59
Bell's palsy
   sarcoidosis, 227
β2 Adrenergic agents
   short-acting
      adult asthma, 141
β2 Agonists
   adult asthma, 140
   exercise-induced bronchospasm, 154, 155
   pediatric asthma, 125
Bitolbuterol
   adult asthma, 141
Blood eosinophilia non-allergic rhinitis syndrome, 51
Blood gas
   arterial, 10
      pulmonary embolism, 295, 296
Breast cancer
   hemoptysis, 309
Breath
   adventitious sounds, 8
   shortness of, 4
      exercise-induced bronchospasm, 150
Breathing
   exercise-induced bronchospasm, 153
   pattern of
      obesity, 276
   work of
      obesity, 275, 276
Bronchi, 12
Bronchial hyperresponsiveness, 134
Bronchiectasis, 211
   adult chronic cough, 180, 181
Bronchioles, 13
Bronchiolitis, 249–259
   case presentation, 249, 250
   causes, 251t
   child acute cough, 164
   diagnosis, 253, 254
   differential diagnosis, 254, 255
   epidemiology, 250, 251
   pathophysiology, 252, 253
   prevention, 255, 256
   treatment, 256–258
Bronchitis
   acute
      adult acute cough, 162
      child acute cough, 164
   chronic
      adult chronic cough, 179, 180
      chronic obstructive pulmonary disease, 193
      smoking, 4, 5
   eosinophilic
      adult chronic cough, 180
Bronchodilators
   bronchiolitis, 256
   chronic obstructive pulmonary disease, 197
   response, 20
Bronchogenic carcinoma
   adult chronic cough, 181
   primary
      hemoptysis, 309
   types, 207
Broncholithiasis
   hemoptysis, 309
Bronchoprovication testing, 20–22
Bronchopulmonary dysplasia
   bronchiolitis, 255
Bronchoscopy, 10
   fiber
      hemoptysis, 313
   hemoptysis, 314
Bronchospasm. *See* Exercise-induced bronchospasm
Budesonide
   non-allergic rhinitis, 59

C

Cachexia, 7
Cancer
   VTE, 303
Carbon monoxide diffusion, 22–25
Carcinoid
   hemoptysis, 309
Cardiopulmonary disease
   laryngitis/hoarseness, 94, 95

Cetuximab
  lung cancer, 218
Chest pain, 5
  lung cancer, 210
  pleuritic
    pulmonary embolism, 292
    sarcoidosis, 224
Chest radiography, 9, 10
  bronchiolitis, 253
  chronic obstructive pulmonary
    disease, 194
  hemoptysis, 312, 314
  lung cancer, 217
  pneumonia, 241
  sarcoidosis, 229
Chest tightness
  exercise-induced bronchospasm, 150
  pediatric asthma, 119
Chest wall
  palpation, 7, 8
  percussion, 8
  syndrome
    pulmonary embolism, 294
Chest X-ray (CXR)
  pulmonary embolism, 296
Child acute cough, 163–165
  bronchiolitis, 164
  bronchitis, 164
  community-acquired pneumonia, 164, 165
  diagnosis, 166, 167
  foreign body aspiration, 165
  influenza, 164
  parainfluenza, 164
  respiratory syncytial virus, 164
  rhinovirus, 164
  tracheobronchitis, 164
Child chronic cough
  asthma, 182
  causes, 182, 183
  chloride sweat test, 185
  congenital heart disease, 182
  24-Esophageal pH monitoring, 185
  foreign body aspiration, 182
  GERD, 182
  habit, 182
  PFT, 185

physical exam, 185
postnasal drip, 182
psychogenic, 182
psychogenic cough, 182
smoking, 182
sweat test, 183
tracheobronchitis, 182
Chlamydial infection
  bronchiolitis, 255
Chlamydia pneumoniae, 237, 239
Chlamydia trachomatis
  bronchiolitis, 255
Chlorambucil
  sarcoidosis, 232
Chloride sweat test
  child chronic cough, 185
Chloroquine
  sarcoidosis, 232
Cholinergic rhinitis, 53
Chronic bronchitis
  adult chronic cough, 179, 180
  chronic obstructive pulmonary
    disease, 193
  smoking, 4, 5
Chronic cough, 173–187
  anatomy, 174–176
  case presentation, 173
  causes, 177t, 186t
    adult, 178–181
    child, 182, 183
  diagnosis, 183–185, 184f
  differential diagnosis, 176–178
  future, 187
  physical exam, 185
  physiology, 174–176
  treatment, 186, 187
Chronic obstructive pulmonary disease
  (COPD), 7, 21, 189–202
  case presentation, 189, 190
  definition, 190
  diagnosis, 194, 195
  differential diagnosis, 193, 194
  flow-volume loop, 21f
  future, 201
  hospital admission criteria, 200t
  medications, 197–201
  pathophysiology, 191–193

Index 329

physical exam, 194, 195
signs of, 6
staging, 195, 196
treatment, 196–201, 198t
Cigarette smoking
  community-acquired pneumonia, 246
  lung cancer, 209
Clarithromycin
  pneumonia, 243
Cocaine
  hemoptysis, 311
  laryngitis/hoarseness, 95
Cockroaches
  allergen avoidance, 40t
Codeine
  chronic cough, 186
Cold intolerance
  laryngitis/hoarseness, 95
Colon cancer
  hemoptysis, 309
Community-acquired pneumonia
  causative organisms, 240t
  causes, 165t
  child acute cough, 164, 165
  epidemiology, 236, 237
  prevention, 245, 246
  risk factors, 238t
  signs and symptoms, 240t
Complete blood count
  sarcoidosis, 230
Compression stockings
  pulmonary embolism, 302
Computed tomography (CT)
  chest, 9, 10
  high-resolution chest
    hemoptysis, 313
  lung cancer, 217
  sarcoidosis, 229
  sinusitis, 71
  spiral, 9, 10
    pulmonary embolism, 297, 298
Conditioning
  exercise-induced bronchospasm, 154
Conducting airways
  anatomy, 12
Congenital heart disease
  child chronic cough, 182

Continuous positive airway pressure (CPAP)
  obstructive sleep apnea, 268–270
COPD. *See* Chronic obstructive pulmonary disease (COPD)
Corticosteroids
  adult asthma, 140
  allergic rhinitis, 41
  bronchiolitis, 257
  chronic obstructive pulmonary disease, 197, 198
  croup, 111
  inhaled
    adult asthma, 142–144
    exercise-induced bronchospasm, 156
    pediatric asthma, 123
    sarcoidosis, 231, 232
  systemic
    adult asthma, 141, 142
  topical
    non-allergic rhinitis, 59, 60
Corynebacterium diphtheriae
  pharyngitis, 79
Coryza, 107
Cost
  acute cough, 160, 161
Costochondritis, 8
  pulmonary embolism, 294
Cough, 4, 5. *See also* Acute cough; Chronic cough
  child, 163–165
    causes, 182, 183
    diagnosis, 166, 167
  differential diagnosis, 121t
  exercise-induced bronchospasm, 150
  GERD, 318, 319
  life-threatening
    signs and symptoms, 167t
  lung cancer, 210
  pediatric asthma, 119
  psychogenic
    child chronic cough, 182
  pulmonary embolism, 292
  receptors, 175
  reflex, 161
  reflex arc, 175, 175f
  reflux, 320f
  sarcoidosis, 224
  subacute, 176

Coumadin®
  pulmonary embolism, 300, 301
CPAP. *See* Continuous positive airway pressure (CPAP)
Crack
  hemoptysis, 311
Crackles, 9
  pediatric asthma, 120
Cranial nerve VII neuropathy
  sarcoidosis, 227
Cromolyn sodium
  adult asthma, 144
  exercise-induced bronchospasm, 155, 156
  pediatric asthma, 125
Croup, 103–113
  adult, 108
    complications, 110
  case presentation, 103, 104
  causes, 106t
  complications, 110
  definition, 104
  diagnosis, 107–110
  differential diagnosis, 105, 106
  epidemiology, 104, 105
  etiology, 105
  future, 112, 113
  pathophysiology, 107
  severity scoring, 109t
  spasmodic, 107
  treatment, 110–112, 112f
Cryptococcosis, 212
CT. *See* Computed tomography (CT)
Cushing syndrome, 211t
CXR. *See* Chest X-ray (CXR)
Cyclophosphamide
  sarcoidosis, 232
Cysts
  laryngitis, 93

D

DALY. *See* Disability-adjusted life year (DALY)
Dander
  animal
    allergen avoidance, 40t
D-dimer tests
  pulmonary embolism, 296

Decongestants
  allergic rhinitis, 41, 42
  non-allergic rhinitis, 59
  sinusitis, 72, 73
Deep vein thrombosis (DVT)
  pulmonary embolism, 290–292
  travel, 292
Dehydration
  bronchiolitis, 252
  croup, 110
Depression
  laryngitis/hoarseness, 95
Dermatitis
  atopic
    rhinitis, 55
Dexamethasone
  croup, 111
Diagnostic testing, 9, 10
Diffusion, 14
Diffusion capacity for carbon monoxide (DLCO), 17, 22–25
  sarcoidosis, 230
Dirithromycin
  pneumonia, 243
Dirofilaria immitis (dog heartworm), 212
Disability-adjusted life year (DALY), 191
Distress
  life-threatening illness, 7
Diuretics
  exercise-induced bronchospasm, 157
DLCO. *See* Diffusion capacity for carbon monoxide (DLCO)
Dog heartworm, 212
Doxycyclin
  pneumonia, 243
Dust mites
  allergen avoidance, 40t
DVT. *See* Deep vein thrombosis (DVT)
Dyspnea, 4
  lung cancer, 210
  pediatric asthma, 119
  pulmonary embolism, 292
  sarcoidosis, 224

E

Echinococcus granulosus, 212
Echocardiogram
  chronic obstructive pulmonary disease, 194

Edema
  laryngeal
    laryngitis/hoarseness, 95
EDS. *See* Excessive daytime
    sleepiness (EDS)
Education
  pediatric asthma, 127, 128
EKG. *See* Electrocardiogram (EKG)
Elderly
  hoarseness, 94
Electrocardiogram (EKG)
  pulmonary embolism, 296
Electrocautery
  hemoptysis, 314
Embolectomy
  pulmonary embolism, 301
Emergency room
  pediatric asthma, 126
Emphysema, 8, 193
Endometriosis
  hemoptysis, 311
Environment
  exercise-induced bronchospasm, 153
Environmental tobacco smoke (ETS)
  lung cancer, 209
Eosinophilic bronchitis
  adult chronic cough, 180
Epidermoid carcinoma
  lungs, 208
Epiglottis
  anatomy, 12
Epiglottitis, 106
ERV. *See* Expiratory reserve volume (ERV)
Erythema nodosum
  sarcoidosis, 226
Erythromycin
  pneumonia, 243
24-Esophageal pH monitoring
  child chronic cough, 185
Essential tremor
  laryngitis/hoarseness, 95
Ethmoid sinuses, 67
Ethnic groups
  sarcoidosis, 223, 228
ETS. *See* Environmental tobacco
    smoke (ETS)
Excessive daytime sleepiness (EDS)
  obstructive sleep apnea, 264, 265

Exercise capacity
  obesity, 276
Exercise-induced bronchospasm, 147–157
  case presentation, 147, 148
  clinical presentation, 150, 151
  diagnosis, 151, 152
  differential diagnosis, 151, 152
  epidemiology, 148, 149
  vs exercise-induced asthma, 149t
  future, 157
  pathophysiology, 149, 150
  pharmacological treatment, 154–156
  treatment, 152–156
Exercise test
  exercise-induced bronchospasm, 152
Expiratory reserve volume (ERV)
  obesity, 275
Extra breath sounds, 8

F

Factor V Leiden defect
  pulmonary embolism, 291, 292
Family history, 6
Fatigue
  bronchiolitis, 252
  exercise-induced bronchospasm, 150
  sarcoidosis, 224
FEF. *See* Forced expiratory flow (FEF)
FEV_1. *See* Forced expiratory volume
    in one second (FEV_1)
Fever
  sarcoidosis, 224
Fiber bronchoscopy (FOB)
  hemoptysis, 313
Firefighters
  sarcoidosis, 223
Flow loops, 21
Fluoroquinolone
  pneumonia, 243
Fluticasone propionate
  non-allergic rhinitis, 59
FOB. *See* Fiber bronchoscopy (FOB)
Fondaparinux
  pulmonary embolism, 303
Food allergy
  rhinitis, 55
Forced expiratory flow (FEF), 20
  adult asthma, 135

Forced expiratory volume in one
second (FEV$_1$), 18
  exercise-induced bronchospasm,
    151, 152
Forced vital capacity (FVC), 18
  adult asthma, 135
  exercise-induced bronchospasm,
    151, 152
  pediatric asthma, 121
Foreign body aspiration
  bronchiolitis, 254
  child acute cough, 165
  child chronic cough, 182
  croup, 105
  hemoptysis, 309
Formoterol
  adult asthma, 143
FRC. *See* Functional residual capacity
    (FRC)
Fremitus, 8
Friction rubs, 9
Frontal sinuses, 67
Functional dysphonia
  laryngitis, 92
Functional residual capacity (FRC), 13
  obesity, 275
Funnel chest, 7
FVC. *See* Forced vital capacity (FVC)

G

GAS. *See* Group A streptococcus (GAS)
Gas exchange
  chronic obstructive pulmonary
    disease, 192
  obesity, 276
Gastroesophageal reflux disease
    (GERD), 317–323
  adult chronic cough, 179
  bronchiolitis, 254
  case presentation, 317
  child chronic cough, 182
  chronic cough, 178, 185
  cost-effectiveness, 322
  diagnosis and treatment, 321, 322
  idiopathic rhinitis, 50
  laryngitis, 92
  pathophysiology, 318–321
  presenting symptoms, 319f
  vocal cord dysfunction, 282

Gatifloxacin
  pneumonia, 243
Gefitinib
  lung cancer, 218
Gemifloxacin
  pneumonia, 243
GERD. *See* Gastroesophageal reflux
    disease (GERD)
Glomerulonephritis, 80
Glottic carcinoma
  laryngitis/hoarseness, 98
Glottic opening, 281, 282
Goodpasture's syndrome, 211
  hemoptysis, 311
Gram stains
  chronic obstructive pulmonary
    disease, 194
Granulomatous vasculitis
  hemoptysis, 311
Grass fever, 32
Grass pollen immunotherapy
  allergic rhinitis, 42–44
Group A streptococcus (GAS)
  pharyngitis, 78, 85
    antibiotics, 84t
Guaifenesin
  chronic cough, 186

H

Habit
  child chronic cough, 182
Haemophilus influenzae, 91
  pneumonia, 237, 239
  sinusitis, 69
Hamartomas, 212
Hampton's hump
  pulmonary embolism, 296
Hay fever, 32
Head and neck morphometric
    examinations
  obstructive sleep apnea, 267
Health care providers
  community-acquired pneumonia, 246
Heerfordt's syndrome
  sarcoidosis, 227
Heliox, 112
  bronchiolitis, 257
  pediatric asthma, 127
  vocal cord dysfunction, 284

Hemoptysis, 4, 5, 5, 307–315, 311
  abscess, 311
  case presentation, 307, 308
  diagnosis, 312, 313
  differential diagnosis, 312
  epidemiology, 308
  etiology, 309, 310t
  lung cancer, 210
  pathophysiology, 308–312
  physical exam, 312
  pulmonary embolism, 292
  surgery of, 315
  treatment, 313–315
Heparin
  exercise-induced bronchospasm, 157
  low-molecular-weight
    pulmonary embolism, 300
  pulmonary embolism, 299, 300
  unfractionated
    pulmonary embolism, 299, 300
Hepatocyte growth factor
  chronic obstructive pulmonary
    disease, 202
Hereditary hemorrhagic telangiectasia
  hemoptysis, 311
Her2/neu protooncogene
  lung cancer, 218
Herpes virus type I
  pharyngitis, 80
Hiatal hernia
  GERD, 321
High-resolution chest computed
    tomography (HRCT)
  hemoptysis, 313
Histoplasmosis, 212
History
  hemoptysis, 312
History of present illness, 3–5
  acute cough, 166, 167
HIV. See Human immunodeficiency
    virus (HIV)
Hoarseness. See Laryngitis/hoarseness
Hormonal rhinitis, 53
Horner syndrome, 210
Hospital employees
  sarcoidosis, 223
HRCT. See High-resolution chest
    computed tomography (HRCT)

Human chorionic gonadotropic-like
    peptide syndrome, 211t
Human immunodeficiency virus (HIV)
  pharyngitis, 80
  Pneumocystis carinii pneumonia, 6
Humidity
  croup, 111
Hydration
  laryngitis/hoarseness, 97
Hydroxychloroquine
  sarcoidosis, 232
Hypercalcemia
  sarcoidosis, 227
Hypercalciuria
  sarcoidosis, 227
Hypercapnia
  obstructive sleep apnea, 266
Hypercoagulable work-up
  pulmonary embolism, 302, 303
Hypertension
  obstructive sleep apnea, 266
Hypochondriasis
  laryngitis/hoarseness, 95
Hypothyroidism
  laryngitis/hoarseness, 95
Hypoxemia
  obstructive sleep apnea, 266
Hypoxia
  bronchiolitis, 252

I

Idiopathic pulmonary hemosiderosis
  hemoptysis, 311
Idiopathic rhinitis, 49–51
Ig. See Immunoglobulin (Ig)
Immunization. See Vaccine
Immunoglobulin (Ig)
  respiratory syncytial virus
    bronchiolitis, 257
Immunoglobulin E (IgE)
  allergen-specific serum
    allergic rhinitis, 38
  allergic rhinitis, 38
Immunotherapy
  allergic rhinitis, 42
  bronchiolitis, 257
  sublingual
    allergic rhinitis, 44

Indomethacin
  inhaled
    exercise-induced bronchospasm, 157
Indoor mold
  allergen avoidance, 40t
Infectious mononucleosis
  pharyngitis, 80
Infectious rhinitis, 53, 54
Inferior vena caval filters
  pulmonary embolism, 301
Inflammation
  adult asthma, 133
  chronic obstructive pulmonary disease, 192
Infliximab
  sarcoidosis, 232
Influenza
  child acute cough, 164
  pharyngitis, 80
Influenza vaccine
  acute cough, 169
  bronchiolitis, 255
  community-acquired pneumonia, 245, 246
Influenza virus
  community-acquired pneumonia, 235–238
Inhaled corticosteroids
  adult asthma, 142–144
  exercise-induced bronchospasm, 156
Inhaled indomethacin
  exercise-induced bronchospasm, 157
Inherited thrombophilas
  pulmonary embolism, 291
In-laboratory polysomnography
  obstructive sleep apnea, 267, 268
Inspection
  thorax, 7
Intercostal arteries
  hemoptysis, 309
Intradermal skin tests
  allergic rhinitis, 38
Intrathoracic obstruction, 22
Ipratropium bromide
  adult asthma, 141
  chronic obstructive pulmonary disease, 197
  pediatric asthma, 126
Iressa®
  lung cancer, 218

J

Japanese
  sarcoidosis, 228

K

Kaposi's sarcoma (KS)
  hemoptysis, 309
Klebsiella
  hemoptysis, 311
KS. *See* Kaposi's sarcoma (KS)
Kulchitsky's (argentaffin) cells, 208
Kyphoscoliosis, 7

L

Laboratory polysomnography
  obstructive sleep apnea, 267, 268
Laboratory testing
  bronchiolitis, 253, 254
  pneumonia, 241
Lamina propria, 91
Large cell carcinoma
  lungs, 207–211
Laryngeal edema
  laryngitis/hoarseness, 95
Laryngitis/hoarseness, 89, 99
  case presentation, 89
  causes, 92t
  diagnosis, 96, 97
  differential diagnosis, 93–96, 94t
  epidemiology, 90
  laryngeal edema, 95
  lung cancer, 210
  pathophysiology, 90–93
  treatment, 97, 98
Laryngoscopy
  croup, 109
  vocal cord dysfunction, 284
Laryngotracheitis
  community-acquired croup, 105
Larynx, 280, 281, 281f
  anatomy, 90
  irritants, 92
Laser therapy
  hemoptysis, 314
Legionella pneumoniae, 237, 239
Leiden defect
  factor V
    pulmonary embolism, 291, 292

Leukopenia
  sarcoidosis, 227
Leukotriene
  modifiers
    adult asthma, 143, 144
    exercise-induced bronchospasm, 156
    pediatric asthma, 125
  receptor antagonists
    allergic rhinitis, 41
Levofloxacin
  pneumonia, 243
LFT. *See* Liver function tests (LFT)
Life-threatening cough
  signs and symptoms, 167t
Lignocaine
  chronic cough, 186
Listlessness
  bronchiolitis, 252
Liver function tests (LFT)
  sarcoidosis, 230
LMWH. *See* Low-molecular-weight heparin (LMWH)
Lobar pneumonia, 8
Löfgren's syndrome
  sarcoidosis, 227
Long-acting β-adrenergic agents
  adult asthma, 143
Low-molecular-weight heparin (LMWH)
  pulmonary embolism, 300
Lung
  open biopsy
    sarcoidosis, 229
  percutaneous biopsy
    hemoptysis, 312
  total capacity, 13
Lung abscess
  hemoptysis, 310
Lung cancer, 205–218
  adult chronic cough, 181
  case presentation, 205
  clinical presentation, 210, 211
  defining characteristics, 213t
  diagnosis, 212, 213
  differential diagnosis, 211, 212
  epidemiology, 207
  future, 218
  management, 212–216

pathogenesis, 207–211
prevention, 216, 217
risk factors, 208, 209
screening, 216, 217
staging and prognosis, 213, 214
treatment, 214–216
types, 207, 208
Lung inflammatory disorders
  hemoptysis, 310
Lung volume, 13f, 19f, 24
Lupus pernio
  sarcoidosis, 226
Lymphadenopathy
  sarcoidosis, 225
Lymphadermatitis
  croup, 110

M

Macrolides
  pneumonia, 243
Magnesium
  pediatric asthma, 126
Magnetic resonance imaging (MRI)
  neurosarcoidosis, 230
Major histocompatibility complex (MHC) class II molecules, 34, 35
Malaise
  sarcoidosis, 224
Malignancy
  laryngitis/hoarseness, 98
  pulmonary embolism, 292
Malignant melanoma
  hemoptysis, 309
Mandibular devices
  obstructive sleep apnea, 270
Maxillary sinuses, 33, 67
Maximal expiratory pressure, 24, 25
Maximal inspiratory pressure, 24, 25
MDI. *See* Metered-dose inhaler (MDI)
Mediastinoscopy
  sarcoidosis, 229
Medical history
  past, 5, 6
Menstrual irregularities
  laryngitis/hoarseness, 95
Menthol
  chronic cough, 186

Metastatic cancer
   hemoptysis, 309
Metered-dose inhaler (MDI)
   exercise-induced bronchospasm, 154, 155
Methacholine challenge, 20
   exercise-induced bronchospasm, 152
Methotrexate
   sarcoidosis, 232
Methylcholine challenge test, 321
Methylprednisolone
   adult asthma, 141, 142
Methylxanthines
   adult asthma, 144
MHC. *See* Major histocompatibility complex (MHC) class II molecules
Microaspiration theory, 320
Mist therapy
   croup, 111
Mites
   dust
      allergen avoidance, 40t
Mitral stenosis
   hemoptysis, 311
Mold
   indoor
      allergen avoidance, 40t
Monoclonal antibodies
   lung cancer, 218
   pediatric asthma, 128
Montelukast
   adult asthma, 144
   allergic rhinitis, 41
Moraxella catarrhalis, 91
Morphine
   chronic cough, 186
Moxifloxacin
   pneumonia, 243, 246
MRI. *See* Magnetic resonance imaging (MRI)
Mucus
   chronic obstructive pulmonary disease, 192
Multiple sclerosis
   laryngitis/hoarseness, 95
Mycobacterium pneumoniae, 239
Mycobacterium tuberculosis, 181
Mycoplasma pneumoniae, 237
Myocardial infarction
   obstructive sleep apnea, 266

N

NAEPP. *See* National Asthma Education and Prevention Program (NAEPP)
Nail beds clubbing, 9
NARES. *See* Non-allergic rhinitis with eosinophilia syndrome (NARES)
Nasal cavity, 33, 34f
Nasal endoscopy
   allergic rhinitis, 36
Nasal mucosa
   allergic rhinitis, 37
Nasal polyps
   rhinitis, 52
Nasal provocation
   allergic rhinitis, 39
Nasal pruritis, 36
Nasal salute, 37
Nasal septum, 33
Nasal specimen
   bronchiolitis, 253
Naso-oropharynx
   anatomy, 12
Nasopharynx, 33
   anatomy, 12
National Asthma Education and Prevention Program (NAEPP)
   pediatric asthma guidelines, 120, 121, 123
Neck morphometric examinations
   obstructive sleep apnea, 267
Nedocromil
   adult asthma, 144
   pediatric asthma, 125
Neisseria
   sinusitis, 69
Nephritic syndrome, 80
Neuropeptide tyrosine (NPY), 50
Neurosarcoidosis, 227
Night sweats
   sarcoidosis, 224
Non-allergic rhinitis, 47–61
   case presentation, 47–48
   clinical testing, 57
   diagnosis, 55–57
   differential diagnosis, 54, 55
   eosinophilic types, 51
   epidemiology, 49f

future, 60, 61
history, 55
pathophysiology, 48–54
physical exam, 57
surgery, 60
treatment, 57–60
Non-allergic rhinitis with eosinophilia syndrome (NARES), 51
Noncaseating granulomas
sarcoidosis, 222, 223
Non-small cell lung cancer (NSCLC), 207–211
staging, 214f
treatment, 214–216
NPY. See Neuropeptide tyrosine (NPY)
NSCLC. See Non-small cell lung cancer (NSCLC)

O

Obesity, 7, 273–278
airflow resistance, 275
case presentation, 273
diagnosis, 277
differential diagnosis, 277
dyspnea, 277t
epidemiology, 274
future, 278
laryngitis/hoarseness, 95
lung compliance, 274, 275
lung volume, 275
obstructive sleep apnea, 264, 265
pathophysiology, 274–277
spirometry, 275
treatment, 277, 278
ventilatory drive, 275, 276
Obstructive lung disease
pulmonary function testing, 17
Obstructive sleep apnea (OSA), 22, 23f, 263–270
case presentation, 263
diagnosis, 266, 267
epidemiology, 264, 265
pathophysiology, 265, 266
signs and symptoms, 267t
treatment, 268–270, 269t
Occupational carcinogens
lung cancer, 209

Occupational rhinitis, 52, 53
Omalizumab
allergic rhinitis, 44
OMC. See Osteomeatal complex (OMC)
Open lung biopsy
sarcoidosis, 229
Opiates
chronic cough, 186
Orthopnea, 4
OSA. See Obstructive sleep apnea (OSA)
Osler-Weber-Rendu syndrome
hemoptysis, 311
Osteomeatal complex (OMC), 67, 68f
OTC. See Over-the-counter (OTC) medications
Otitis media
croup, 110
Overeating
GERD, 321
Over-the-counter (OTC) medications
acute cough, 167, 168t
bronchiolitis, 256
Oxygen therapy
chronic obstructive pulmonary disease, 201
Oxymetazoline
sinusitis, 72

P

Pain
chest, 5
lung cancer, 210
sarcoidosis, 224
Palivizumab
bronchiolitis, 255, 257
Palpation
sinusitis, 70
thorax, 7
Pancoast tumors, 210
Panting
vocal cord dysfunction, 284
Paragonimiasis
hemoptysis, 311
Parainfluenza
child acute cough, 164
virus type I
croup, 105

Paranasal sinuses, 67
Paraneoplastic syndrome, 210, 211t
Parasitic infection
   hemoptysis, 310
Parathormone, 211t
Parathyroid hormone-related peptide excess, 211t
Parkinson's disease
   laryngitis/hoarseness, 95
Paroxysmal nocturnal dyspnea, 4
Past medical history, 5, 6
Pattern of breathing
   obesity, 276
Peak expiratory flow (PEF)
   adult asthma, 135
   exercise-induced bronchospasm, 151, 152
   pediatric asthma, 121
Peak-flow monitoring
   adult asthma, 137
Pectus excavatum (funnel chest), 7
Pediatric asthma, 115–128
   case presentation, 115
   classification system, 123t
   clinical presentation, 119, 120
   diagnosis, 120–122, 122t
   differential diagnosis, 120
   epidemiology, 116, 117
   future, 128
   pathophysiology, 117–119
   treatment, 122–128, 124t
   triggers, 121t
PEF. *See* Peak expiratory flow (PEF)
Penicillin
   pharyngitis, 84
Pentoxifylline
   sarcoidosis, 232
Percussion
   sinusitis, 70
   thorax, 7
Percutaneous lung biopsy
   hemoptysis, 312
Perennial allergic rhinitis, 32
Perfusion, 14, 15
Pertussis
   adult acute cough, 163
   bronchiolitis, 255

PET. *See* Positron emission tomography (PET)
PFT. *See* Pulmonary function testing (PFT)
Pharyngitis, 77–85
   case presentation, 77
   causes, 81t
   diagnosis, 82, 83
   differential diagnosis, 80–82
   epidemiology, 78
   future, 85
   GAS, 78
   pathophysiology, 79, 80
   treatment, 83–85
Phenylephrine
   sinusitis, 72
Phosphodiesterase 4 inhibitors
   chronic obstructive pulmonary disease, 202
Physical exam, 7–9
   acute cough, 166, 167
   child chronic cough, 185
   chronic obstructive pulmonary disease, 194, 195
   hemoptysis, 312
   pulmonary embolism, 294
   sinusitis, 70
Pirbuterol
   adult asthma, 141
Pirodavir
   acute cough, 170
Pleconaril
   acute cough, 170
Pleural effusion, 8
Pleurisy
   pulmonary embolism, 294
Pleuritic chest pain
   pulmonary embolism, 292
Pneumococcal vaccine
   community-acquired pneumonia, 246
Pneumoconiosis, 212
Pneumocystis carinii, 212
Pneumomediastinum
   croup, 110
Pneumonia, 235–246. *See also* Community-acquired pneumonia
   adult acute cough, 163

bacterial
  bronchiolitis, 254
  hemoptysis, 311
case presentation, 235
clinical presentation, 239–241
diagnosis, 239–241
differential diagnosis, 239
epidemiology, 236, 237
future, 246
hemoptysis, 310
inpatient treatment, 244
lobar, 8
outpatient treatment, 243, 244
pathophysiology, 237–239
treatment, 241–246, 245t
Pneumonia severity index (PSI), 241, 242f
Pneumothorax, 8
  croup, 110
Pneumovax
  acute cough, 169
Pollen, 32
Polyps
  laryngitis, 93
Polysomnography
  in-laboratory
    obstructive sleep apnea, 267, 268
Positron emission tomography (PET)
  neurosarcoidosis, 230
Postnasal drip
  adult chronic cough, 178
  child chronic cough, 182
  chronic cough, 178
  laryngitis, 92
Poststreptococcal glomerulonephritis, 80
PPI. *See* Proton pump inhibitors (PPI)
Prednisolone
  adult asthma, 141, 142
Prednisone
  adult asthma, 141,142
Pregnancy
  non-allergic rhinitis, 59
Presbylaryngeus
  elderly, 94
Primary bronchogenic carcinoma
  hemoptysis, 309
Proteinase inhibitors
  chronic obstructive pulmonary
    disease, 201

Proton pump inhibitors (PPI), 321, 322f
Pseudoephedrine
  non-allergic rhinitis, 59
PSI. *See* Pneumonia severity index (PSI)
Psychogenic cough
  child chronic cough, 182
Psychological counseling
  vocal cord dysfunction, 285
Psychological disorders
  laryngitis/hoarseness, 95
Puerto Ricans
  sarcoidosis, 228
Pulmonary angiogram
  pulmonary embolism, 298
Pulmonary arterial catheters
  hemoptysis, 312
Pulmonary arteries
  hemoptysis, 309
Pulmonary arteriography
  hemoptysis, 315
Pulmonary arteriovenous malformation
  hemoptysis, 311
Pulmonary embolism, 289–303
  case presentation, 289
  clinical manifestations, 292, 293
  diagnosis, 294–299
  differential diagnosis, 294, 295t
  epidemiology, 290
  future, 303
  hemoptysis, 310
  inherited thrombophilas, 291
  pathophysiology, 290–292
  physical exam, 294
  prophylaxis, 302
  treatment, 299–303
Pulmonary function testing (PFT), 9,
    10, 17–26
  child chronic cough, 185
  chronic obstructive pulmonary
    disease, 195t
  pediatric asthma, 121
  preoperatively, 25
  sarcoidosis, 230
  types, 18–20
Pulmonary infection
  hemoptysis, 310
Pulmonary rehabilitation
  chronic obstructive pulmonary
    disease, 201

Pulmonary sarcoidosis
  adult chronic cough, 181
Pulse oximetry, 10
  bronchiolitis, 253
  croup, 109
  obstructive sleep apnea, 267, 268

R

Racemic epinephrine
  bronchiolitis, 256, 257
  croup, 111
Racial groups
  sarcoidosis, 223, 228
Radiographs
  sinusitis, 71
Rales, 8
Ramirez criteria, 244
Rapid antigen test (RAT)
  pharyngitis, 82
Rasmussen's aneurysm
  rupture, 311
RAT. *See* Rapid antigen test (RAT)
Recurrent laryngeal nerve, 90
Red flags
  physical exam
    acute cough, 166, 167
Remicade
  sarcoidosis, 232
Renal cell cancer
  hemoptysis, 309
Respiratory disorder
  agents, 162t
  approach to patient, 3–10
Respiratory syncytial virus (RSV)
  bronchiolitis, 250, 251
  child acute cough, 164
  immune globulin
    bronchiolitis, 257
Respiratory tract
  anatomy, 11–13
  physiology, 13–15
Restrictive lung disease
  pulmonary function testing, 18
Retention cysts
  laryngitis, 93
Retinoic acids
  chronic obstructive pulmonary
    disease, 201

Retroagnathia
  obstructive sleep apnea, 270
Rheumatic fever
  acute
    pharyngitis, 79
Rheumatoid arthritis
  laryngitis/hoarseness, 95
Rhinitis. *See also* Allergic rhinitis;
    Non-allergic rhinitis
  adult asthma, 133
  cholinergic, 53
  drug-induced, 52
  idiopathic, 49–51
  infectious, 53, 54
  irritative-toxic, 52, 53
  occupational, 52, 53
  perennial allergic, 32
  questionnaire, 56f
  seasonal allergic, 32
Rhinoscopy
  anterior
    allergic rhinitis, 36
Rhinosinusitis, 66
  bacterial
    adult acute cough, 162
Rhinovirus
  child acute cough, 164
  pharyngitis, 80
Rhonchi, 8, 9
  pediatric asthma, 120
Ribivirin
  bronchiolitis, 257
Rienke's space, 91
Risk factors
  community-acquired pneumonia,
    236, 237
  lung cancer, 208, 209
  VTE, 293t
RSV. *See* Respiratory syncytial virus
    (RSV)

S

Salmeterol
  adult asthma, 143
Sarcoidosis, 221–233
  adult chronic cough, 181
  case presentation, 221, 222

clinical course, 227, 228
clinical presentation, 224, 225
    poor prognosis, 226t
diagnosis, 229–231
differential diagnosis, 228, 229
epidemiology, 222, 223
future, 233
laryngitis/hoarseness, 95
organs, 225t
pathophysiology, 223, 224
pulmonary
    adult chronic cough, 181
staging, 229t
treatment, 231–233
SCLC. *See* Small-cell lung cancer (SCLC)
Screening
    pediatric asthma, 120
Seasonal allergic rhinitis, 32
Secondhand smoke
    lung cancer, 209
Septum
    deviated, 68f
Short-acting β2-adrenergic agents
    adult asthma, 141
Shortness of breath, 4
    exercise-induced bronchospasm, 150
Sinuses, 67f
Sinusitis, 65–74
    case presentation, 65
    diagnosis, 69–72, 71t
        differential diagnosis, 69
    epidemiology, 66
    future, 74
    microbiology, 69
    pathophysiology, 66–69
    physical exam, 70
    treatment, 72–74
Skin-prick-puncture tests
    allergic rhinitis, 37, 38
Skin-prick test
    non-allergic rhinitis, 57
Skin tests
    intradermal
        allergic rhinitis, 38
    non-allergic rhinitis, 54
    tuberculin, 181
Sleep apnea. *See* Obstructive sleep
    apnea (OSA)

Sleepiness
    excessive daytime
        obstructive sleep apnea, 264, 265
Sleep study
    obstructive sleep apnea, 266, 267
Small-cell lung cancer (SCLC), 207–211
    treatment, 215, 216
Smoking. *See also* Tobacco smoke
    cessation, 196, 196t, 216
    child chronic cough, 182
    cigarette
        community-acquired pneumonia, 246
        lung cancer, 209
    history, 6
Social history, 6
Solitary pulmonary nodule, 211
    evaluation, 212, 213
Sore throat, 80
Spasmodic croup, 107
Spasmodic dysphonia
    laryngitis/hoarseness, 95
Speech therapy
    vocal cord dysfunction, 285
Sphenoid sinuses, 67
Spiral computed tomography (CT), 9, 10
    pulmonary embolism, 297, 298
Spirometry, 18, 19
    acceptability, 18
    adult asthma, 137
    chronic obstructive pulmonary
        disease, 194
    exercise-induced bronchospasm,
        151, 152
    interpreting results, 18, 19
    sarcoidosis, 230
    terms, 19f
Spondylitis
    ankylosing, 7
Sputum
    bacterial infections, 5
    chronic bronchitis, 5
    chronic obstructive pulmonary
        disease, 194
    cytology
        lung cancer, 217
Squamous cell carcinoma
    lungs, 207–211

Staphylococcus aureus
  hemoptysis, 311
  sinusitis, 69
Steeple sign, 108
Steroids
  pediatric safety, 125
Streptococcal group C
  pharyngitis, 81
Streptococcal group G
  pharyngitis, 81
Streptococcal toxic shock syndrome
  pharyngitis, 79
Streptococcus pneumoniae, 237, 239
  sinusitis, 69
Stridor, 9
  differential diagnosis, 106t
Stroke
  laryngitis/hoarseness, 95
  obstructive sleep apnea, 266
Subacute cough, 176
Subglottic stenosis
  croup, 110
Sublingual immunotherapy
  allergic rhinitis, 44
Substance abuse
  laryngitis/hoarseness, 95
Superficial laryngeal nerve, 90
Superior vena cava syndrome, 210
Surfactant
  bronchiolitis, 257
Sweat test
  child chronic cough, 183
Sympathomimetics
  non-allergic rhinitis, 59
Syndrome of inappropriate antidiuretic
    hormone secretion, 211t
Systemic corticosteroids
  adult asthma, 141, 142
Systemic lupus erythematosus
  hemoptysis, 311
  laryngitis/hoarseness, 95

T

Terbutaline
  adult asthma, 141
Thalidomide
  lung cancer, 218
Theophylline
  adult asthma, 144
  pediatric asthma, 125

Thoracic inlet, 22
Thorax
  examination, 7
Throat
  culture
    pharyngitis, 83
  sore, 80
Thrombocytopenia
  sarcoidosis, 227
Thrombolysis
  pulmonary embolism, 301
Thrush
  laryngitis/hoarseness, 95
Tidal volume, 13
Tiotropium bromide
  chronic obstructive pulmonary
    disease, 197, 199
Tobacco smoke
  bronchiolitis, 255
  environmental
    lung cancer, 209
  laryngitis/hoarseness, 92, 95
  lung cancer, 208
  secondhand
    lung cancer, 209
Topical corticosteroids
  non-allergic rhinitis, 59, 60
Total lung capacity, 13
Trachea, 12
Tracheitis
  bacterial, 107
  croup, 105
Tracheobronchitis
  child acute cough, 164
  child chronic cough, 182
Tracheostomy tube
  hemoptysis, 312
Transfer function, 22–25
Tremacamra
  acute cough, 170
True vocal folds, 91
Tuberculin skin test, 181
Tuberculosis
  adult chronic cough, 181
  hemoptysis, 310
Turbinates
  allergic rhinitis, 37
Tympanic membrane, 9

Index

U

Unfractionated heparin (UH)
    pulmonary embolism, 299, 300
Upper airway obstruction, 7, 22f, 23
Uveitis
    anterior
        sarcoidosis, 226
Uveoparotid fever
    sarcoidosis, 227
Uvulopalatopharyngoplasty
    obstructive sleep apnea, 270

V

Vaccine
    bronchiolitis, 258
        influenza, 255
    community-acquired pneumonia
        influenza, 245, 246
        pneumococcal, 246
    influenza
        acute cough, 169
        bronchiolitis, 255
        community-acquired pneumonia, 245, 246
Vagal medicated reflex
    GERD, 319
Venous thromboembolism (VTE)
    risk factors, 293t
Ventilation, 14
Ventilation-perfusion (V/Q) scan
    pulmonary embolism, 296
Ventilatory drive, 14
Ventricular prolapse
    laryngitis, 93
Vesicular breath sounds, 8
Virchow's triad, 290
Vital capacity, 13
Vitamin C
    exercise-induced bronchospasm, 157
Vitamin K antagonist
    pulmonary embolism, 300, 301
Vocal cord dysfunction, 279–287
    case presentation, 279, 280
    diagnosis, 282–284
    differential diagnosis, 284, 285f
    etiology, 282
    future, 286, 287
    management, 286t
    pathophysiology, 280–282
    treatment, 284, 285
Vocal cord paralysis, 93, 94, 98
Vocalis muscle, 91
Vocal ligament, 91
V/Q. *See* Ventilation-perfusion (V/Q) scan
VTE. *See* Venous thromboembolism (VTE)

W

Warfarin
    pulmonary embolism, 300, 301
Wegener's granulomatosis, 212
    hemoptysis, 311, 312
    laryngitis/hoarseness, 95
Weight loss
    lung cancer, 210
    obesity, 277–278
    obstructive sleep apnea, 268
    sarcoidosis, 224
Wells system
    pulmonary embolism, 298, 299
Westermark's sign
    pulmonary embolism, 296
Wheezing, 8
    differential diagnosis, 121t
    exercise-induced bronchospasm, 150
    pediatric asthma, 119
Work of breathing
    obesity, 275, 276

X

Ximelagatran
    pulmonary embolism, 303

Z

Zyrtec®
    exercise-induced bronchospasm, 154

```
RC       Disorders of the
731       respiratory tract.
.D58
2006
```

48707

$79.50

DATE			

SOUTH UNIVERSITY
709 MALL BLVD.
SAVANNAH, GA 31406

BAKER & TAYLOR